Emergency Procedures

Emergency Procedures

MICHAEL S. JASTREMSKI, MD, EDITOR
Professor and Director
Program in Multidisciplinary Critical Care
State University of New York Health Science Center
Syracuse, New York

MARC DUMAS, MD, EDITOR/ILLUSTRATOR
Department of Emergency Medicine
Fairbanks Memorial Hospital
Fairbanks, Alaska

LISA PEÑALVER, AMI, ILLUSTRATOR
Fairbanks, Alaska

W. B. SAUNDERS COMPANY
Harcourt Brace Jovanovich, Inc.
Philadelphia London Toronto Montreal Sydney Tokyo

W. B. SAUNDERS COMPANY
Harcourt Brace Jovanovich, Inc.

The Curtis Center
Independence Square West
Philadelphia, PA 19106

Library of Congress Cataloging-in-Publication Data

Emergency procedures / [edited by] Michael S. Jastremski, Marc Dumas.

p. cm.

Includes index.

ISBN 0–7216–5127–5

1. Emergency medicine. 2. Traumatology. I. Jastremski, Michael S. II. Dumas, Marc
[DNLM: 1. Emergencies. 2. Emergency Medicine—methods. WB 105 E5582]

RC86.7.E589 1992 616.02′5—dc20

DNLM/DLC 92–7626

Editor: Raymond R. Kersey
Developmental Editor: David Kilmer
Designer: Ellen Bodner-Zanolle
Cover Artist: Joseph Kulka
Production Manager: Ken Neimeister
Manuscript Editor: Jeanne Carper
Illustration Specialist: Brett MacNaughton
Indexer: Nancy Newman

EMERGENCY PROCEDURES ISBN 0–7216–5127–5

Printed in MEXICO

Last digit is the print number: 9 8 7 6 5 4 3 2 1

To John Dyson,
who in his many years as an editor at the W. B. Saunders Company
has made extensive contributions to the literature of medicine.
His behind-the-scenes advice, guidance, invaluable encouragement,
and occasional patient prodding
have helped many authors, including this one,
bring their dreams into print.

MSJ

Contributors

RICHARD CANTOR, MD
Assistant Professor, Departments of Emergency Medicine and Pediatrics, State University of New York Health Science Center at Syracuse; Attending Physician, University Hospital; Medical Director, Central New York Poison Control Center, Syracuse, New York
Intraosseous Infusions

RICHARD A. CHERRY, MEd, NREMT-P
Director of Paramedic Training, Program in Multidisciplinary Critical Care, State University of New York Health Science Center at Syracuse, Syracuse, New York
Traction Splinting; Pneumatic Antishock Garment

KEVIN FERGUSON, MD
Lecturer, Emergency Medicine Section, Department of Surgery, University of Michigan Medical School; Attending, University of Michigan Hospital, Ann Arbor, Michigan
Ankle Dislocation Reduction; Hip Dislocation Reduction; Knee Dislocation Reduction; Emergency Thoracotomy; Thoracentesis

DENISE P. GAVULA, DO
Assistant Professor, Pediatrics and Emergency Medicine, State University of New York Health Science Center at Syracuse; Pediatric Emergency Department Staff Physician, University Hospital, Syracuse, New York
Bladder Catheterization; Slit Lamp Examination

DAVID G. HEISIG, MD
Assistant Professor, Medicine and Emergency Medicine, State University of New York Health Science Center at Syracuse; Attending Physician, University Hospital and Veterans Affairs Medical Center, Syracuse, New York
Anoscopy; Balloon Tamponade of Bleeding Gastroesophageal Varices

MICHAEL S. JASTREMSKI, MD, FCCM, FACEP, FCCP
Professor and Director, Program in Multidisciplinary Critical Care, State University of New York Health Science Center at Syracuse; Attending Physician, University Hospital, Syracuse, New York
Analgesia and Anesthesia; Emergency Childbirth; Fishhook Removal; Removal of Protective Headgear; Ring Removal; Tooth Reimplantation; Zipper Removal; Laceration Repair; Nasal Packing; Ocular Tonometry; Amputations; Reduction of Dislocated Mandible; Emergency External Pacing; Temporary Transvenous Pacing; Pericardiocentesis; Arterial Blood Drawing; Arterial Cannulation; Peripheral Venous Cannulation

GARY A. JOHNSON, MD
Assistant Professor, Department of Emergency Medicine, State University of New York Health Science Center at Syracuse; Attending Physician, University Hospital, Syracuse, New York
Paracentesis; Transthoracic Pacing

JUDY L. KILPATRICK, RN, MSN, CCRN
Adjunct Faculty, College of Nursing, State University of New York Health Science Center at Syracuse; Clinical Nurse Specialist, Critical Care and Emergency Nursing, University Hospital, Syracuse, New York
Implantable Venous Access Devices

DAVID M. KRUGER, MD
Clinical Assistant Professor, University of Connecticut; Orthopaedic Surgeon, Saint Francis Hospital, Hartford, Connecticut
Paronychial Drainage

MARCY LAYTON, MD
Infectious Disease Fellow, Yale University, New Haven, Connecticut
Bone Marrow Aspiration; Nasogastric Tube Insertion; Lumbar Puncture; Subclavian Vein Catheterization; Writing Prescriptions

JODY RIVA LEWINTER, MD
Clinical Assistant Professor, University of Connecticut School of Medicine, Farmington; Emergency Department Physician, Hartford Hospital, Hartford, Connecticut
Cricothyroidotomy; Tube Thoracostomy

CELESTE M. MADDEN, MD, FAAP, FACEP
Assistant Professor of Pediatrics and Emergency Medicine, State University of New York Health Science Center at Syracuse, Syracuse, New York
Sexual Assault Examination

PETER MARIANI, MD, FACEP
Assistant Professor and Vice Chairman, Department of Emergency Medicine, State University of New York Health Science Center at Syracuse; Attending Physician, University Hospital, Syracuse, New York
Endotracheal Intubation; Internal Jugular Vein Catheterization

TIMOTHY PAGE, MD
Assistant Professor, Program in Multidisciplinary Critical Care, State University of New York Health Science Center at Syracuse; Attending Physician, University Hospital, Syracuse, New York
Airway Suctioning

E. JAMES RADIN, MD
Clinical Assistant Professor, Program in Multidisciplinary Critical Care, State University of New York Health Science Center at Syracuse, Syracuse, New York; Associate in Critical Care Medicine, Guthrie Clinic/Robert Packer Hospital, Sayre, Pennsylvania
Rigid Sigmoidoscopy; Arthrocentesis

GREGORY D. RIEBEL, MD
Clinical Instructor in Orthopedics, State University of New York Health Science Center at Syracuse; Chief Resident, Department of Orthopedic Surgery, University Hospital, Syracuse, New York
Reduction of Dislocated Shoulder

LEO ROTELLO, MD
Assistant Professor/Co-Fellowship Director, Program in Multidisciplinary Critical Care, State University of New York Health Science Center at Syracuse; Attending Physician, University Hospital, Syracuse, New York
Removal of Foreign Bodies from the Ear; Removal of a Foreign Body from the Eye; Removal of Foreign Bodies from the Nose; Removal of Rectal Foreign Bodies; Removal of Vaginal Foreign Bodies

RAE NADINE SMITH, RN, MS
Clinical Nurse Specialist; President, Medical Communicators and Associates, Salt Lake City, Utah
Invasive Vascular Pressure Monitoring

SAMMY F. SURIANI, RPA-C, EMT-P
Clinical Physician Assistant, Department of Emergency Medicine, State University of New York Health Science Center at Syracuse; Paramedic and Resource Hospital EMS Field Liaison, Central New York Emergency Medical System Program, Syracuse, New York
Incision and Drainage of a Subcutaneous Abscess; Synchronized Cardioversion

THOMAS TERNDRUP, MD, FACEP
Assistant Professor, Departments of Emergency Medicine and Pediatrics, State University of New York Health Science Center at Syracuse; Attending Physician, Emergency Department, University Hospital, Syracuse, New York
Needle Cricothyroidotomy; Radial Head Subluxation (Nursemaid's Elbow); Reduction of Finger Dislocations; Femoral Vein Catheterization; Venous Cutdowns

CONNIE WALLECK, RN, MS, FCCM
Adjunct Assistant Professor, State University of New York Health Science Center at Syracuse College of Nursing; Senior Associate Director of Nursing, University Hospital, Syracuse, New York
Universal Precautions; Gastric Lavage; Intracranial Pressure Monitoring; Defibrillation; Hickman Catheter

JONATHAN WARREN, MD, FCCM
Clinical Assistant Professor of Medicine, University of Pittsburgh; Director, Critical Care Medicine, Western Pennsylvania Hospital, Pittsburgh, Pennsylvania
Pulmonary Artery Catheterization; Percutaneous Femoral Artery Cannulation; Percutaneous Axillary Artery Cannulation

JEFFREY WINFIELD, MD, PhD
Associate Professor of Neurosurgery/Pediatrics, Section Head of Neuro-Oncology, Director of Pediatric Neurosurgery, Neurosurgical Director of Stereotactic Linear Radiosurgery Program, State University of New York Health Science Center at Syracuse; Attending Physician, University Hospital, Crouse-Irving Memorial Hospital, and Syracuse Veterans Affairs Hospital, Syracuse, New York
Emergency Temporal Burr Hole in Patients with Clinical Signs of Progressive Tentorial Herniation; Ventriculoperitoneal/Atrial Shunt Tap

LUKE YIP, MD
Assistant Professor, Department of Emergency Medicine, State University of New York Health Science Center at Syracuse; Attending Physician, Emergency Medicine, University Hospital, Syracuse, New York
Culdocentesis; Peritoneal Lavage

W. JOHN ZEHNER, MD
Assistant Professor, Emergency Medicine, State University of New York Health Science Center at Syracuse; Attending Physician, University Hospital, Syracuse, New York
Ankle Block; Dental Blocks; Digital Nerve Block; Wrist Blocks; Incision and Drainage of a Felon; Incision and Drainage of External Hemorrhoids

Preface

Emergency Procedures is designed primarily for the beginning physician who is learning patient management. It presents a single, tried-and-true technique for performing each of a variety of diagnostic and therapeutic procedures. Each is presented in a simple stepwise description supplemented by photos and drawings. However, even experienced clinicians should find some useful pearls in this manual.

Procedural skills are learned by doing, and you will not become competent at performing any of these procedures until you have had adequate practice under the watchful eye of a skilled mentor. This book will provide you with the basic theory and concepts that are the necessary foundation you must master before you begin practicing on patients. You will find it most valuable if you initially develop a general familiarity with its content and then use it for a quick, specific review before you perform each procedure.

MICHAEL S. JASTREMSKI, MD

Acknowledgments

A number of individuals deserve special thanks for their contributions to this volume. In spite of my handwriting, Debra Boyle, Mary Garvey, Kelly Bunch, and Diane Barsh cheerfully and competently typed multiple drafts of the manuscript. Ken Peek produced the photo illustrations. David Dexter, MSIV, allowed himself to be shanghaied from the Emergency Department one afternoon to model for the photos.

Contents

1

Universal Precautions

CONNIE WALLECK, RN, MS

Indication

To protect all health care workers from contagious diseases that may be contracted by exposure to blood and body fluids of all patients. Throughout this book, each procedure description includes specific recommendations for the universal precautions that are indicated for that procedure.

Contraindications

None

Equipment

Gloves
Gowns and/or aprons
Masks
Goggles (protective eye wear)
Resuscitation masks

Technique

Universal precautions should be used for all patient contacts if the health care provider may be exposed to blood, certain other body fluids (amniotic fluid, pericardial fluid, peritoneal fluid, pleural fluid, synovial fluid, cerebrospinal fluid, semen, and vaginal secretions), or any body fluid visibly contaminated with blood. Generally, universal precautions do not apply to feces, nasal secretions, sputum, sweat, tears, urine, and vomitus unless these secretions are contaminated with blood. Universal precautions assume that *all* patients are carriers of infectious, contagious diseases, since there is no reliable, immediate means to identify infected patients. Thus, we should be equally cautious when caring for all patients.

Gloves

Gloves should be worn when handling blood, body fluids, mucous membranes, nonintact skin, body tissues, and specimens. New gloves should be worn for each patient contact. Hands must be washed after glove removal and between patient contacts.

Gowns

Sterile gowns may be necessary during specific procedures. If the health care provider anticipates the possibility of soiling his or her clothing with patient material, a protective garment should be worn.

Apron

An apron can be worn if a large amount of bleeding is anticipated.

Masks

If a splash of blood or body fluid to the face is anticipated, a full face shield or goggles and face mask should be worn.

Resuscitation Mask

If emergency ventilatory support is necessary, a resuscitation mask should be used.

Other Precautions

1. Do not recap needles.
2. Promptly place disposable sharps in a designated puncture-resistant container. Pick them up with a hemostat, not with your fingers.
3. Place all soiled linen in a clear plastic bag before sending it to the laundry.
4. Use a solution of 1 part household bleach to 10 parts of water to clean equipment, clean up spills, and decontaminate walls and other objects soiled with blood and body fluids.
5. If skin has a cut, break, abrasion, or dermatitis, use gloves and avoid any contact with blood or body fluids.

Pearls and Pitfalls

Have you had your hepatitis B vaccination yet? Hepatitis B, which causes several hundred deaths annually, is a much greater threat to health care workers than is AIDS, yet it can be prevented by a simple, safe vaccine.

Reference

Centers for Disease Control: Recommendations for prevention of HIV transmission in health-care settings. MMWR 36(Suppl 25):3S–18S, 1987.

Anesthesia

2

Analgesia and Anesthesia

MICHAEL S. JASTREMSKI, MD

He that relieves pain is blessed, but he that causes none is doubly so.
Anonymous

All of the procedures described in this book are painful and/or unpleasant and anxiety producing. Appropriate and adequate analgesia and anesthesia, in addition to being a basic human kindness, will both facilitate the successful completion of the procedure and endear you to the patient. Topical, local (by direct infiltration or regional block), and systemic techniques, alone or in combination, are recommended in this book. In this chapter general recommendations are provided concerning the choice of agents (Tables 2–1 and 2–2 and Figures 2–1 and 2–2) and an overview is presented of the features of the various agents we use for analgesia and anesthesia (Table 2–3). You should be familiar with the dosing, pharmacokinetics, and toxicity of these agents and be able to manage any acute life-threatening toxic reactions before administering them. The focus here is on one or two tried and tested agents for each use. Do not forget to ask the patient about allergies and previous allergic reactions before administering any drug. You should also determine whether your female patients are pregnant or breast feeding.

Allergy to local anesthetics can be approached in several ways:

1. There are two chemically unrelated classes of local anesthetics: the amides and the esters. If there is a clear-cut history of reactions to agents of only one class, then a drug in the other class may be used.
2. Diphenhydramine (Benadryl), given by infiltration, usually provides adequate analgesia for minor procedures on the skin. It is not effective for regional blocks or deep procedures.
3. Skin testing and progressive challenge with lidocaine are performed as follows:
   a. Prick test with lidocaine 1%, diluted 1:100
   b. Prick test with lidocaine 1%, full strength
   c. Intradermal skin test with 0.02 ml lidocaine 1%, diluted 1:100
   d. Intradermal skin test with 0.02 ml lidocaine 1%
   e. Subcutaneous injection of 0.1 ml lidocaine 1%
   f. Subcutaneous injection of 0.5 ml lidocaine 1%
4. A systemic technique can be used.
5. Remember that very few persons are truly allergic to local anesthetics. Their reported "allergic" reactions are actually an epinephrine effect, hyperventilation or a vasovagal response to a procedure or injury, or toxic effects from an excessive dose of the local anesthetic. Therefore, if a careful history of the prior "allergic" reaction does not include any of the usual elements of allergy (e.g., anaphylaxis, hives, stridor, wheezing) and does fit one of the other entities listed above, it is almost certainly safe to use the local anesthetic.

TABLE 2–1. Anesthetic and Analgesic Drugs

Topical
- Benzocaine (Cetacaine)
- Cocaine
- Lidocaine (Xylocaine)
- Proparacaine (Ophthetic)
- TAC (tetracaine, epinephrine [Adrenalin], cocaine)

Local and Regional
- Amides
  - Bupivacaine (Marcaine)
  - Lidocaine (Xylocaine)
- Esters
  - Procaine (Novocain)
  - Tetracaine (Pontocaine)
- Other (as an option in allergic patients)
  - Diphenhydramine (Benadryl)

Systemic
- Diazepam (Valium)
- DPT (meperidine [Demerol], promethazine [Phenergan], chlorpromazine [Thorazine])
- Fentanyl (Innovar, Sublimaze)
- Meperidine (Demerol)
- Midazolam (Versed)
- Morphine
- Nitrous oxide (Nitronox)

TABLE 2–2. Recommended Agents for Each Anesthetic Technique

Technique	Situation	Agent
Topical	Ear	Nothing works well
	Eye	Proparacaine
	Mucosa	Lidocaine 4%
	Nose	Cocaine
	Pharynx	Benzocaine
	Skin	TAC
Infiltrative	Short procedure (<45 minutes)	Lidocaine
	Long procedure (>45 minutes)	Bupivacaine
Regional block	Short procedure	Lidocaine
	Long procedure	Bupivacaine
Systemic	Adult	Nitrous oxide or midazolam and morphine
	Child	DPT

TABLE 2–3. Characteristics of Anesthetic and Analgesic Drugs

		Dose		Action				
Drug	**How Supplied**	***Usual***	***Maximum***	***Onset***	***Duration***	**Side Effects**	**Management**	**Cautions**
Benzocaine	Spray with tetracaine (Cetocaine) delivering 200 mg benzocaine and 20 mg tetracaine per second	One second spray	Two second spray	30–60 sec	Variable up to 1 hr	Poor absorption prevents systemic toxicity. Damage to mucous membranes	Avoid prolonged contact, especially at a localized site	Not for injection. Not for ocular use.
Bupivacaine*	0.25% (2.5 mg/ml) 0.5% (5 mg/ml)	Infiltrative: use 0.25% solution in volume necessary for size of lesion up to maximal dose	2.5 mg (1 ml)/kg	Several minutes	4–6 hr	Coma	Airway and ventilation	
						Seizures	Diazepam	
						Hypotension	IV fluids Vasopressors	
						Dysrhythmias	ACLS protocols	
		Blocks: use 0.5% solution. Volume will vary with site of block.	2.5 mg (0.5 ml)/kg	5–20 min				
Cocaine	4% topical solution (40 mg/ml)	Minimal necessary	Lesser of 3 mg/kg or 200 mg	2–5 min	45–60 min	Agitation Seizures	Diazepam	If toxicity occurs, remember to remove the pledget and flush the nasal passage to prevent further absorption.
						Coma	Airway and ventilation	
						Hypertension	Propranolol or nitroprusside	
						Tachydysrhythmias	Propranolol, then ACLS protocols	
						Hyperthermia	Vigorous surface cooling	
DPT	IM cocktail of meperidine (demerol), promethazine, chlorpromazine (Thorazine) mixed in same syringe	2 mg/kg IM meperidine 1 mg/kg IM promethazine 1 mg/kg IM chlorpromazine	50 mg meperidine 25 mg prometha-zine 25 mg chlorproma-zine	30 min	4–24 hr	Respiratory depression	Observe patients until fully awake Ventilatory support	Do not administer intravenously.
						Hypotension	Raise legs IV fluids	
						Dystonic reactions	Diphenhydramine	
Diazepam	Solution for IV use of 5 mg/ml	0.1 mg/kg IV	2.5 mg (children)	2–5 min	4–6 hr	Coma	Airway and ventilation	
						Hypotension	Raise legs IV fluids	
Diphen-hydramine	10 mg/ml solution	Local IV infiltration based on size of area	Lesser of 100 mg (10 ml) or 5 mg/kg	5–10 min	Variable	Sedation	Make sure patient is fully awake before discharge	
Fentanyl	Solution for IV use of 50 μg/ml	2 μg/kg IV (slow push over 3–5 min)	4 μg/kg (in divided doses over 10 min)	1 min	30–60 min	Respiratory depression	Naloxone Airway and ventilation	
						Hypotension	Raise legs IV fluids Naloxone	
Lidocaine*	Solutions of 1% (10 mg/ml), 2% (20 mg/ml), and 4% (40 mg/ml)	Topical: 4% solution	Lesser of 300 mg or 4 mg/kg	1–2 min	30–60 min	Seizures	Diazepam	
		Infiltrative: use 1% or 2% solution in volume necessary for size of lesion up to maximal dose		1–2 min	30–60 min	Respiratory depression	Airway and ventilation	
		Blocks: use 1% or 2% solution. Volume will vary with site of block.		5–20 min	30–60 min			

TABLE 2–3. Characteristics of Anesthetic and Analgesic Drugs *Continued*

		Dose		Action				
Drug	**How Supplied**	***Usual***	***Maximum***	***Onset***	***Duration***	**Side Effects**	**Management**	**Cautions**
Midazolam	Solution of 1 mg/ml	1–2 mg IV	5 mg (in divided doses over 10 min)	1–5 min	30–60 min	Coma Hypotension	Airway and ventilation Raise legs IV fluids Vasopressors	
Morphine	Use 5 mg/ml diluted to 5 ml for final concentration of 1 mg/ml	3–5 mg (0.1 mg/kg in children)	0.2 mg/kg (in divided doses over 10 min)	Several minutes	1–2 hr	Respiratory depression Hypotension	Naloxone Airway and ventilation Raise legs IV fluids Vasopressor	
Nitrous oxide	Premixed delivery system 50:50 with oxygen (Nitronox)	Self-administered continuous inhalation of 50:50 mixture until procedure completed	30 min	1–2 min	1–2 min after inhalation ceases	Excessive sedation Nausea and vomiting	Stop administering	Do not use in children, during pregnancy, or in patients with sickle cell disease.
Procaine*	Solutions of 1% (10 mg/ml) and 2% (20 mg/ml)	Infiltrative: use 1% solution in volume necessary for size of lesion up to maximal dose	Lesser of 1000 mg or 14 mg/kg	5–10 min	60–90 min	Seizures Respiratory depression Hypotension	Diazepam Airway and ventilation Raise legs IV fluids Vasopressor	Do not use in patients receiving sulfonamides.
		Blocks: use 2% solution. Volume will vary with site of block.		10–20 min	60–90 min			
Proparacaine	0.5% solution	1–2 drops	7–10 drops	Seconds	15–30 min	Has no serious side effects with single use; may cause acute hypersensitivity reaction of cornea		Do not give any to the patient for repetitive instillation. Do not use if the solution is amber colored.
TAC	Solution containing tetracaine 0.5%, 5 mg/ml, epinephrine (Adrenalin) 1:2000, 0.5 mg/ml, and cocaine 11.8%, 118 mg/ml	3–5 ml applied to wound for 10–15 min	5 ml	10–15 min	Several hours	Seizures Hypertension Tachydysrhythmias Hyperthermia	Diazepam Nitroprusside Propranolol, then ACLS protocols Surface cooling	FOR TOPICAL USE ONLY. Do not use on mucous membranes, large burns, or abrasions—increased absorption may cause systemic toxicity. Do not use on digits, ears, penis, nose, lips—may cause ischemia.

*These local anesthetics are also available with various concentrations of epinephrine. The vasoconstriction induced by epinephrine reduces bleeding and increases the duration of anesthetic effect. Epinephrine may increase the incidence of wound infection, delay wound healing, and should not be used on digits, ears, or the penis since the vasoconstriction it induces may cause ischemia of these appendages.

DRUG TREATMENT: SHORT, PAINFUL PROCEDURES—COOPERATIVE ADULT PATIENT

First-Line Drug
Nitrous Oxide

Initial Dose	50:50 with oxygen by continuous inhalation
Repeat Dose	Maximum usage time—30 minutes
End-Points	Successful procedure No respiratory or cardiac side effects

Second-Line Drugs
Midazolam and Morphine

Initial Dose	Midazolam, 1–2 mg IV *and* Morphine, 3–5 mg IV (in same syringe over 5 minutes)
Repeat Dose	Midazolam, 1–2 mg IV in 30–40 minutes Morphine, one-half of initial dose in 10 minutes
End-Points	Successful procedure No respiratory or cardiac side effects

Third-Line Drugs
Meperidine and Hydroxyzine

Initial Dose	Meperidine, 1–1.5 mg/kg IM Hydroxyzine, 25–50 mg IM
Repeat Dose	50% of initial dose of both drugs in 45 minutes
End-Points	Successful procedure No respiratory or cardiac side effects

FIGURE 2–1. Recommended approach for systemic analgesia in adults. (From Barsan WG, Jastremski MS, Syverud SA: Emergency Drug Therapy. Philadelphia, WB Saunders, 1991, p 110.)

DRUG TREATMENT: SHORT, PAINFUL PROCEDURES—PEDIATRIC PATIENT

First-Line Drugs
Meperidine, Promethazine, and Chlorpromazine

Initial Dose	Meperidine, 2 mg/kg IM (≤50 mg) Promethazine, 1 mg/kg IM (≤25 mg) Chlorpromazine, 1 mg/kg IM (≤25 mg)
Repeat Dose	Not recommended
End-Points	Successful procedure No respiratory or cardiac side effects

Second-Line Drug
Fentanyl

Initial Dose	0.001 mg/kg by slow IV push
Repeat Dose	One-half the initial dose in 10 minutes
End-Points	Successful procedure No respiratory or cardiac side effects

Third-Line Drugs
Meperidine and Diazepam

Initial Dose	Meperidine, 1–1.5 mg/kg IM (maximum dose, 50 mg) Diazepam, 0.1 mg/kg by slow IV push (maximum dose, 2.5 mg)
Repeat Dose	One-half the initial dose of only diazepam in 15 minutes IV
End-Points	Successful procedure No respiratory or cardiac side effects

FIGURE 2–2. Recommended approach for systemic analgesia in children. (From Barsan WG, Jastremski MS, Syverud SA: Emergency Drug Therapy. Philadelphia, WB Saunders, 1991, p 111.)

References

Altman RS, Smith-Coggins R, Ampel LL: Local anesthetics. Ann Emerg Med 14:1209, 1985.

Barsan W, Jastremski M, Syverud S (eds): Emergency Drug Therapy. Philadelphia, WB Saunders, 1990.

Nelson HS: Allergic reactions to drugs. Adv Asthma Allergy 3:29, 1976.

Physician's Desk Reference. Oradell, NJ, Medical Economics Company, 1990.

Ankle Block

W. JOHN ZEHNER, MD

Indication

To anesthetize the foot, most commonly for laceration repair, reduction of fractures or dislocations, or abscess drainage

Contraindications

Allergy to local anesthetics
Infection in the region of the injection site

Equipment

Gloves
12-ml syringe
22-gauge, 2½-inch needle
25- or 27-gauge, 1-inch needle
Local anesthetic
Betadine swab

Universal Precautions

1. Wear gloves.
2. Dispose of needles and syringe properly.

Technique

The foot is innervated by five nerves, and thus complete anesthesia of the foot requires blocks of all five nerves (Figure 2–3).

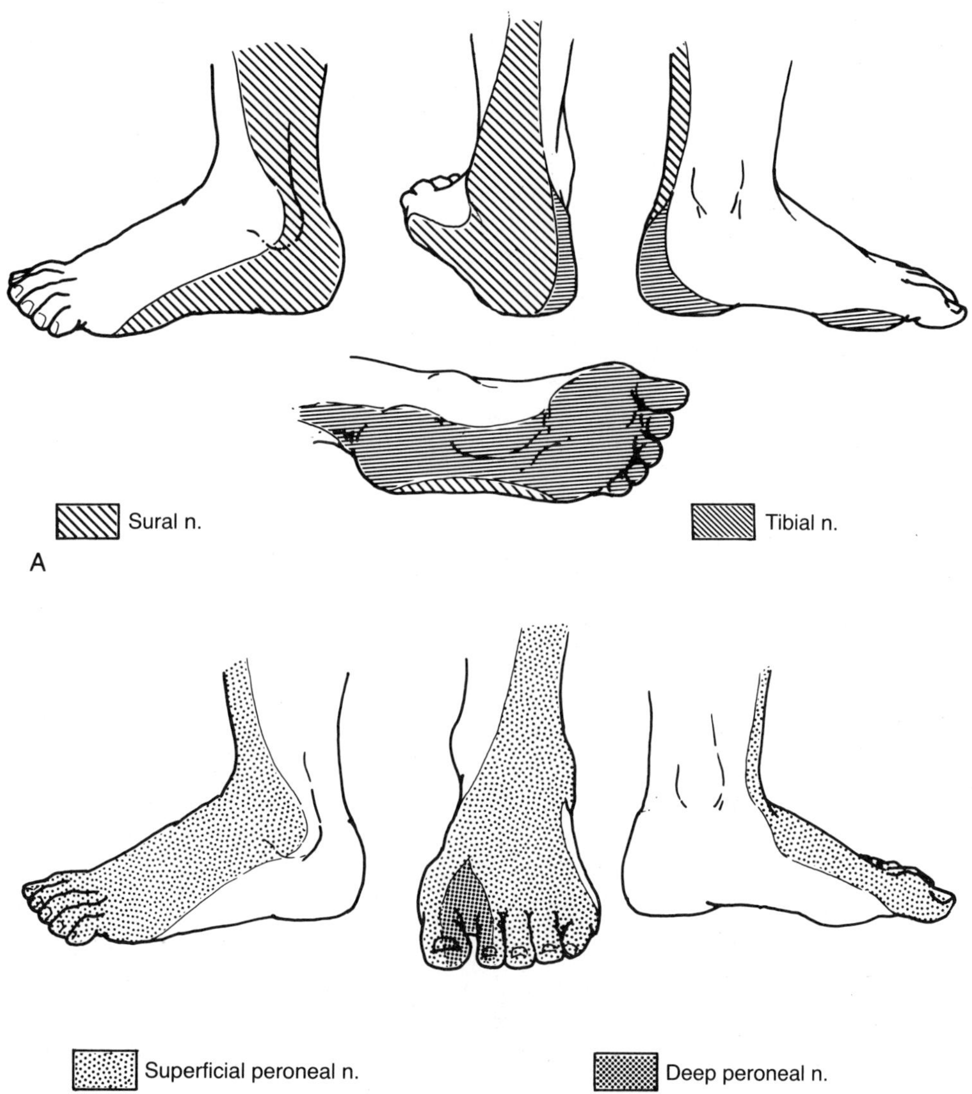

FIGURE 2–3. Nerve distribution of the foot. The area innervated by the saphenous nerve is delineated by the clear area on the medial aspect of the foot.

Anterior Tibial (Deep Peroneal) Block

1. Explain the procedure to the patient and obtain consent.
2. Position the patient supine on a stretcher.
3. Stand at the foot of the stretcher facing the patient.
4. Locate the injection site by having the patient dorsiflex the great toe and foot to identify the extensor hallucis longus tendon and the tibialis anterior tendon. The injection site over the anterior tibial nerve lies between these two tendons, on the line joining the medial and lateral malleoli (the anterior ankle crease) (Figure 2–4).
5. Prep the area with Betadine.
6. Put on gloves.
7. Fill the syringe with 10 ml of anesthetic solution.
8. Attach the 25- or 27-gauge needle to the syringe and inject a small amount of anesthesia under the skin at the injection site.
9. Change to the 22-gauge, 2½-inch needle and insert it perpendicular to the skin at the injection site. Advance the needle until bone is reached. Then withdraw the needle 2 or 3 mm, aspirate, and, if no blood returns, slowly inject 5 or 6 ml of the anesthetic solution (see Figure 2–4).
10. Wait several minutes, then test for effective anesthesia in the area needing it.

Posterior Tibial Nerve

1. Explain the procedure to the patient and obtain consent.
2. Position the patient prone on a stretcher with a pillow supporting the lower leg and the legs spread apart.
3. Stand at the side of the stretcher opposite the ankle to be anesthetized so you are facing the medial side of the patient's ankle.
4. Locate the injection site by finding a point at the level of the superior border of the medial malleolus posterior to the posterior tibial artery and anterior to the Achilles tendon (Figure 2–5).
5. Cleanse the area with Betadine.
6. Put on gloves.
7. Fill the syringe with 10 ml of anesthetic solution.
8. Attach the 25- or 27-gauge needle to the syringe and inject a small amount of anesthesia under the skin at the injection site.
9. Change to the 22-gauge, 2½-inch needle and advance the needle toward the second toe until paresthesia of the sole occurs. The needle may need to be withdrawn and readvanced at different angles in the mediolateral plane before paresthesia occurs. When paresthesia occurs, withdraw the needle a tiny bit, aspirate to ensure it is not in a vessel, and then slowly inject 5 to 6 ml of anesthetic.

   If paresthesia is not elicited, then slowly inject 10 to 12 ml of anesthetic in a fan distribution approximately 1 inch under the skin. Remember to aspirate before injection. It may take 20 to 30 minutes before complete anesthesia occurs with this technique.
10. Wait several minutes, then test for effective anesthesia in the area needing it.

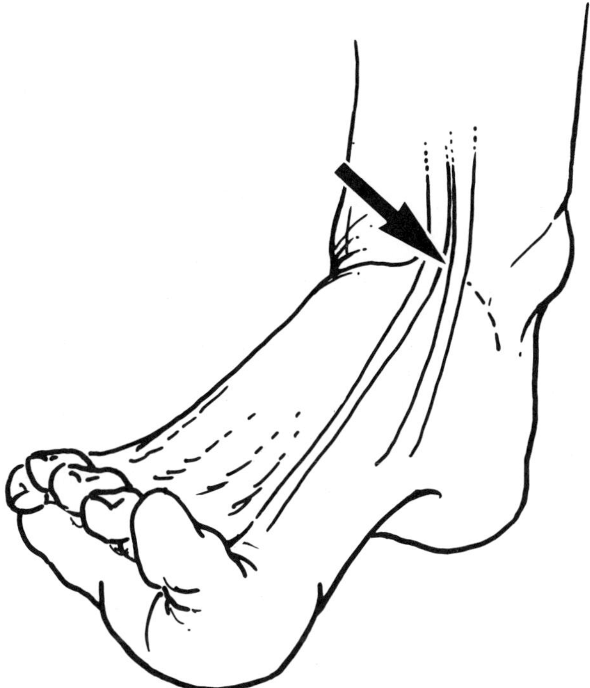

FIGURE 2–4. Anterior tibial nerve block.

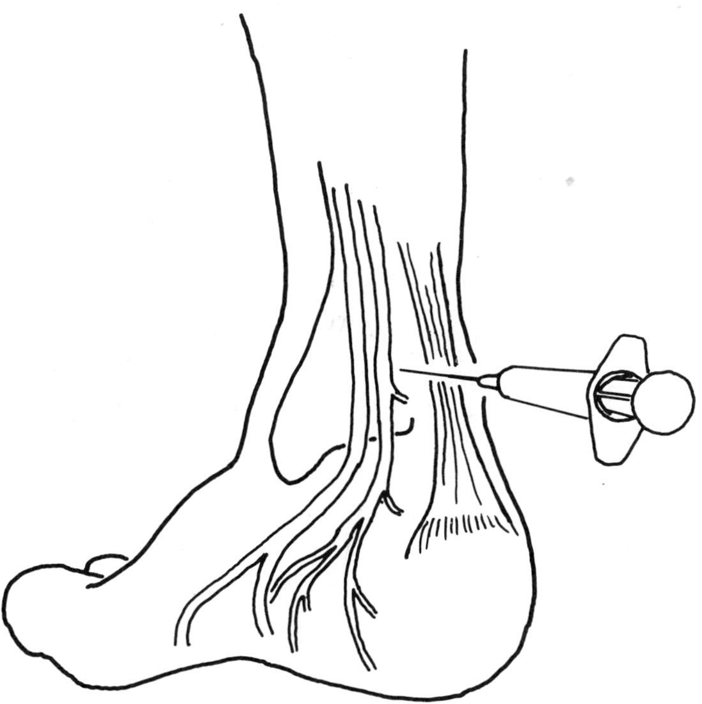

FIGURE 2–5. Posterior tibial nerve block.

Saphenous and Superficial Peroneal Nerves

1. Explain the procedure to the patient and obtain consent.
2. Position the patient supine on a stretcher.
3. Stand at the foot of the stretcher facing the patient.
4. Locate the injection site by finding the midpoint of a line connecting the superior borders of the medial and lateral malleoli on the dorsum of the foot (Figure 2–6).
5. Prep this area with Betadine.
6. Put on gloves.
7. Fill the syringe with 10 ml of anesthetic solution.
8. Attach the 25- or 27-gauge needle to the syringe and inject a small amount of anesthetic under the skin at the injection site.
9. Change to the 22-gauge, 2½-inch needle and advance the needle through the skin into the subcutaneous tissue at an angle that aims toward the lateral malleolus. Slowly advance the needle through the subcutaneous tissue toward the lateral malleolus while injecting the local anesthetic. A total of 5 to 6 ml should be deposited along the tract.
10. Withdraw the needle and reinsert it at the same site, only now aiming toward the medial malleolus. Deposit 5 to 6 ml of anesthetic solution in the subcutaneous tissue as the needle is advanced to the malleolus.
11. Wait several minutes, then test for effective anesthesia in the area needing it.

Sural Nerve

1. Explain the procedure to the patient and obtain consent.
2. Position the patient prone on a stretcher with a pillow supporting the lower leg and the legs spread apart.
3. Stand at the foot of the stretcher facing the ankle to be anesthetized.
4. Locate the injection site at the lateral border of the Achilles tendon in the same plane as the superior border of the lateral malleolus (Figure 2–7).
5. Cleanse the area with Betadine.
6. Put on gloves.
7. Fill the syringe with 10 ml of anesthetic solution.
8. Attach the 25- or 27-gauge needle to the syringe and inject a small amount of anesthetic under the skin at the injection site.
9. Change to the 22-gauge, 2½-inch needle. Slowly advance the needle from the injection site through the subcutaneous tissue toward the superior border of the lateral malleolus. Deposit 6 to 8 ml of anesthetic along the needle's tract as the needle is being advanced (see Figure 2–6).
10. Wait several minutes, then test for effective anesthesia in the area needing it.

Complications

Intravascular injection

Nerve trauma from the needle

Hematoma

Inadequate anesthesia

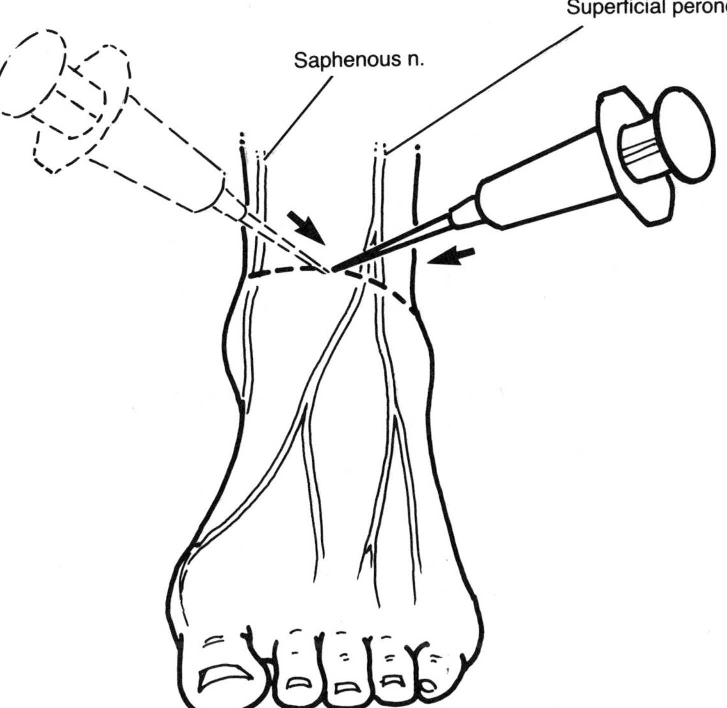

FIGURE 2–6. Saphenous and superficial peroneal nerve block.

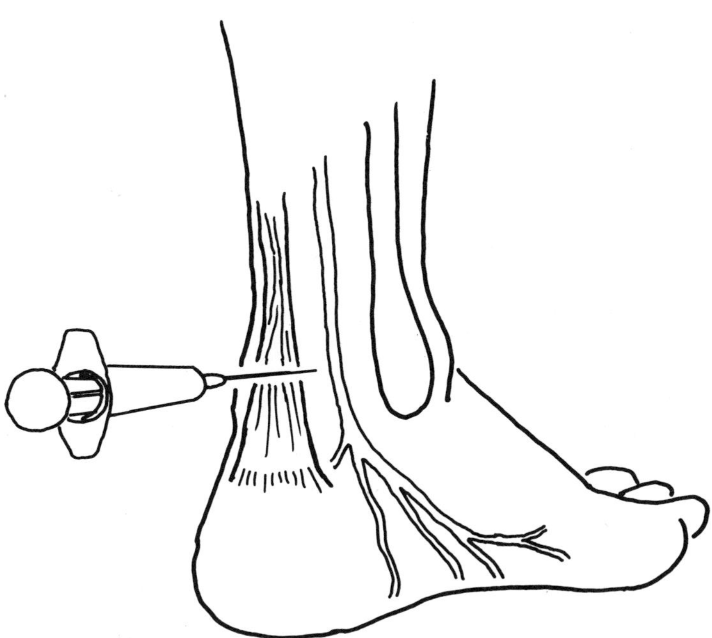

FIGURE 2–7. Sural nerve block.

Pearls and Pitfalls

The block is performed in two phases: on the anterior aspect of the ankle and on the posterior aspect of the ankle. However, it is usually not necessary to block all the nerves of the ankle. Match the area needing anesthesia to the nerve most likely to supply that area using Figure 2–3. Then block that nerve and test for adequate anesthesia. If adequate anesthesia is not achieved, then add blocks of contiguous nerves.

Do not forget to test for neurologic function *before* doing the nerve block.

References

Carron H, Korbon GA, Rowlingson JC: Regional Anesthesia, pp 116–121. Orlando, FL, Grune & Stratton, 1984.

Moore KL: Clinically Oriented Anatomy, pp 538–542. Baltimore, Williams & Wilkins, 1980.

Dental Blocks

W. JOHN ZEHNER, MD

INFRAORBITAL NERVE BLOCK

Indications

To anesthetize the skin below the eye to the upper lip including the maxillary incisors, cuspids, and bicuspids on that side

Use primarily for suturing facial and upper lip lacerations when local infiltrations would cause tissue distention and make laceration repair more difficult.

Contraindications

Facial cellulitis

Allergy to local anesthetics

Coagulopathy

Equipment

Gloves

Aspirating dental syringe with capsules of anesthetic or 5-ml syringe with 25- or 27-gauge, 1½-inch needle

2% lidocaine or bupivacaine with epinephrine

Topical anesthetic such as cetacaine, cocaine, or lidocaine

Cotton-tipped applicator

Headlight (optional, but very useful)

Universal Precautions

1. Wear gloves.
2. Use a face shield.
3. Dispose of syringe and needles properly.

Technique

Intraoral

1. Explain the procedure to the patient and obtain consent.
2. Position the patient sitting in an examining chair.
3. Stand at the side of the patient to be injected, facing the patient.
4. Put on gloves.
5. Prepare anesthetic solutions by soaking a cotton-tipped applicator with the topical agent and filling the syringe with attached 25-gauge, 1½-inch needle with the local anesthetic.
6. Use your left thumb to palpate the infraorbital foramen, which is located approximately 0.5 cm below the infraorbital rim in line with the pupil when the patient stares straight ahead (Figure 2–8).
7. While keeping your thumb in place, grasp the patient's upper lip with your index finger, retracting out and up (see Figure 2–8).
8. Apply a topical anesthetic to the mucosa of the needle entry site—the mucolabial fold above the second bicuspid in the same plane as the inner canthus of the eye. Wait several minutes for the topical anesthetic to take effect.
9. Again palpate the foramen and retract the lip with the thumb and index finger of your left hand. Insert the needle attached to the syringe containing the anesthetic at the site described in No. 8 and direct it upward and laterally toward the infraorbital foramen (which is under your left thumb) until you can feel the needle with your left thumb. Do not advance the needle more than 2 cm.
10. Aspirate and if there is no blood return inject 1 to 2 ml of local anesthetic over 1 minute. Then massage the area with your thumb to force the anesthetic into the foramen.

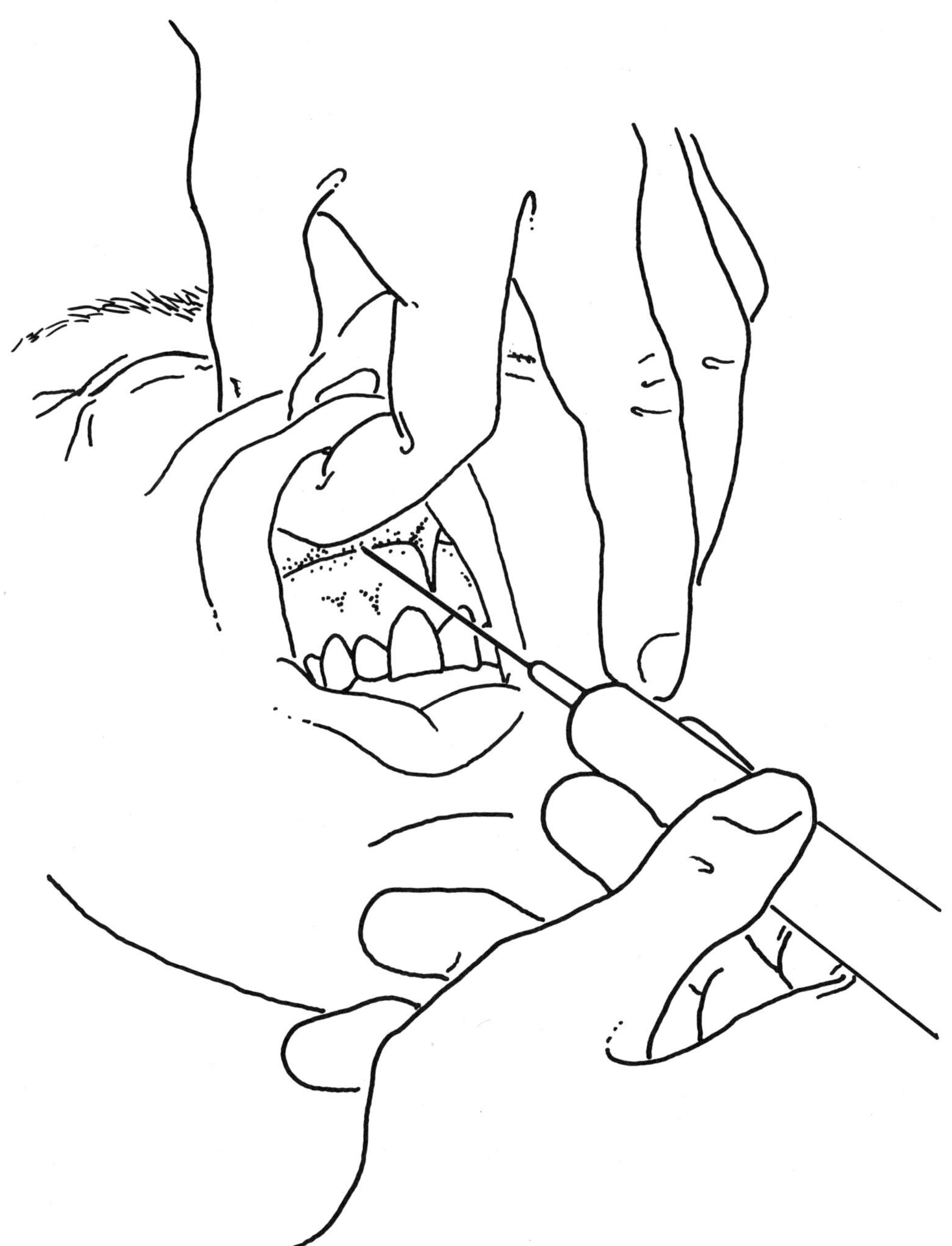

FIGURE 2–8. Infraorbital nerve block: intraoral approach.

Extraoral

1. Explain the procedure to the patient and obtain consent.
2. Position the patient sitting in an examining chair.
3. Stand at the side of the patient to be injected, facing the patient.
4. Put on gloves.
5. Prepare anesthetic solution by filling the syringe with attached 25-gauge, 1½-inch needle with the local anesthetic.
6. Use your left thumb to palpate the infraorbital foramen located approximately 0.5 cm below the infraorbital rim in line with the pupil when the patient stares straight ahead (Figure 2–9).
7. Cleanse the skin with alcohol or Betadine.
8. Enter the skin slightly medially and inferiorly to the infraorbital foramen with the 25-gauge needle attached to a syringe containing the anesthetic.
9. Advance the needle to the foramen (see Figure 2–9).
10. Aspirate, and if no blood returns inject 1 to 2 ml of the anesthetic over 1 minute. Then massage the area with your thumb.

Complications

Intravascular injection
Entering the orbit with the needle
Hematoma
Facial cellulitis
Broken needle

Pearls and Pitfalls

Because of the proximity of the orbit to the foramen, always be sure of the location of your needle. Keep a finger on the foramen when you localize it. Do not inject if you are unsure of the location of your needle. Do not advance the needle more than 2 cm.

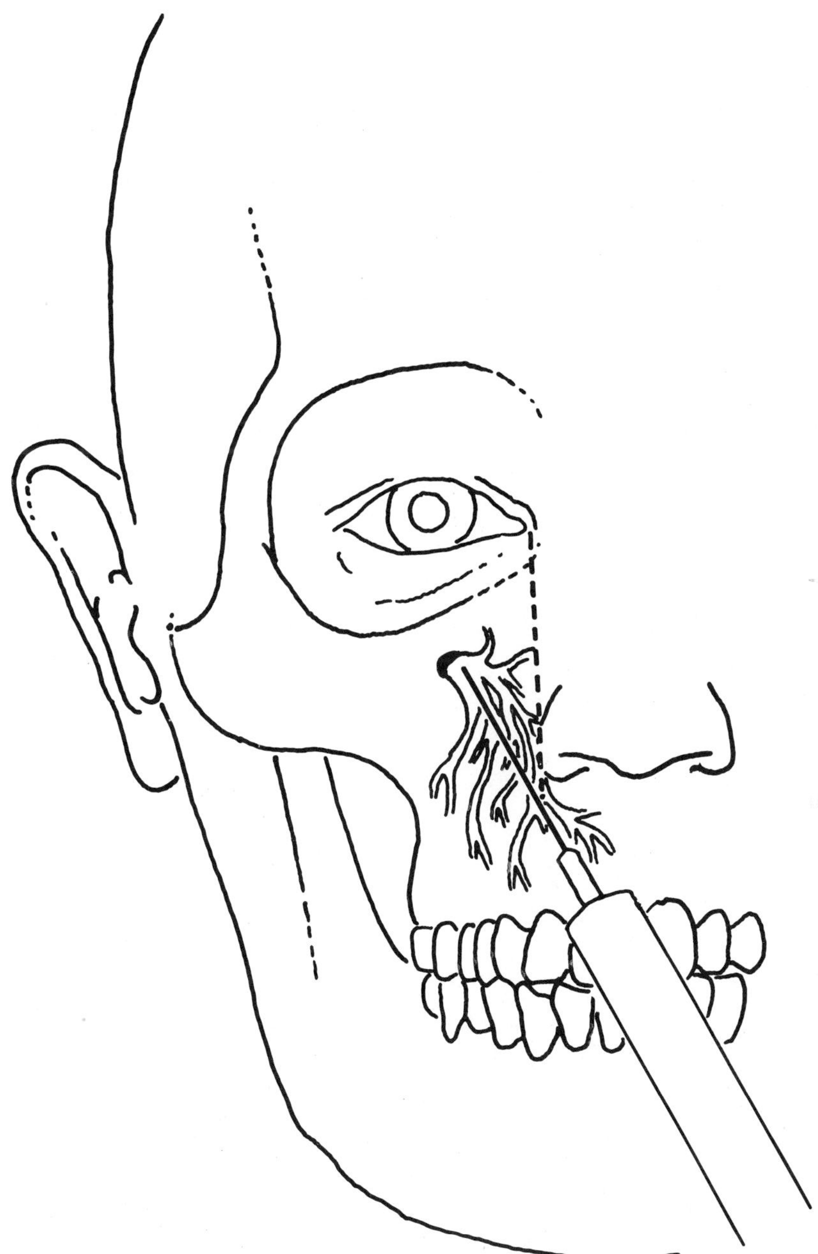

FIGURE 2–9. Infraorbital nerve block: extraoral approach.

INFERIOR ALVEOLAR BLOCK

Indications

To anesthetize all the teeth on one side of the mandible, which is useful in patients with postextraction pain, dry socket (alveolar osteitis), or periapical abscess

To anesthetize the ipsilateral lower lip, chin, and tongue, which aids in repairing lacerations in this region

Contraindications

Obvious infection at the site of the injection

Coagulopathy

Allergy to local anesthetics

Equipment

Gloves

Aspirating dental syringe with capsules of anesthetic or 5-ml syringe with 25- or 27-gauge, 1½-inch needle

2% lidocaine or bupivacaine with epinephrine

Topical anesthetic such as cetacaine, cocaine, or lidocaine

Cotton-tipped applicator

Headlight (optional, but very useful)

Universal Precautions

1. Wear gloves.
2. Use a face shield.
3. Dispose of needle and syringe properly.

Technique

1. Explain the procedure to the patient and obtain consent.
2. Position the patient sitting in an examining chair.
3. Right-handed physicians should stand at the patient's right, facing the patient, when injecting right-sided teeth, and when injecting the left side should stand behind the patient to the patient's right, facing in the same direction as the patient, bending forward to look in the patient's mouth. Left-handed physicians should reverse these directions.
4. Ensure that the oral cavity is well lighted.
5. Put on gloves.
6. Prepare anesthetic solution by soaking a cotton-tipped applicator with the topical agent and filling the syringe with attached 25-gauge, 1½-inch needle with the local anesthetic.

7. With the patient's mouth open, palpate the mandibular ramus on the side you wish to anesthetize with the index finger of your left hand. Locate the coronoid notch (the deepest part of the anterior border of the mandibular ramus) with the tip of your index finger. Retract both the cheek and the mucosa over the notch laterally with your index finger (Figure 2–10).

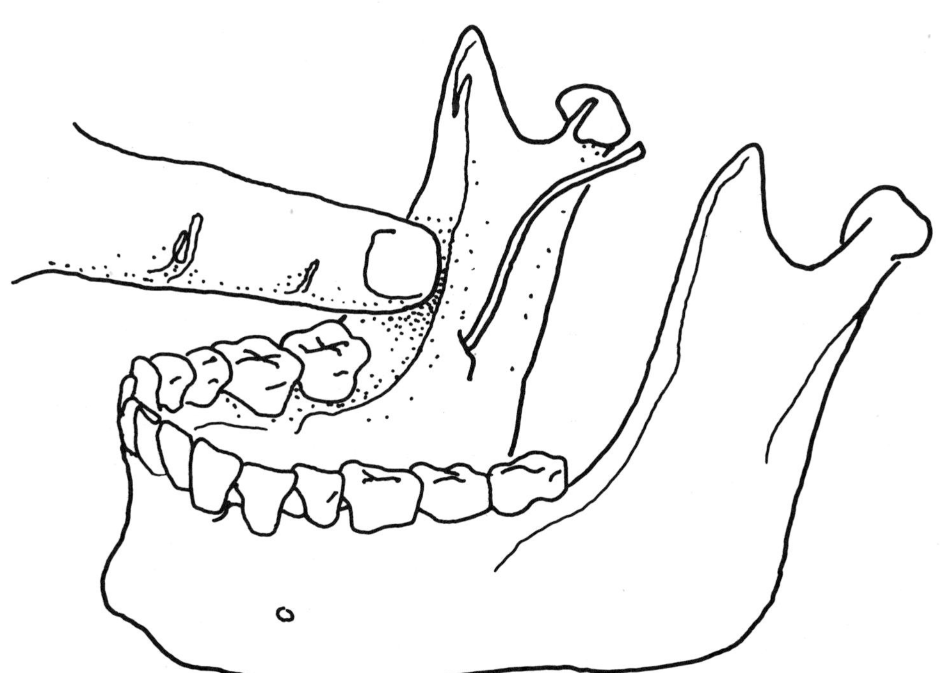

FIGURE 2–10. Inferior alveolar block.

8. Visualize the pterygomandibular triangle located posterior and cephalad to the last molar next to the tip of your index finger.
9. Approach the pterygomandibular triangle with your anesthetic-filled syringe and needle on a line from the first and second bicuspids on the opposite side and parallel to the surface of the lower teeth. Advance the needle into the triangle until the needle hits the periosteum of the mandible (Figure 2–11).
10. Aspirate, and if there is no blood return inject 2 to 3 ml of anesthetic over at least 2 minutes.
11. Withdraw the needle until about ¼ inch remains in the tissue. Aspirate, and if there is no blood return inject an additional 0.5 ml of anesthetic to anesthetize the lingual nerve.

Complications

Spread of localized infection

Anesthesia of the facial nerve, which may affect the patient's ability to close the eyelid

Intravascular injection

Hematoma

Broken needle

Pearls and Pitfalls

1. If the needle does not hit bone within 5 to 10 mm, the syringe is angulated either too anteriorly or too posteriorly and should be redirected.
2. Anesthetizing the facial nerve and the orbicularis muscle must be recognized and the eye protected with an eye patch and artificial tears until function is restored (which may take several hours depending on the type of anesthetic).
3. If the inferior alveolar block does not provide adequate anesthesia, you may anesthetize individual teeth using a supraperiosteal block.
4. Do not insert the needle up to the bevel since a broken needle completely embedded in the tissue of the oral cavity can be very difficult to retrieve.

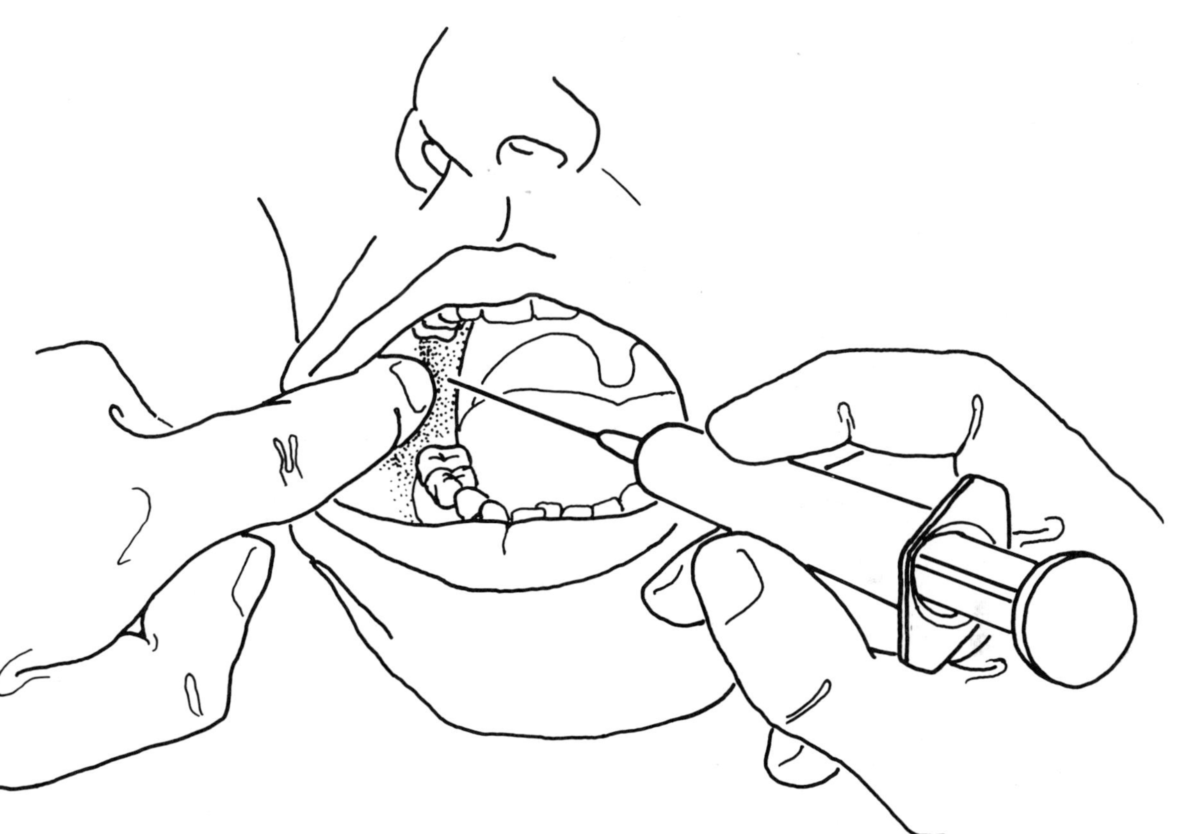

FIGURE 2–11. Inferior alveolar block.

POSTERIOR SUPERIOR ALVEOLAR BLOCK

Indication

To anesthetize the first, second, and third molars of the maxilla

Contraindications

Infection in the region of the injection site
Coagulopathy
Allergy to local anesthetics

Equipment

Gloves
Aspirating dental syringe with anesthetic capsules or a 5-ml syringe with a 25- or 27-gauge, 1-inch needle
Lidocaine (2%) or bupivacaine with epinephrine
Topical anesthetic such as cetacaine, cocaine, or lidocaine
Cotton-tipped applicator
Headlight (optional, but very useful)

Universal Precautions

1. Wear gloves.
2. Use a face shield.
3. Dispose of needles properly.

Technique

1. Explain the procedure to the patient and obtain consent.
2. Position the patient sitting in an examining chair.
3. Right-handed physicians should stand at the patient's right, facing the patient, when injecting right-sided teeth, and when injecting the left side should stand behind the patient to the patient's right, facing in the same direction as the patient, bending forward to look in the patient's mouth. Left-handed physicians should reverse these directions.
4. Ensure that the oral cavity is well lighted.
5. Put on gloves.
6. Prepare the anesthetic solutions by soaking a cotton-tipped applicator with the topical agent and filling the syringe with attached 25-gauge, 1-inch needle with the local anesthetic.
7. Use your left index finger to palpate the posteroinferior surface of the malar prominence in the mucobuccal fold, opposite the tricuspids (Figure 2–12).

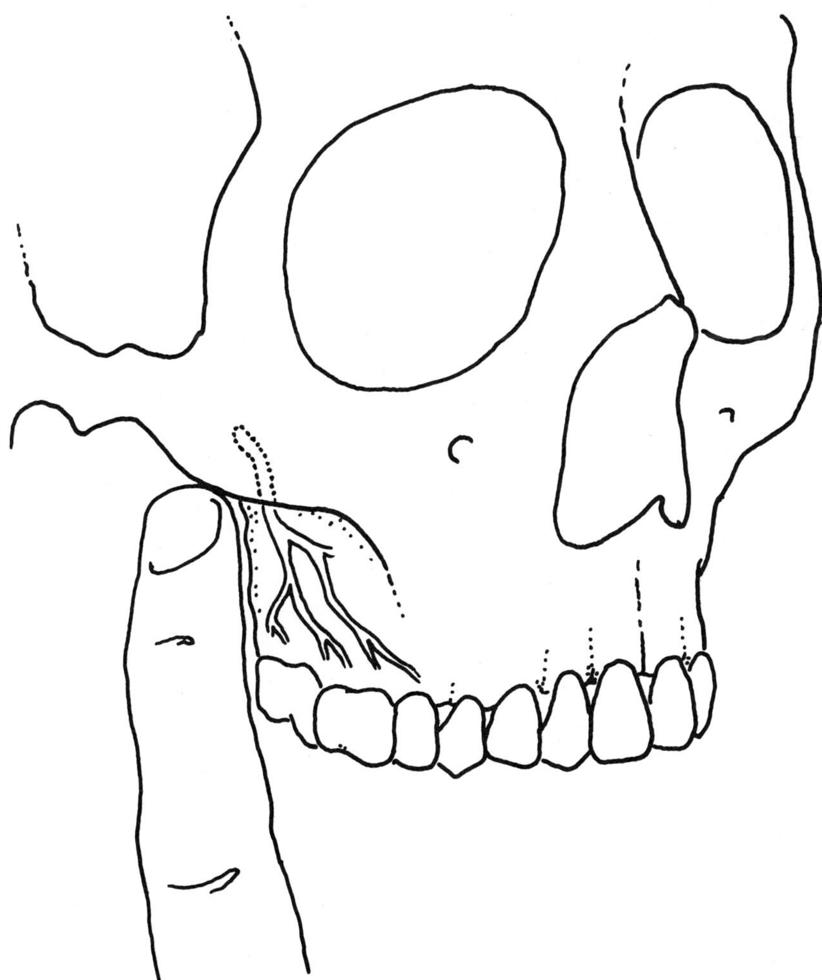

FIGURE 2–12. Posterior superior alveolar block.

8. Pull the patient's lip and cheek outward with your left index finger while keeping your fingertip on the malar prominence (Figure 2–13).
9. Apply topical anesthetic to the injection site located at the apex of the buccolabial fold medial and a little forward of your fingertip. Wait 1 or 2 minutes for it to take effect.
10. Advance the needle attached to the syringe filled with anesthetic upward and medially from the injection site to a depth of ¾ inch (see Figure 2–13).
11. Aspirate, and if no blood returns slowly inject 2 to 3 ml of anesthetic.

Complications

Hematoma
Infection
Broken needle
Unsuccessful anesthesia

Pearls and Pitfalls

Complete anesthesia of the first molar requires that an additional 0.25 ml of anesthetic be injected at its apex using the supraperiosteal technique.

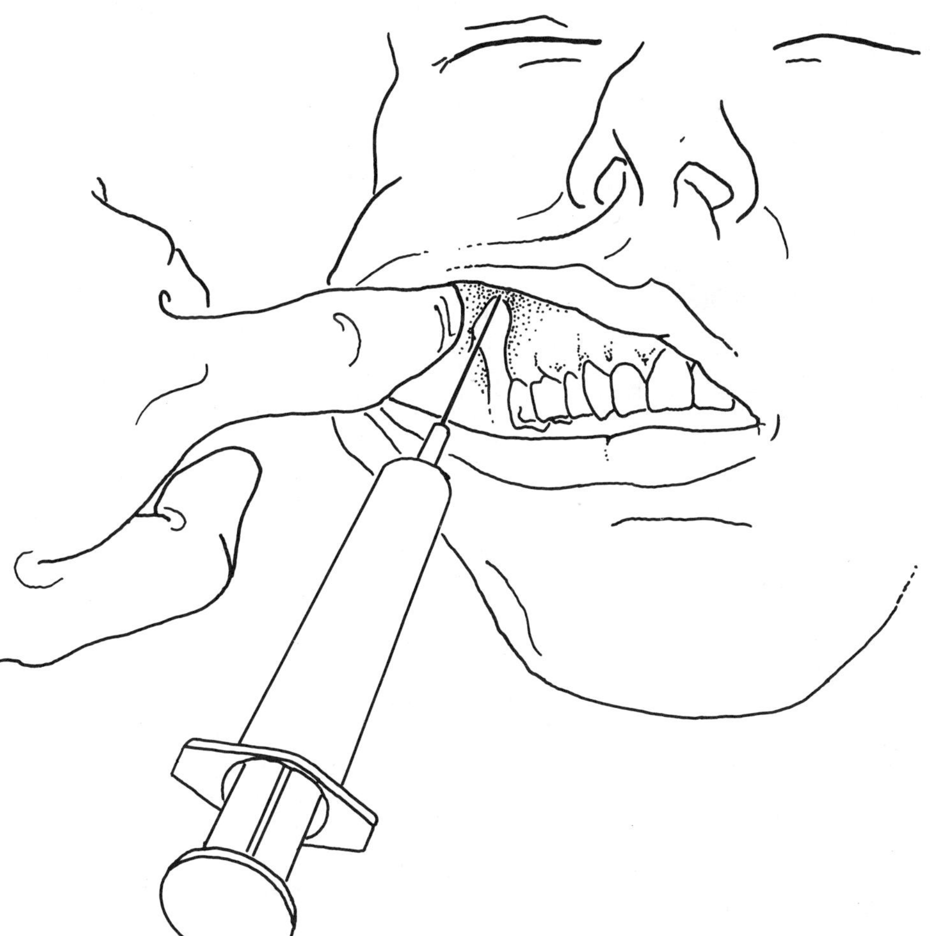

FIGURE 2–13. Posterior superior alveolar block.

SUPRAPERIOSTEAL INFILTRATION

Indication

To anesthetize an individual tooth, which is useful for pain relief from a periapical tooth abscess

Contraindications

Localized infection of the soft tissue at the site of injection
Allergy to local anesthetics

Equipment

Gloves
Aspirating dental syringe with capsules of anesthetic or 5-ml syringe with 27-gauge, 1-inch needle
2% lidocaine or bupivacaine with epinephrine
Topical anesthetic such as cetacaine, cocaine, or lidocaine
Cotton-tipped applicator
Headlight (optional, but very useful)

Universal Precautions

1. Wear gloves.
2. Use a face shield.
3. Dispose of needle and syringe properly.

Technique

1. Explain the procedure to the patient and obtain consent.
2. Position the patient sitting in an examining chair.
3. Right-handed physicians should stand at the patient's right, facing the patient, when injecting right-sided teeth, and when injecting left-sided teeth should stand behind the patient to the patient's right, facing in the same direction as the patient, bending forward to look in the patient's mouth. Left-handed physicians should reverse these directions.
4. Ensure that the oral cavity is well lighted.
5. Put on gloves.
6. Prepare the anesthetic solutions by soaking a cotton-tipped applicator with the topical agent and filling the syringe with attached 27-gauge, 1-inch needle with the local anesthetic.
7. Grasp the patient's lip near the involved tooth and pull the lip downward and out from the mandible or upward and out from the maxilla.
8. Identify the involved tooth and apply a topical anesthetic to the mucosa in the gingivobuccal fold at its base.

9. Wait several minutes for the topical anesthetic to take effect, and then insert the needle attached to the syringe containing the local anesthesia at the gingivobuccal fold adjacent to the tooth to be anesthetized with the bevel toward the tooth. Direct the needle toward the periapical region of the tooth until it touches bone.
10. Aspirate, and if there is no blood return inject 1 to 2 ml of anesthetic at the apex of the tooth.

Complications

Spread of localized infection
Unsuccessful anesthesia
Hematoma
Broken needle

Pearls and Pitfalls

1. The anesthetic must be absorbed by the bone (hence the name "supraperiosteal") to reach the nerve.
2. It may take 5 to 10 minutes to achieve anesthesia, so be patient.
3. It may not be effective for the posterior molars because of their thicker bone.
4. Any needle smaller than a 27-gauge will prevent aspiration of blood when in a vessel and may lead to inadvertent intravascular injection of anesthetic.

References

Amsterdam JT: Anesthetic nerve block. In Tintanelli J, Rothstein R, Krome R (eds): Emergency Medicine—A Comprehensive Study Guide, pp 763–766. New York, McGraw-Hill Book Company, 1985.
Amsterdam JT, Hendler BH, Rose LF: Emergency dental procedures. In Roberts J, Hedges J (eds): Clinical Procedures in Emergency Medicine, pp 946–973. Philadelphia, WB Saunders, 1985.
Bennett CR: Monheim's Local Anesthesia and Pain Control in Dental Practice, pp 69–123. St. Louis, CV Mosby, 1984.
Olson C: Oral anesthesia. In Jastremski M, Cantor R, Olson C, Smith R, Tyndall G (eds): The Whole Emergency Medicine Catalog, pp 370–374. Philadelphia, WB Saunders, 1985.

Digital Nerve Block

W. JOHN ZEHNER, MD

Indication

To anesthetize an individual finger or toe. It is most successful with second, third, and fourth digits. The small digit, thumb, and great toe require a proximal block.

Contraindications

Uncooperative patient
Localized infection at the injection site
Allergy to local anesthetics

Equipment

Gloves
10-ml syringe
25-gauge, 1-inch needle
Betadine skin prep
Local anesthetic without epinephrine

Universal Precautions

1. Wear gloves.
2. Dispose of needle and syringe properly.

Technique—Finger Block

1. Explain the procedure to the patient and obtain consent.
2. Position the patient supine on a stretcher with the arm to be treated abducted on an armboard with the palm up and fingers abducted.
3. Stand at the end of the arm board facing the hand.
4. Wipe an area on either side of the metacarpophalangeal joint and contiguous palm of the finger or fingers to be anesthetized with Betadine.
5. Put on sterile gloves.
6. Attach the 25-gauge, 1-inch needle to the syringe and fill the syringe with the chosen anesthetic solution.

7. Enter the skin at the palmar digital junction in the middle of the finger, aiming toward the base of the proximal phalanx. Advance the needle to one side of the proximal phalanx and just before the needle tip is at the proximal edge of the bone, aspirate; then inject 1 to 1.5 ml of anesthetic solution. Advance the needle to the distal margin of the bone, aspirate, and then inject an additional 1 ml of anesthetic solution (Figure 2–14).

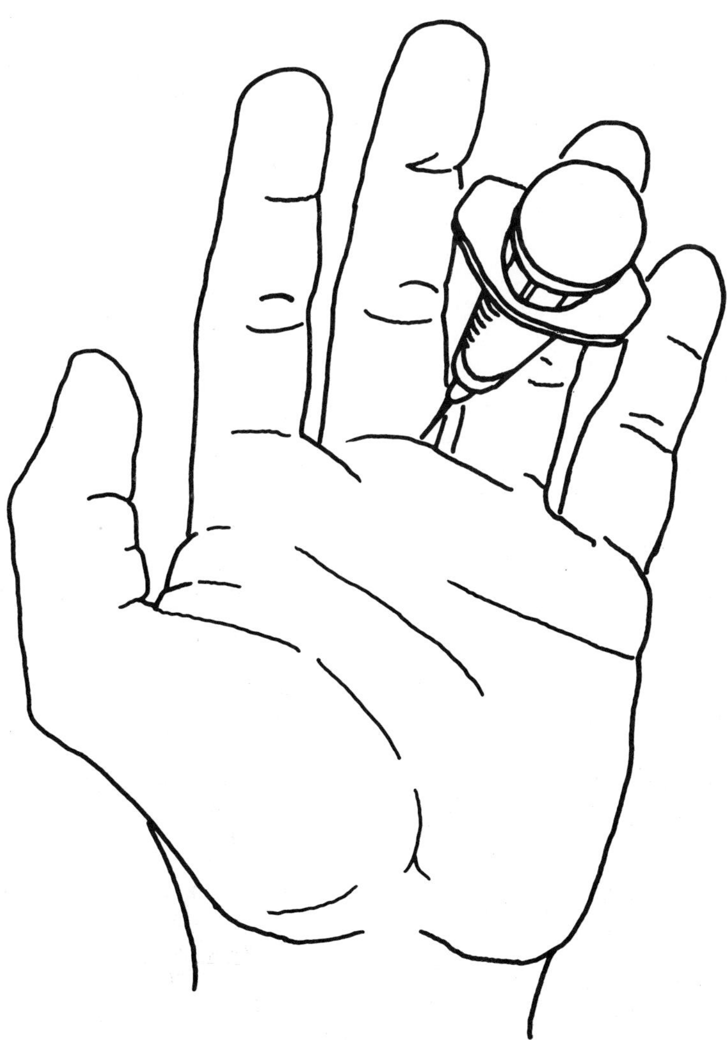

FIGURE 2–14. Digital block: palmar approach.

8. Withdraw the needle so the tip is just below the palmar skin, redirect it to the other side of the digit, and repeat the procedure on the other side of the finger.
9. Wait 5 minutes, then test the area you wish to work on to ensure adequate anesthesia. If anesthesia is not adequate, massage the area of injection and wait a few more minutes. If anesthesia is still not adequate, repeat the block, but do not exceed a total volume of anesthetic solution of 5 ml per digit.

Technique—Toe Block

1. Explain the procedure to the patient and obtain consent.
2. Position the patient supine on a stretcher with the ankle plantar-flexed.
3. Stand at the side of the patient's foot to be anesthetized, facing the foot.
4. Use Betadine to cleanse an area on either side of the metatarsophalangeal joint. If the foot is particularly dirty, soak it and scrub it in a Betadine-saline solution first.
5. Put on sterile gloves.
6. Attach the 1-inch 25-gauge needle to the syringe and fill the syringe with the chosen anesthetic solution.
7. Hold the patient's foot with the index finger of your nondominant hand at the plantar side of the metatarsophalangeal joint of the toe to be anesthetized.
8. Insert the needle on the dorsum of the digit just distal to the metatarsophalangeal joint, several millimeters off the midline of the toe, aiming for the sole in the web space. Slowly advance the needle along the side of the proximal phalanx until resistance is felt from the plantar skin or you can

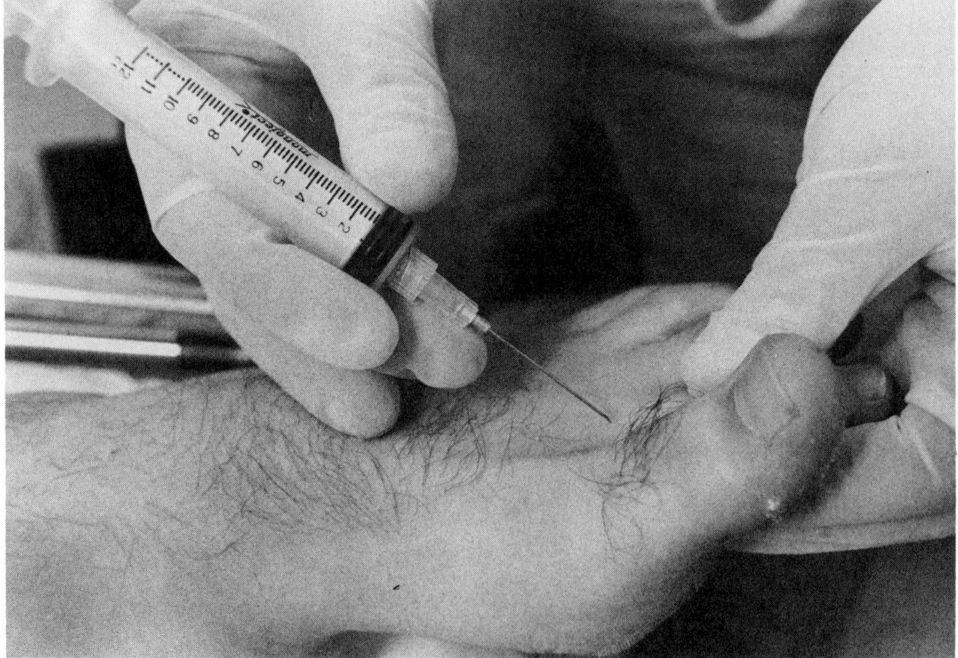

FIGURE 2–15. Digital block: dorsal approach.

palpate the needle with your index finger. Do not exit the plantar skin. If you encounter bone, redirect the needle lateral to it (Figure 2–15).

9. When the needle tip is palpated or reaches the plantar skin, aspirate and then inject 1 to 2 ml of anesthetic.
10. Withdraw the needle until the tip is at the level of the top of the bone, aspirate, and then inject another 1 ml of anesthetic.
11. Repeat steps 8, 9, and 10 for the other side of the digit.
12. Wait 5 minutes and then test the area you wish to work on to ensure adequate anesthesia. If anesthesia is not adequate, massage the area of injection and wait a few more minutes. If anesthesia is still not adequate, repeat the block, but do not exceed a total volume of anesthetic solution of 5 ml per digit.

Complications

Intravascular injection

Vascular compromise from arterial compression (likelihood increases with increasing volume of anesthetic solution)

Nerve injury

Reaction to the anesthetic agent

Pearls and Pitfalls

1. Never use epinephrine-containing anesthetic solutions since this may lead to arterial spasm and ischemia of the digit.
2. This is a painful procedure and the patient should know this initially.
3. A circumferential subcutaneous injection at the base of the digit often works best for the first and fifth digits.
4. Many clinicians prefer the dorsal approach, as described for the toes, for the fingers also (Figure 2–15).

References

Carron H, Karbon G, Rowlinger J: Regional Anesthesia—Techniques and Clinical Applications, pp 100–105. Orlando, FL, Grune & Stratton, 1989.

Carter P: Injuries of wrist and hand. In Tintanelli J, Rothstein R, Krome R (eds): Emergency Medicine—A Comprehensive Study Guide, p 854. New York, McGraw-Hill Book Company, 1985.

Moore KL: Clinically Oriented Anatomy, pp 758–769. Baltimore, Williams & Wilkins, 1980.

Wrist Blocks

W. JOHN ZEHNER, MD

Major procedures on the hand usually require all three nerves to be blocked.

MEDIAN NERVE BLOCK

Indication

To facilitate performance of painful procedures in the region of the hand supplied by the median nerve. This usually includes the radial side of the palm, thumb, and fingers from a line bisecting the fourth finger to the wrist and the dorsum of the index and middle fingers and radial half of the fourth finger distal to the proximal interphalangeal joint (Figure 2–16).

Contraindications

Uncooperative patient
Allergy to local anesthetics
Localized infection at the injection site

Equipment

Gloves
10-ml syringe with 25-gauge, 1-inch needle
Local anesthetic
Betadine skin prep

Universal Precautions

1. Wear gloves.
2. Dispose of needle and syringe properly.

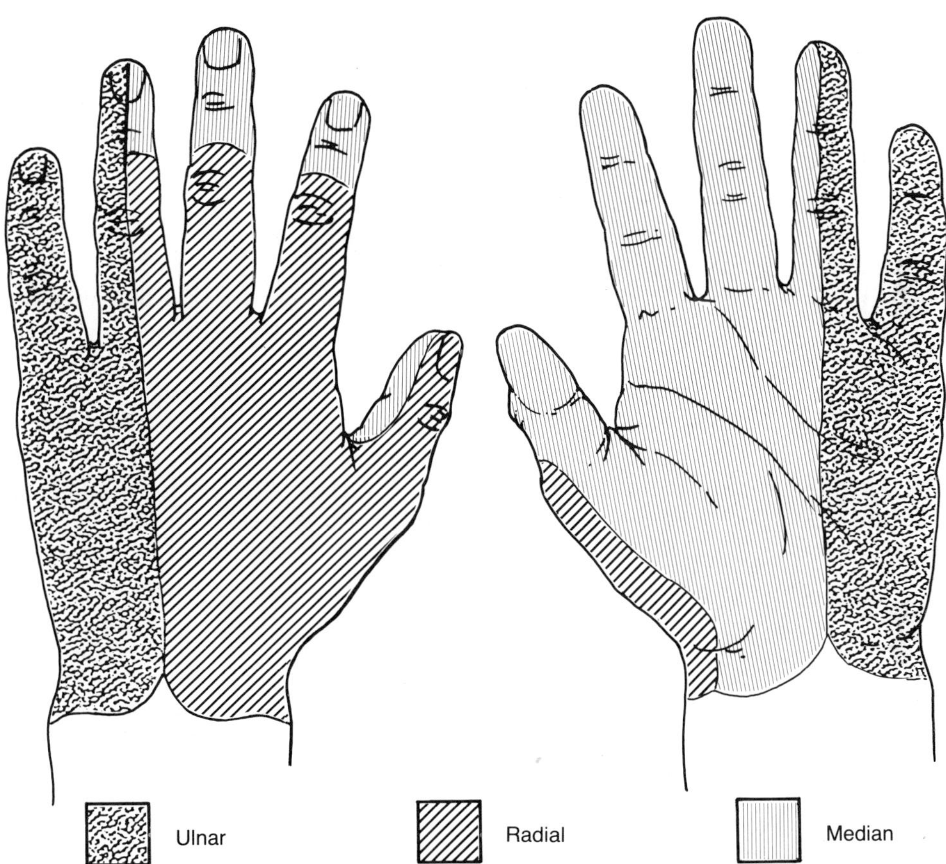

FIGURE 2–16. Nerve distribution of the hand.

Techniques

1. Explain the procedure to the patient and obtain consent. Remember to test motor and sensory function *before* administering the block. Warn the patient that he or she will have both anesthesia and temporary paralysis as a result of the block.
2. Position the patient supine on a stretcher with the arm to be blocked abducted away from the body on an armboard and the hand palm up with the wrist neutral (neither flexed nor extended).
3. Stand on the side to be anesthetized, at the patient's elbow, facing the hand.
4. The median nerve is located between the palmaris longus and the flexor carpi radialis tendons. Locate these tendons by having the patient flex the wrist against resistance. The flexor carpi radialis is slightly radial to the palmaris longus tendon. The injection site is between these two tendons at the level of the flexion crease (Figure 2–17).
5. Prep this area with Betadine.
6. Put on sterile gloves.
7. Attach the 25-gauge, 1-inch needle to the syringe and fill the syringe with the chosen anesthetic solution.
8. At the level of the proximal flexor crease, puncture the skin between the two tendons with the needle held perpendicular to the skin (see Figure 2–17).
9. Advance the needle 0.5 to 1.0 cm, aspirate to ensure the needle is not in a blood vessel, and then inject 3 to 5 ml of anesthetic.
10. Wait 5 minutes, and then test the area you wish to work on for adequacy of anesthesia. Because there is individual variation in the innervation of the hand, it may be necessary to additionally block the contiguous nerve.

Complications

Intravascular injection

Trauma/laceration of nerve leading to pain and paresthesia in that nerve's distribution

Unsuccessful block

Reaction to the local anesthetic

Pearls and Pitfalls

1. Attempt only one puncture. Multiple attempts may lacerate the nerve.
2. Always perform and document a neurovascular examination prior to the block.
3. Do not use anesthetics that contain epinephrine.

References

Carron H, Karbon G, Rowlinger J: Regional Anesthesia—Techniques and Clinical Applications, pp 100–105. Orlando, FL, Grune & Stratton, 1989.

Carter P: Injuries of the wrist and hand. In Tintanelli J, Rothstein R, Krome R (eds): Emergency Medicine—A Comprehensive Study Guide, p 854. New York, McGraw-Hill Book Company, 1985.

Moore KL: Clinically Oriented Anatomy, pp 758–769. Baltimore, Williams & Wilkins, 1980.

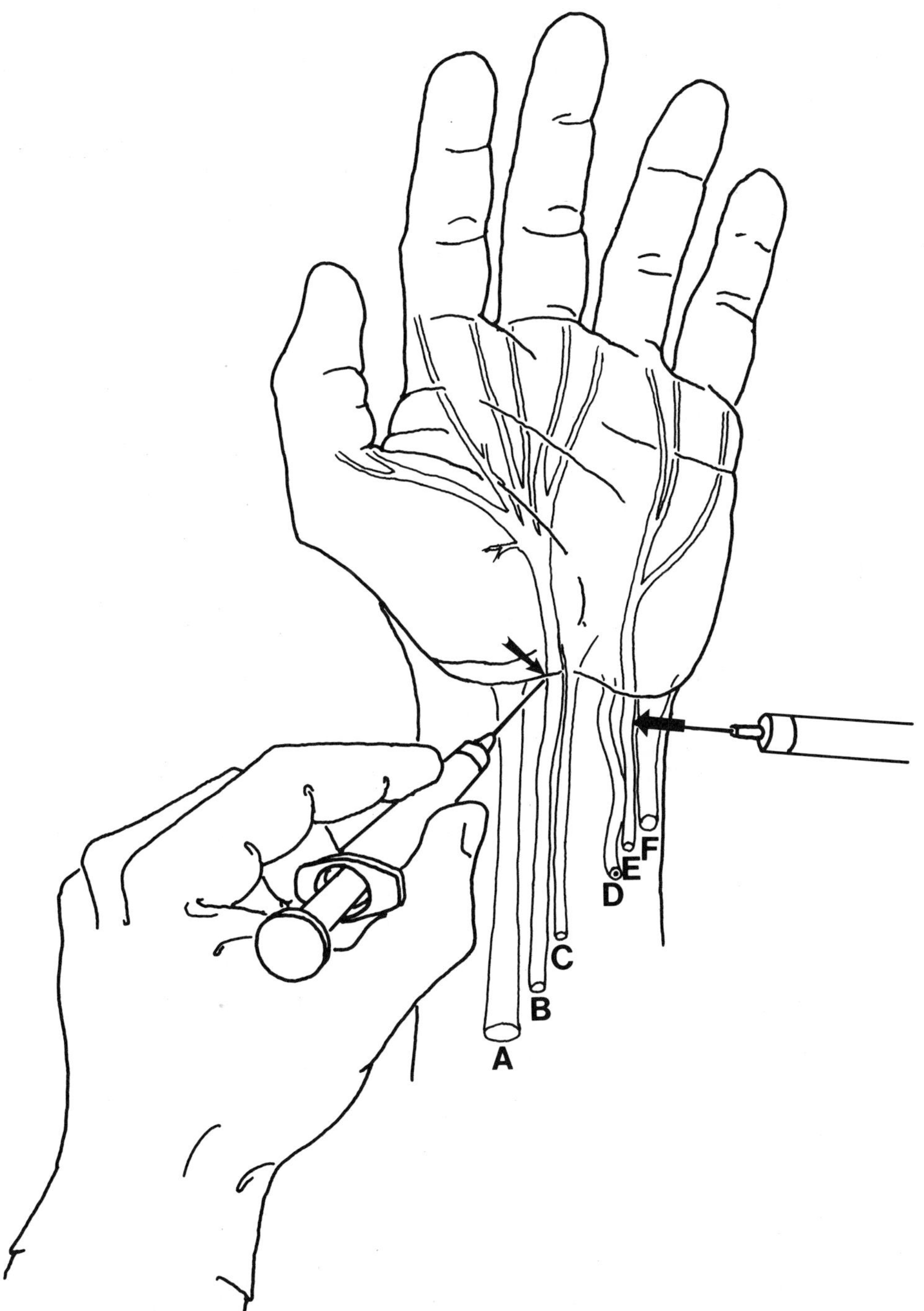

FIGURE 2–17. Injection sites for median *(small arrow)* and ulnar *(large arrow)* nerve blocks. *A,* Flexor carpi radialis tendon; *B,* median nerve; *C,* palmaris longus tendon; *D,* ulnar artery; *E,* ulnar nerve; *F,* flexor carpi ulnaris tendon. (We illustrated this one using a left-handed operator so all the lefties using this book wouldn't feel totally left out.)

RADIAL NERVE BLOCK

Indication

To facilitate performance of painful procedures in the area of distribution of the radial nerve. This usually includes the dorsum of the thumb, the radial aspect of the dorsum of the hand from a line down the middle of the fourth finger to the wrist, and the dorsum of the index and middle fingers and radial half of the fourth finger proximal to the proximal interphalangeal joint (Figure 2–16).

Contraindications

Uncooperative patient
Localized infection at the injection site
Allergy to local anesthetics

Equipment

Gloves
12-ml syringe
25-gauge, 1-inch needle
Local anesthetic
Betadine skin prep

Universal Precautions

1. Wear gloves.
2. Dispose of needle and syringe properly.

Technique

1. Explain the procedure to the patient and obtain consent. Remember to test motor and sensory function *before* administering the block. Warn the patient that he or she will have both anesthesia and temporary paralysis as a result of the block.
2. Position the patient supine on a stretcher with the arm to be blocked abducted from the body on an armboard and the hand positioned with the palm up so the palm is at approximately 45 degrees to the armboard.
3. Stand on the same side, facing the hand to be blocked.
4. Locate the injection site by palpating the radial artery at the flexion crease of the wrist.
5. Prepare the skin around the injection site with Betadine.
6. Put on sterile gloves.
7. Puncture the skin, and enter the subcutaneous tissue just lateral to the radial artery 1 cm or so proximal to the wrist flexor crease. Aspirate to ensure that the needle is not in a vessel, and then inject 2 ml of anesthetic solution.
8. Make four or five additional subcutaneous injections extending laterally and dorsally around the radial styloid to the mid dorsum of the wrist to block all the sensory branches of the radial nerve (Figure 2–18).

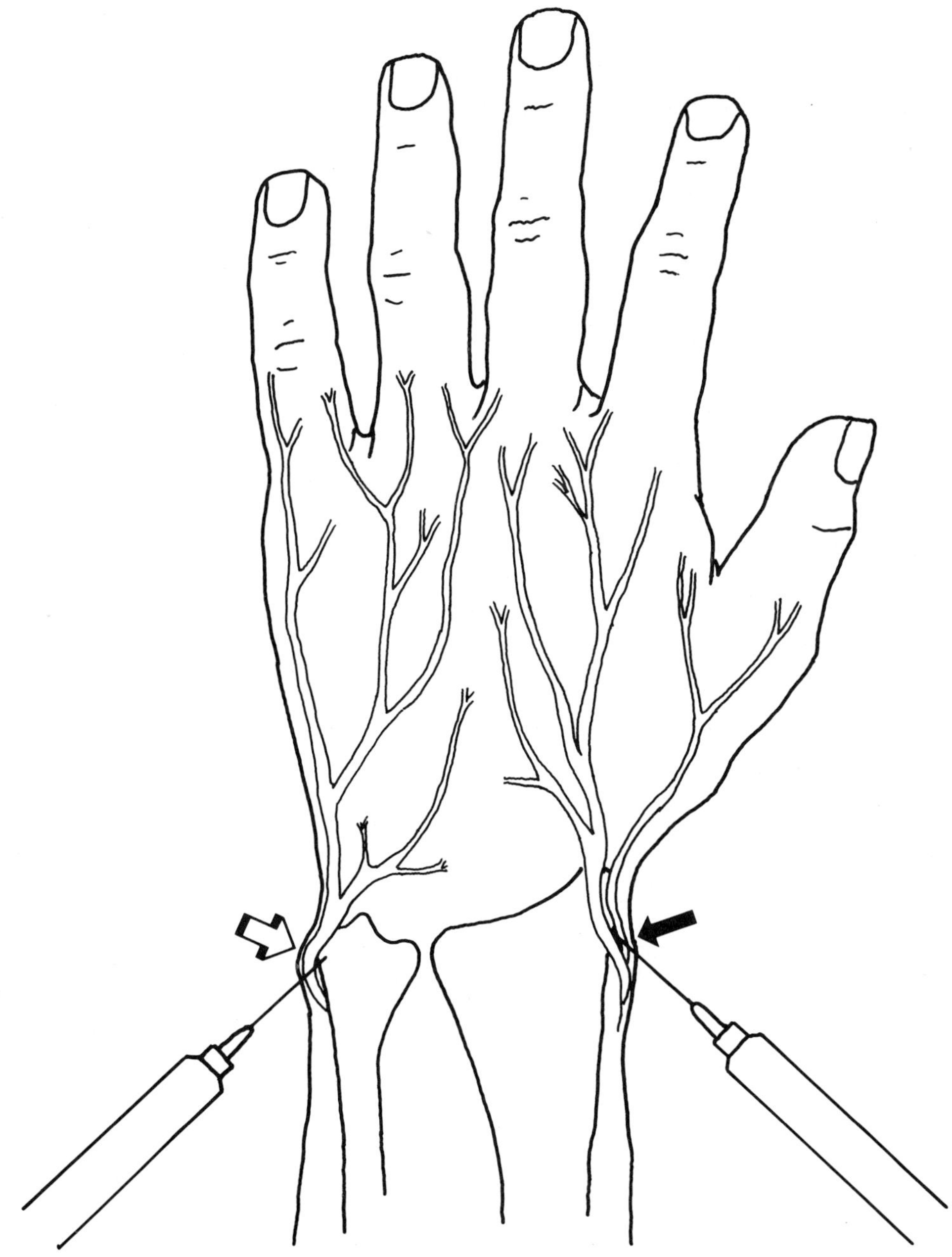

FIGURE 2–18. Injection sites for dorsal ulnar *(open arrow)* and dorsal radial *(black arrow)* nerve blocks.

9. Wait 5 minutes, and then test the area you wish to work on for adequacy of anesthesia. Because there is individual variation in the innervation of the hand, it may be necessary to additionally block the contiguous nerve.

Complications

Intravascular injection

Damage to radial nerve or its branches, leading to pain and/or paresthesia of the nerve

Unsuccessful block

Reaction to the anesthetic agent

Pearls and Pitfalls

1. Always perform and document a neurovascular examination prior to a block.
2. It will require multiple injections totaling 10 to 12 ml of anesthetic to fully block the radial nerve.
3. Do not use anesthetics that contain epinephrine.

References

Carron H, Karbon G, Rowlinger J: Regional Anesthesia—Techniques and Clinical Applications, pp 100–105. Orlando, FL, Grune & Stratton, 1989.

Carter P: Injuries of the wrist and hand. In Tintanelli J, Rothstein R, Krome R (eds): Emergency Medicine—A Comprehensive Study Guide, p 854. New York, McGraw-Hill Book Company, 1985.

Moore KL: Clinically Oriented Anatomy, pp 758–769. Baltimore, Williams & Wilkins, 1980.

ULNAR NERVE BLOCK

Indication

To facilitate performance of painful procedures in the region of the hand supplied by the ulnar nerve. An ulnar block will usually provide anesthesia of an area from the middle of the fourth finger laterally to the ulnar border of the hand, including both the dorsum and the palm, and proximally to the wrist (see Figure 2–16).

Contraindications

Uncooperative patient
Allergy to local anesthetics
Localized infection at the site of injection

Equipment

Gloves
10-ml syringe
25-gauge, 1-inch needle
Betadine skin prep
Local anesthetic

Universal Precautions

1. Wear gloves.
2. Dispose of needle and syringe properly.

Technique

1. Explain the procedure to the patient and obtain consent. Remember to test motor and sensory function *before* administering the block. Warn the patient that he or she will have both anesthesia and temporary paralysis as a result of the block.
2. Position the patient supine on a stretcher with the arm to be blocked abducted away from the body on an armboard and the hand palm up with the wrist neutral (neither flexed nor extended).
3. Stand on the same side, facing the hand to be blocked.
4. The injection site will be between the flexor carpi ulnaris tendon and the ulnar artery at the distal flexion crease of the wrist. Locate this site by palpating the ulnar artery and identifying the flexor carpi ulnaris tendon by having the patient ulnar deviate the hand against resistance (see Figure 2–17).
5. Prep the skin around the injection site with Betadine.
6. Put on sterile gloves.
7. Attach the 25-gauge, 1-inch needle to the syringe and fill the syringe with the chosen anesthetic solution.

8. Insert the needle perpendicular to the skin at the injection site between the flexor carpi ulnaris tendon and ulnar artery at the level of the distal flexor crease of the wrist (Figure 2–17).
9. Advance the needle to a depth of 0.5 inch, aspirate to ensure the needle is not in a blood vessel, and then inject 2 to 3 ml of the anesthetic solution.
10. You must also block the superficial branch of the ulnar nerve at the dorsal aspect of the ulnar styloid process. This is accomplished as follows:
    a. Have the patient turn his or her hand over so the dorsum is up.
    b. Prep the region of the ulnar styloid with Betadine.
    c. Using the same 1-inch, 25-gauge needle on the 10-ml syringe with the anesthetic solution, inject 3 to 5 ml of anesthetic in the subcutaneous tissue along the side and top of the ulnar styloid (see Figure 2–18).
11. Wait 5 minutes, and then test the area you wish to work on for adequacy of anesthesia. Because there is individual variation in the innervation of the hand it may be necessary to additionally block the contiguous nerve.

Complications

Intravascular injection

Trauma/laceration of nerve leading to pain and/or paresthesias in the distribution of that nerve

Unsuccessful block

Reaction to the anesthetic agent

Pearls and Pitfalls

1. The flexor carpi ulnaris muscle extends to a point quite distal on the forearm and inserts on the pisiform bone. It is important to inject the anesthetic at the distal flexor crease or you will inject the muscle and not obtain anesthesia.
2. Always perform and document a neurovascular examination prior to performing your block.
3. Do not use anesthetics that contain epinephrine.

References

Carron H, Karbon G, Rowlinger J: Regional Anesthesia—Techniques and Clinical Applications, pp 100–105. Orlando, FL, Grune & Stratton, 1989.

Carter P: Injuries of the wrist and hand. In Tintanelli J, Rothstein R, Krome R (eds): Emergency Medicine—A Comprehensive Study Guide, p 854. New York, McGraw-Hill Book Company, 1985.

Moore KL: Clinically Oriented Anatomy, pp 758–769. Baltimore, Williams & Wilkins, 1980.

3

Airway Management

Airway Suctioning

TIMOTHY PAGE, MD

Indications

To remove lung secretions
To stimulate coughing, thus moving secretions from small to larger airways
To prevent mucus obstruction and secondary atelectasis
To obtain samples of sputum for laboratory analysis
For patient education, in that most alert, cooperative patients realize after one session with the "pink python" that they would much rather cough on their own than endure tracheal suctioning.

Contraindications

Absolute

Absence of retained secretions

Relative

Airway trauma
Recent airway surgery
Bleeding disorder
Prior complication from suctioning
Recent myocardial infarction

Equipment

- Suction apparatus includes the following:
  - Gauge to indicate amount of negative pressure
  - Collection receptacle
  - Connecting tubing
- Two sterile gloves*
- Sterile container to hold a few ounces of sterile saline*
- Sterile saline
- Water-soluble lubricant
- Sterile 4 × 4-inch gauze pads
- Sterile suction catheter*
  - Soft, pliable, noncollapsible with negative pressure
  - Disposable clear plastic or red rubber (the "pink python")
  - Small enough to pass through airway
  - For nasotracheal suctioning:
    - Adult: 12–14 F
    - Pediatric: 10 F
    - Infants: 5 or 8 F
  - Thumb control valve
  - Several suction ports at tip
- Supplemental oxygen delivery system

Universal Precautions

1. Wear two sterile gloves.
2. Use a face shield or mask.
3. Use protective eye wear.

Technique

Airway suctioning may be accomplished by passing the catheter through the mouth, the nose, or an endotracheal or tracheostomy tube. We prefer the oral route for nonintubated patients since this is less painful than the nasal approach.

1. Explain the procedure to the patient.
2. Check that all equipment is present.
3. If the patient is being monitored, check to ensure that the monitoring devices (for pulse oximetry, electrocardiography, blood pressure, and intracranial pressure) are functioning properly. Since hypoxia is the major complication of airway suctioning, it is recommended that whenever possible all patients undergoing this procedure be monitored by pulse oximetry.
4. Premedicate patient as necessary (vasoconstrictive sprays, topical analgesics, inhaled bronchodilators).

---

*Catheter, gloves, and sterile container are in prepackaged kits.

5. Preoxygenate the patient with 40% to 90% oxygen, depending on the patient's degree of lung dysfunction.
6. Set suction gauge to proper negative suction pressure (adult, 80–120 mm Hg; child, 80–100 mm Hg; infant, 60–80 mm Hg).
7. Wash your hands.
8. Open the catheter package and put on sterile gloves. The dominant (sterile) hand will hold and advance the catheter. The nondominant hand connects the catheter to the suction apparatus and becomes nonsterile.
9. Remove sterile container from package. Pour sterile saline with nondominant hand into the sterile container.
10. Suction some saline to ensure that the apparatus is functioning properly.

In the intubated patient (Figure 3–1):

11. Position the patient supine in bed.
12. Stand at either side of the patient.
13. Have a bag-valve device connected to high-flow oxygen in easy reach of your nondominant hand on the patient's chest. Make sure that the oxygen is turned on.
14. Hold the suction catheter looped in your dominant, sterile hand.
15. With your nondominant, nonsterile hand, disconnect the ventilator tubing from the tube and place it on the clean packaging that the catheter was in.
16. Secure the tube with your nonsterile, nondominant hand.
17. Introduce the catheter into the airway without suctioning.
18. Advance the catheter until you feel resistance. Do not force it.
19. While withdrawing the catheter, intermittently occlude with your thumb the valve that applies suction, not exceeding 15 seconds per suctioning. Continually scan the monitoring equipment while suctioning.

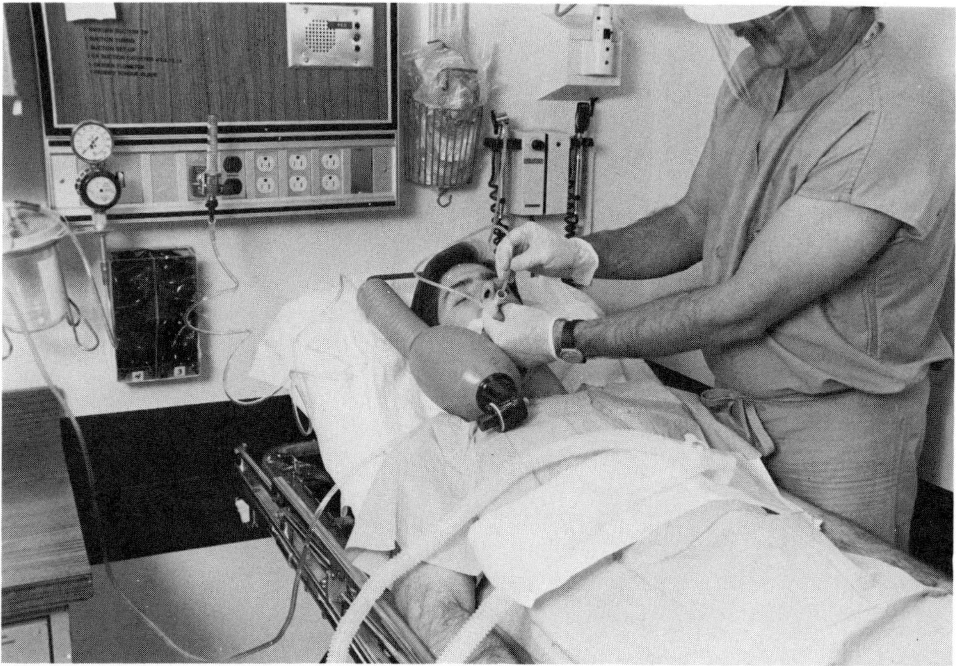

FIGURE 3–1. Airway suctioning: intubated patient.

20. Rotate the catheter while withdrawing it.
21. Hold the suction catheter looped in your sterile, dominant hand. Use your nonsterile hand to attach the bag-valve device with oxygen to the endotracheal tube and use it to give the patient 8 to 10 large breaths.
22. Clear catheter of secretions by suctioning sterile saline.
23. Repeat the suctioning sequence outlined above two or three more times.
24. Reconnect the ventilator.
25. When finished, coil the catheter in your dominant hand, pull glove inside out over catheter, and dispose of both properly.
26. Wash your hands.

In the nonintubated patient (Figure 3–2):

11. Position the patient sitting with the head of the bed elevated. Ask the patient to assume the sniffing position—neck mildly hyperextended and face forward.
12. Stand at either side of the patient.
13. Have the patient hold the oxygen mask and take 10 to 12 deep breaths.
14. Use your nondominant, nonsterile hand to connect the *oxygen* tubing to the suction catheter.
15. Ask the patient to open his or her mouth and stick out the tongue.
16. Hold the tongue with a 4 × 4-inch gauze pad in your nondominant hand.
17. Advance the suction catheter through the patient's mouth into the larynx and trachea. This will be facilitated by having the patient take a deep breath as the catheter is advanced. Remember to keep the suction activation port occluded with your thumb so the oxygen will flow out the tip of the catheter into the patient.

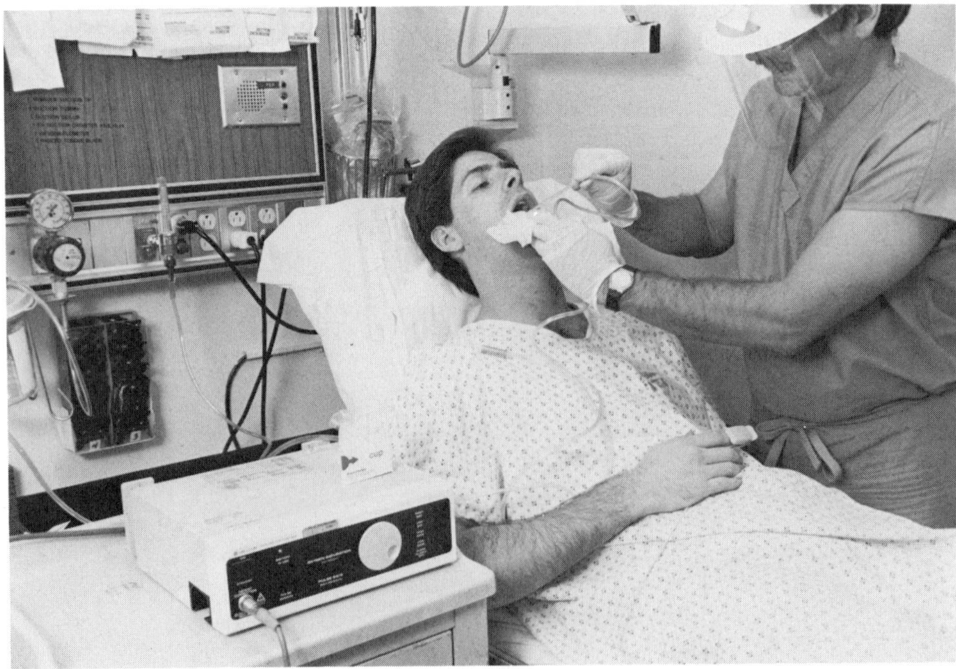

FIGURE 3–2. Airway suctioning: nonintubated patient.

18. Advance the catheter until the patient begins to cough or resistance is encountered. Do not force the catheter if you meet resistance.
19. With your nonsterile, nondominant hand remove the oxygen tubing from the suction catheter and attach the suction tubing.
20. While withdrawing the catheter, intermittently occlude the valve that applies suction with your thumb, not exceeding 15 seconds per suctioning.
21. Rotate the catheter while withdrawing it.
22. Have the patient apply the oxygen mask (yes, you do need to let go of the tongue so they can do this) and take 10 to 12 deep breaths.
23. Clear catheter of secretions by suctioning sterile saline.
24. Repeat the above sequence once or twice more.
25. Remind the patient how unpleasant that was and point out that further sessions with the "pink python" would not be necessary if he or she would just cough and deep breathe on his or her own.
26. Have the patient work out with the incentive spirometer. Substitute intermittent positive-pressure breathing in those patients who are unable to do incentive spirometry (neuromuscular disease, altered level of consciousness) or are uncooperative.

Complications

Death
Bleeding
Hypoxia
Dysrhythmias
Mucosal trauma including nasopharyngeal perforation and subcutaneous emphysema
Infection
Bronchospasm
Hypertension/hypotension
Increase in intracranial pressure
Vomiting and subsequent aspiration
Atelectasis
Pneumothorax

Pearls and Pitfalls

1. Position patient with mild neck hypertension.
2. Reuse decontaminated, resterilized red rubber catheters.
3. Use new sterile gloves for each procedure.
4. *Do not* apply suction during insertion.
5. *Do not* suction for more than 10 to 15 seconds each time.
6. Rotate catheter during removal.
7. Reventilate with oxygen between insertions.
8. If using the nasal route:
   a. Visually inspect for the larger nasal passage
   b. Pretreat with a topical vasoconstrictor and analgesic
9. Suction mouth and/or above endotracheal/tracheostomy tube balloon with same catheter at end of procedure.

This is *not* a routine procedure in nonintubated patients. It is uncomfortable and can cause serious complications.

---

10. Catheter may follow path of nasogastric/orogastric tube.
11. Keep your dominant hand sterile at all times.
12. Ensure that an endotracheal or tracheostomy tube is secure during the procedure.
13. Listen for bilateral breath sounds at end of the procedure.
14. Use a curved-tip catheter to attempt selective left bronchus suctioning. Head turning, body positioning, rotating, and a twisting artificial airway have limited value in facilitating entry into the left bronchus.
15. For tenacious secretions, 5 to 10 ml of sterile saline may be introduced into the trachea with a syringe without a needle through an endotracheal tube or through ultrasonic nebulization in a nonintubated patient.
16. Frequent airway suctioning in a nonintubated patient is best accomplished by inserting a nasopharyngeal airway, which can be left in place and used as an easy passageway to the larynx.
17. Red rubber catheters (pink pythons) are stiffer and thus less likely to coil in the nasopharynx and more likely to enter the trachea.

Reference

Extensive experience.

Cricothyroidotomy

JODY RIVA LEWINTER, MD

Indication

For immediate airway management in a patient in whom oral or nasal intubation is contraindicated or cannot be established. It may be needed for maxillofacial or laryngeal trauma, upper airway obstruction (edema, foreign body, mass lesion), or cervical spine precautions.

Contraindications

For children younger than 8 years of age who need a surgical airway, needle cricothyroidotomy (see page 88) may be preferred.
Coagulopathy
Neck trauma with distortion of landmarks

Equipment

Minimum equipment: Surgical gloves, scalpel and blade, tube

Usually required equipment:

Antiseptic solution
Local anesthetic
Drapes
Scalpel with No. 11 and No. 20 blades
Tracheostomy tube or endotracheal tube (Nos. 5–7)
Trousseau dilator (optional)
Mask
Gown
Goggles
5-ml syringe
10-ml syringe
25-gauge, 1-inch needle
20-gauge, 1-inch needle
Curved hemostats
Tracheostomy ties
Mayo scissors

Universal Precautions

1. Wear mask.
2. Use an eye shield.
3. Wear sterile gloves.

Technique

1. Explain procedure to patient and obtain informed consent, if circumstances permit (they probably will not).
2. Select the appropriate size tracheostomy or endotracheal tube (external diameter approximately equal to patient's thumbnail).
3. Check to ensure that all necessary equipment is present and test the tube's cuff.
4. Position patient:
   a. Neutral with immobilization if cervical spine fracture is possible
   b. Neck extended if there is *no* risk of cervical spine fracture
5. Put on gown, mask, goggles, and sterile gloves.
6. Surgically prepare area with Betadine, drape, and anesthetize, if the situation permits.
7. Locate the cricothyroid membrane directly below the thyroid cartilage and above the cricoid ring. Place thumb and second finger on either side of the larynx to immobilize it. Use first finger to maintain identification of the cricothyroid membrane (Figure 3–3).
8. Make a 2- to 3-cm transverse skin incision over the cricothyroid membrane and then through the membrane into the trachea. Aim all instruments at a 30- to 40-degree angle caudally to avoid injury to vocal cords. *Note:* You may place a large-bore needle through the membrane first to guide the incision and provide temporary ventilation (see page 88).
9. Dilate opening by inserting blunt end of scalpel horizontally and twisting it vertically or by using a hemostat or tracheal dilator to dilate the opening horizontally.
10. Insert tracheostomy tube or endotracheal tube and inflate cuff.
11. Ventilate patient with 100% oxygen and auscultate breath sounds.
12. If adequate ventilation and oxygenation is not immediately established after insertion of the tracheal tube, the tube should be removed immediately, followed by bag-mask ventilation or transtracheal needle ventilation (see page 88) and reinsertion of the tracheal tube.
13. Secure tube with tracheal ties passed around the neck.
14. Obtain a chest x-ray film and look at it.

Complications (Rate = 6% to 7%)

Prolonged hypoxia secondary to prolonged unsuccessful attempts at tracheal cannulation

Hemorrhage

Infection

Subcutaneous or mediastinal emphysema

Right mainstem bronchus intubation (especially if an endotracheal tube is used)

Creation of a paratracheal tract

Damage to vocal cords or voice change

Pneumothorax

Laceration of the trachea or esophagus

Persistent stoma

Subglottic or laryngeal stenosis

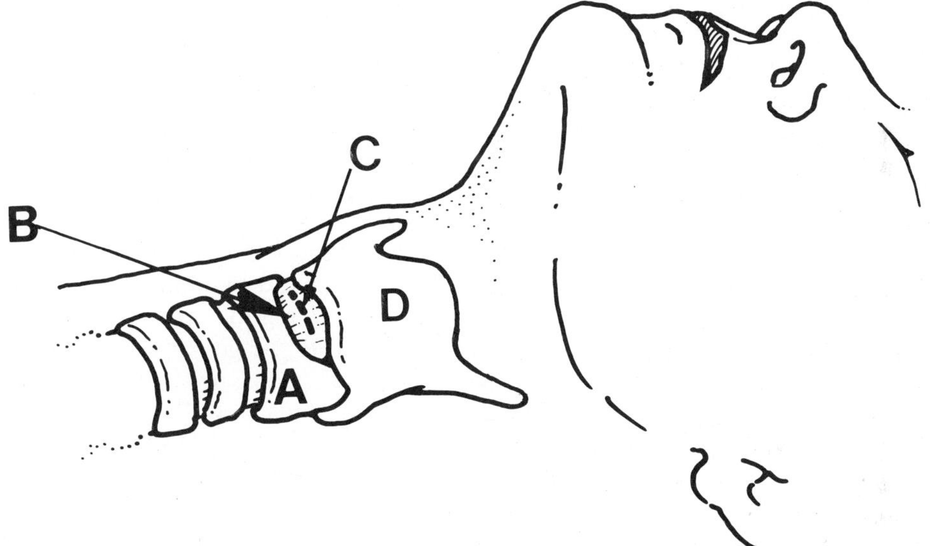

FIGURE 3–3. *A,* Cricoid ring; *B,* cricothyroid membrane; *C,* incision; *D,* thyroid cartilage.

Aspiration

Damage to the carotid artery, internal jugular vein, or vagus nerve secondary to over lateralization of the incision

Pearls and Pitfalls

There are now commercially available prepackaged percutaneous cricothyroidotomy kits that use a needle, guidewire, dilator/tube over guidewire technique. Their effectiveness and ease compared with surgical cricothyroidotomy have not been tested.

The tube is less likely to become dislodged if it is sutured to the skin.

In patients *in extremis,* little time should be spent on skin preparation, local anesthesia, and hemostasis until an endotracheal or tracheostomy tube is in place. In less urgent circumstances, adequate skin preparation, local anesthesia, attention to asepsis, and a separate skin incision and dissection allowing direct visualization of the cricothyroid membrane may reduce complications. Also, a Trousseau or other dilator may be used to prevent having to enlarge the cricothyroid membrane incision with the scalpel. This may reduce the risk for perforation of the posterior trachea and damage to overlying thyroid vessels in the vicinity.

In patients *in extremis,* the incision is enlarged in a transverse fashion in both directions laterally from the midline, allowing for the insertion of a probing finger, followed immediately by the tracheal tube. Should great difficulty be likely to be encountered in identifying anatomic structures, a vertical skin incision to identify underlying anatomy should be considered. This may be indicated in a patient with massive subcutaneous emphysema or hematoma overlying the cricothyroid membrane. In this unusual circumstance, a vertical incision of generous proportion, with dissection and identification of anatomic structures, may be lifesaving. However, whenever possible, a transverse incision is preferred.

If substantial bleeding is encountered following insertion of the tracheal tube, gentle pressure over these structures may result in adequate hemostasis. If not, attempts to identify the bleeding vessel should be made and ligation or cauterization of small vessel injuries can be performed. This should be done in the operating room by the appropriate consultant.

References

American College of Surgeons Committee on Trauma: Advanced Trauma Life Support Program. Chicago, American College of Surgeons, 1989.

Kress TD, Balasubramanian S: Cricothyroidotomy. Ann Emerg Med 11:197–201, 1982.

Endotracheal Intubation

PETER MARIANI, MD

GENERAL CONCEPTS

Indications for Intubating the Trachea

- Airway protection
  - Loss of gag reflex (e.g., cerebrovascular accident, drug overdose)
  - Obstruction of large airways (e.g., epiglottitis, foreign body, vocal cord paralysis)
  - Pharyngeal hemorrhage (e.g., stab wound or gunshot wound to neck)
  - Prophylactic (e.g., obtunded patient for Ewald lavage, computed tomography, or interhospital transfer)
- Airway optimization
  - Conduit for emergent pulmonary toilet (e.g., suctioning and/or bronchoscopy for acute aspiration or severe bacterial tracheitis)
  - Provision of high, continuous positive airway pressure (e.g., adult respiratory distress syndrome, hyaline membrane disease)
- Mechanical ventilation
  - Respiratory failure unrelated to large airway obstruction
    - Pulmonary—asthma, chronic obstructive pulmonary disease, pulmonary embolism, pneumonia
    - Cardiac—pulmonary edema
    - Neurologic—decreased respiratory drive
    - Mechanical—bellows dysfunction in flail chest or neuromuscular disease
  - Decrease work of breathing per se (e.g., "mild" congestive heart failure in the brittle cardiac patient or adult respiratory distress syndrome in the hypermetabolic multiple trauma patient)
  - Therapeutic hyperventilation for patients with elevated intracranial pressure (e.g., head injury)
- Drug administration in absence of intravenous access

Contraindications

NONE! If the patient needs an artificial airway, he or she needs it. The only issue is the technique of obtaining it.

Intubation Attempt is Diagnostic as Well as Therapeutic

Q: "Who needs to be intubated?"
A: "Anyone who will let you."

The patient whose level of consciousness or gag reflex is depressed to the point at which little resistance is offered to attempted intubation probably requires it. Conversely, if the stimulus of an intubation attempt results in significant patient arousal and improved respiration, perhaps the patient can be closely monitored with intubation deferred.

Common Impediments to Optimal Airway Management

1. Lack of training, skill, and facility with standard equipment
2. Undue reliance on arterial blood gas analysis over clinical assessment
3. Underuse of preintubation bag and mask assisted ventilation with 100% oxygen
4. Justified concern for cervical spine in trauma patients
5. Unjustified concern for facial bones and basal skull fracture in trauma patients
6. Lack of facility with neuromuscular blocking agents
7. Dependence on gadgetry
8. Inadequate preparation prior to undertaking any airway procedure:
   a. Has the patient been preoxygenated with 100% oxygen?
   b. Is endotracheal tube balloon competent and is inflation syringe inserted?
   c. Are alternate endotracheal tubes, laryngoscope blades, and stylets at hand?
   d. Are laryngoscope light bulbs functional?
   e. Is all equipment within easy reach of the operator at the head of the bed?
   f. Is respiratory therapist ready with working suction?
   g. Is nurse ready with sedating or paralyzing agents should the need arise?
   h. Is patient restrained if required?
   i. Are dental prostheses removed?
   j. Is x-ray technician on call for portable chest film?
   k. Is mechanical ventilator available as needed?
   l. Is intubator protected with gloves, mask, and eye shield?

Methods of Endotracheal Tube Position Confirmation

1. Observe passage of the tube through the cords.
2. Auscultate good, equal chest breath sounds.
3. Auscultate absent epigastric breath sounds.
4. Observe good chest excursion and lack of abdominal excursion.
5. Auscultate and palpate balloon cuff air movement over the anterior neck on injection and withdrawal.
6. Fiberoptically confirm tracheal rings distal to the tube.
7. Obtain clinical improvement in the patient.
8. Obtain improvement in the patient's pulse oximetry.
9. Perform colorimetric or electronic expiratory capnometry.
10. Note tube end position on chest x-ray film (should be between clavicles and carina).

TABLE 3–1. Guidelines for Endotracheal Tube Diameters and Insertion Distances

Age	Endotracheal Tube Size (mm)	Distance at Lips (cm)	Laryngoscope Size and Blade
Newborn	3.0	10	1 Miller
6 mo	3.5	12	1 Miller
18 mo	4.0	13	1 Miller
3 yr	4.5	14	1 Miller
5 yr	5.0	15	2 MacIntosh
6 yr	5.5	16	2 MacIntosh
8 yr	6.0	17	2 MacIntosh
12 yr	6.5	18	3 MacIntosh
16 yr	7.0	20	3 MacIntosh
Adult (F)	7.5	22	3 MacIntosh
Adult (M)	8.5	23	3–4 MacIntosh

Equipment

Endotracheal Tube

Rules of thumb for endotracheal tube size selection are as follows:

tube diameter = (patient age + 16/4)
= diameter of patient's pinky finger
= width of patient's thumbnail (truly, a rule of thumb)

Alternatively, guidelines for tube diameters and insertion distances have been promulgated by the American Heart Association (Table 3–1).

Normal adult women and men should accommodate 7- to 8-mm and 8- to 9-mm tubes, respectively, but you should allow for individual variation. Children younger than 6 years of age do not require cuffed tubes.

Laryngoscope

Instruments with high-intensity lights are preferred. Curved blades (MacIntosh) are favored by anesthesiologists, while many emergency physicians prefer straight blades (Miller). The upper airway anatomy of children younger than 3 years of age makes the straight blade theoretically easier to use in such patients.

Rather than rely on predetermined standards for "average patients" (see Table 3–1), an appropriately sized blade can be selected at the bedside in a manner similar to the selection of an oral airway: the distance from the patient's lips to the angle of the jaw is the minimal blade length required (Figure 3–4).

Complications

Unrecognized esophageal intubation
Unrecognized right mainstem bronchus intubation
Tension pneumothorax owing to positive-pressure ventilation
Pharyngeal laceration
Vocal cord damage
Tracheal laceration
Vomiting with aspiration
Transient increase in intracranial pressure
Transient hypertension and bradycardia
Hypoxia resulting from prolonged attempt times

Universal Precautions

1. Wear mask.
2. Use an eye shield.
3. Wear gloves.

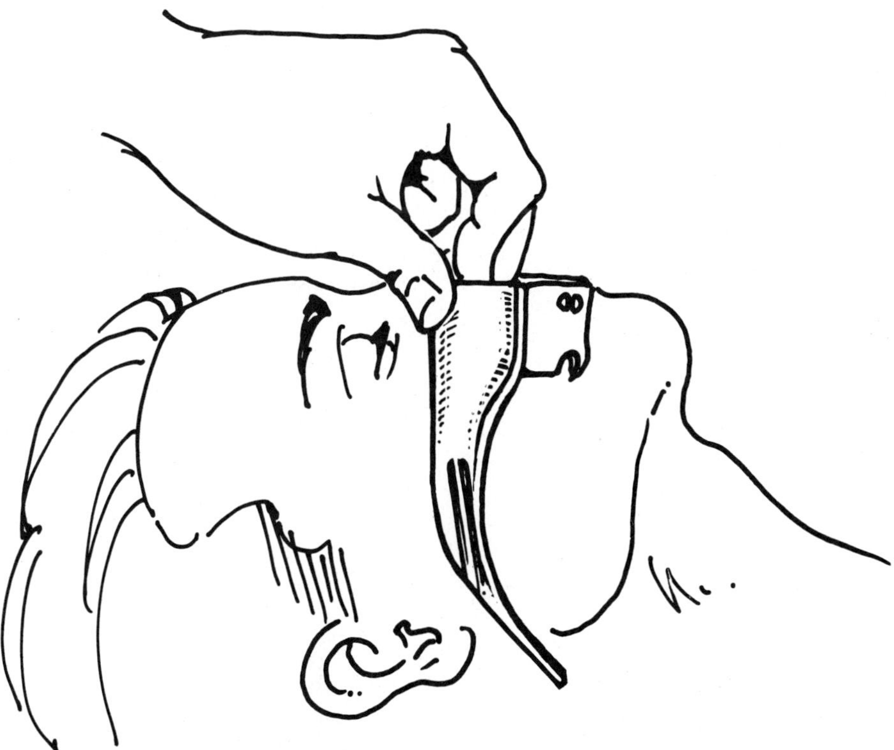

FIGURE 3–4. Laryngoscope blade selection.

OROTRACHEAL INTUBATION

This is the standard technique of endotracheal tube insertion. It may be performed on apneic patients. It allows for direct visualization of tube passage through the vocal cords.

Possible Contraindications

1. Confirmed or suspected cervical spine fracture. Whether risk of fracture displacement constitutes a procedure contraindication (rather than just a need for additional caution) is a matter of ongoing controversy in emergency medicine.
2. Suspicion of tracheal disruption in the setting of blunt laryngeal trauma. Concern over turning a partial tracheal tear into a complete one leads some to advocate exclusive use of fiberoptic intubation or tracheostomy (not cricothyrotomy) in this setting.

Equipment

Endotracheal tubes
Stylet
10-ml syringe
Laryngoscope handle
Laryngoscope blades—straight and curved, various sizes
Yankhauer suction apparatus
Benzocaine/tetracaine topical anesthetic spray
Lidocaine jelly
Tincture of benzoin
Cloth tape
Mask
Eye shield
Gloves
Pulse oximeter

Technique

1. Adequately prepare for the procedure (see No. 8 in Common Impediments).
2. Briefly explain the procedure to the conscious patient, and obtain consent if circumstances allow. Have the conscious, spontaneously breathing patient breathing oxygen through a high FiO_2 mask to begin preoxygenation.
3. Monitor the patient with a pulse oximeter if possible.
4. Put on mask, eye shield, and gloves.
5. Unless the patient is deeply obtunded, spray benzocaine/tetracaine onto the posterior pharynx and base of the tongue.
6. Insert the stylet into the endotracheal tube, making sure no protrusion occurs through the balloon end. Fabricate a "hockey stick" bend to the tube and stylet (Figure 3–5). Test the integrity of the tube balloon by inflating it with 10 ml of air. Deflate the balloon and leave the air-filled syringe attached to the tube.
7. Apply lidocaine jelly to the balloon end of the tube.
8. Taking position at the head of the bed, lay the patient supine and bring the head and neck to the "sniffs position" using towel props as needed (Figure 3–6). Do not do this if there is a possibility of a cervical spine fracture (see Pearls and Pitfalls No. 3).

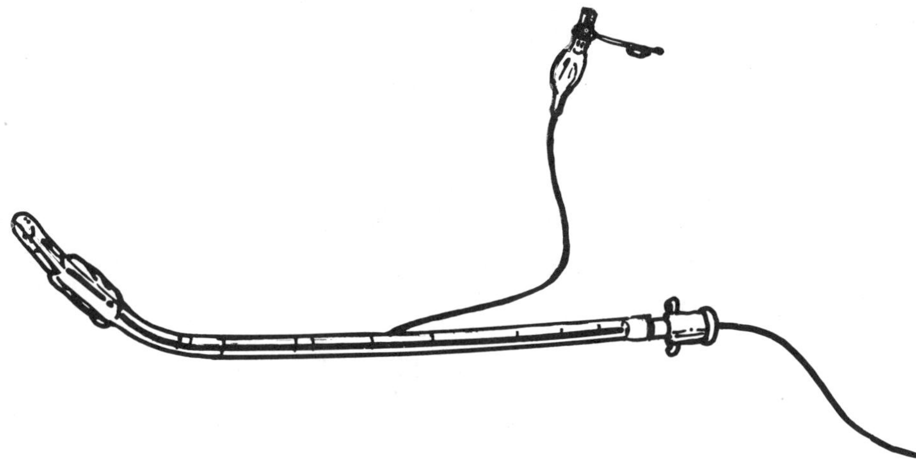

FIGURE 3–5. Endotracheal tube.

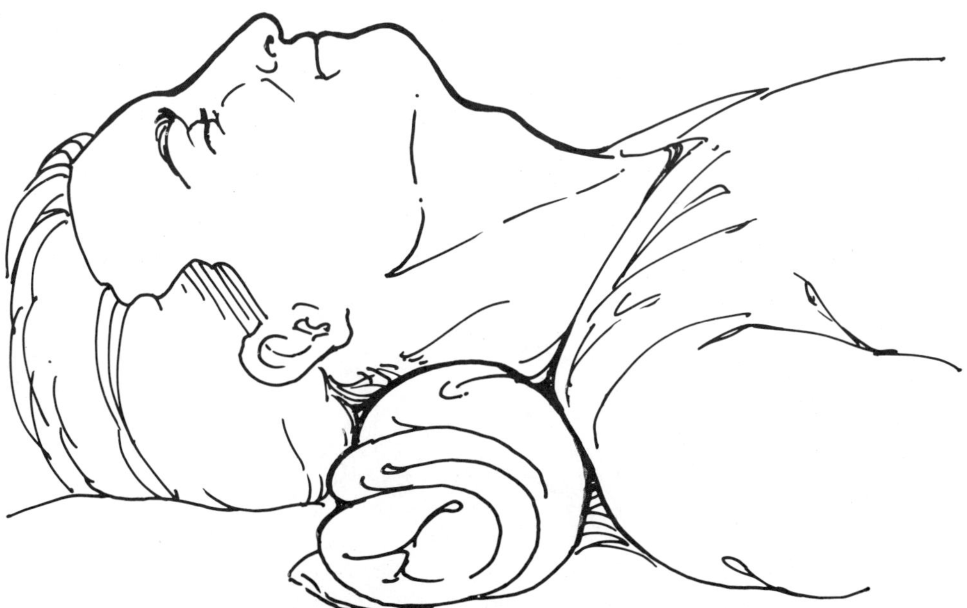

FIGURE 3–6. Position for endotracheal intubation.

9. Use bag and mask to preoxygenate the patient for at least 30 seconds with 100% FiO_2.
10. Grasp the endotracheal tube with the right hand in such a way as to leave the thumb and index finger free. Introduce with the left hand the curved blade laryngoscope into the patient's mouth along the right side of the tongue, then move the laryngoscope to the midline (Figure 3–7).

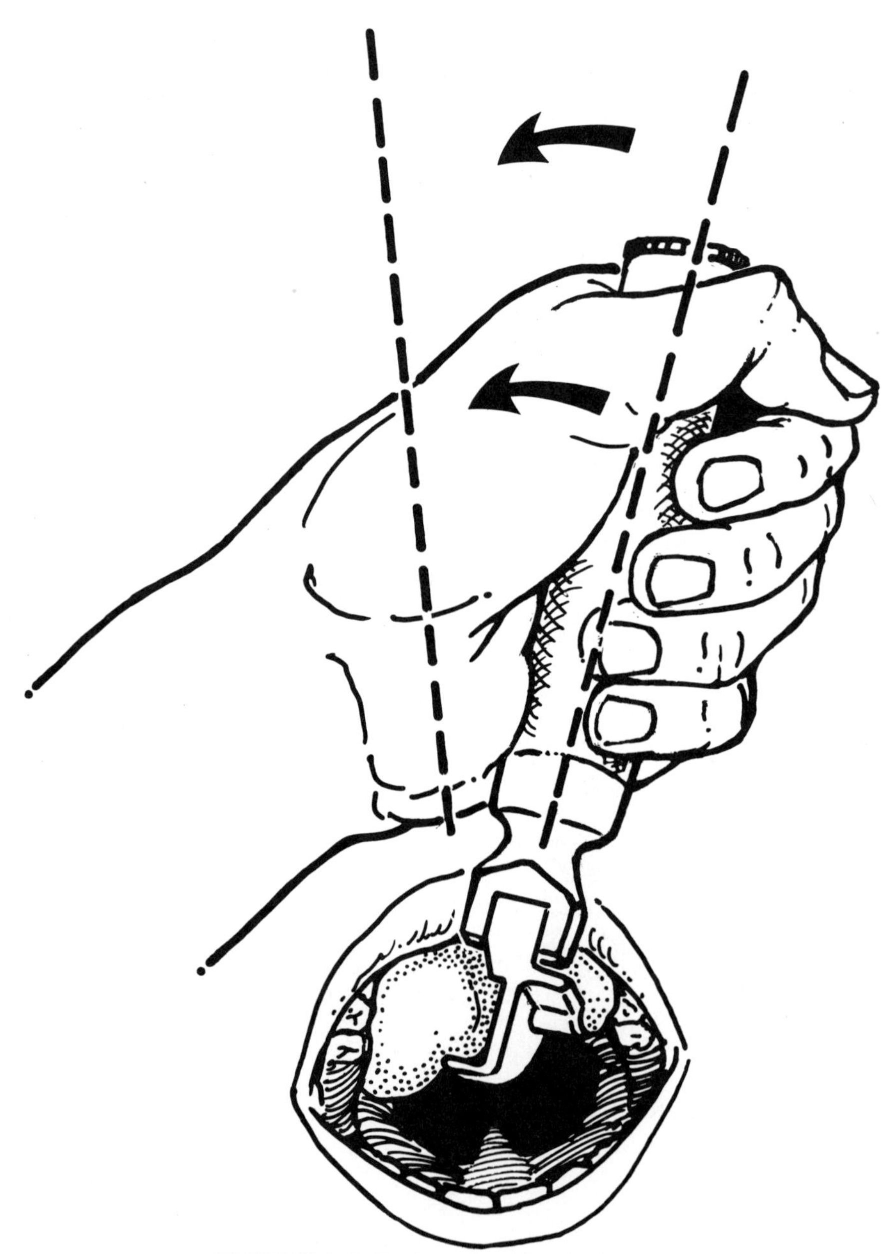

FIGURE 3–7. Endotracheal intubation.

11. Advance the blade to the vallecula, and lift the laryngoscope leftward and upward with a force directed parallel to the long axis of the handle (Figure 3–8*A*). Resist the temptation to use angulating force with the wrist (Figure 3–8*B*).

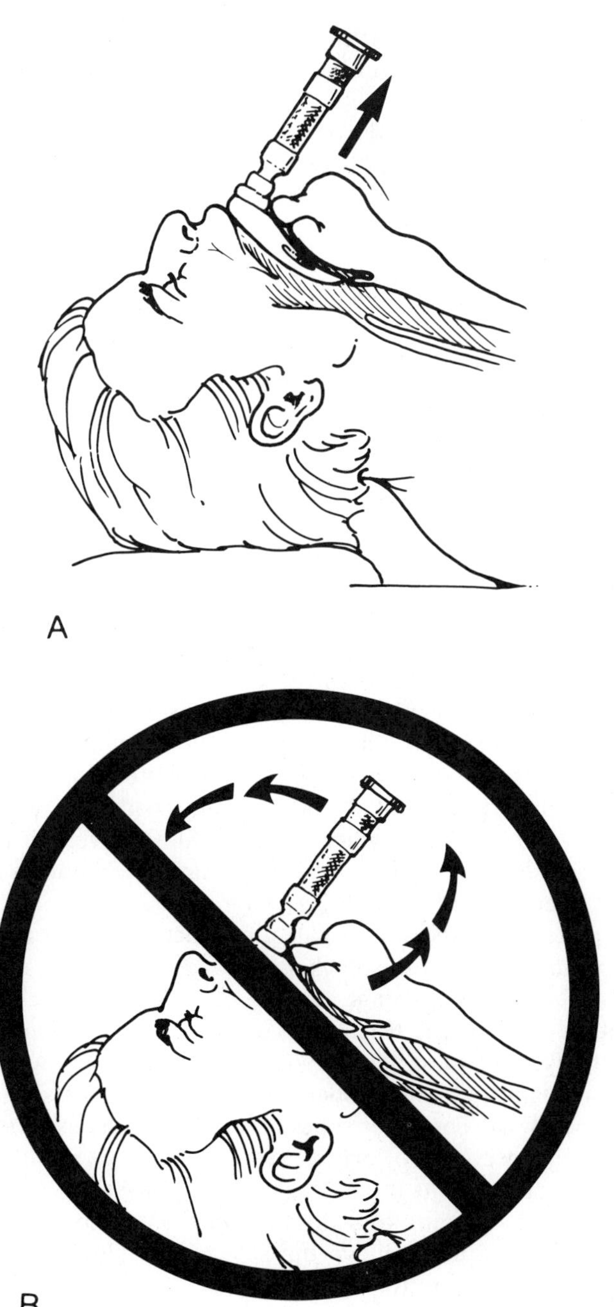

FIGURE 3–8. Endotracheal intubation.

12. View the patient's larynx (Figure 3–9). Should secretions obscure the view, hold the Yankhauer suction apparatus with the free thumb and index finger of the right hand, clear the airway, and return the apparatus to your assistant.
13. Insert the endotracheal tube into the right side of the patient's mouth, advancing it through the pharynx and finally, through the cords.
14. Remove the laryngoscope and the endotracheal tube stylet, and inflate the balloon with 5 to 10 ml of air.
15. Bag-ventilate through the tube while auscultating the hemithoraces and epigastrum. (Diminished breath sounds over the left chest usually indicate excessive tube advancement into the right mainstem bronchus and require balloon deflation, a few centimeters of tube withdrawal, and then reinflation.)
16. After optimal breath sounds are achieved, secure the tube in position with benzoin and tape and then obtain and examine a chest x-ray film. Inserting an oral airway will prevent the patient from biting down on the tube.

Specific Potential Complications

Cervical spine fracture displacement
Dental trauma

Pearls and Pitfalls

1. The most common errors committed by novice intubators are
   a. Inadequate preprocedure preparation
   b. Suboptimal patient positioning
   c. Blade introduction mid mouth and not right sided
   d. Handle traction not axially directed
2. On discontinuing bag and mask preoxygenation of the apneic patient, the intubator should begin to hold his or her own breath as he or she intubates the patient. If the tube has not been passed by the time the intubator's own breath runs out, the attempt should be abandoned and the patient reoxygenated before undertaking another attempt. Alternatively, if the patient has a pulse and pulse oximetry is available, O_2 saturation during attempts should not be allowed to fall below 85% to 90%.
3. Trauma patients at risk of cervical spine fracture and in need of intubation should be intubated in the neck neutral position with an immobilization collar in place. An assistant should provide additional head and neck stabilization (*not* "in-line traction"), especially for the combative patient.
4. The combative patient in need of intubation may have the risks of traumatic intubation minimized with prudent use of intravenous sedation and neuromuscular paralysis. The latter should be used only by experienced physicians or under the supervision of experienced physicians.
5. If laryngospasm prevents the passage of an appropriately sized tube through the vocal cords, spraying topical anesthetic onto the cords under laryngoscopic visualization may relieve the spasm and allow passage on constant, even pressure applied to the tube.
6. The proportionately larger head of the small child tends to force the neck

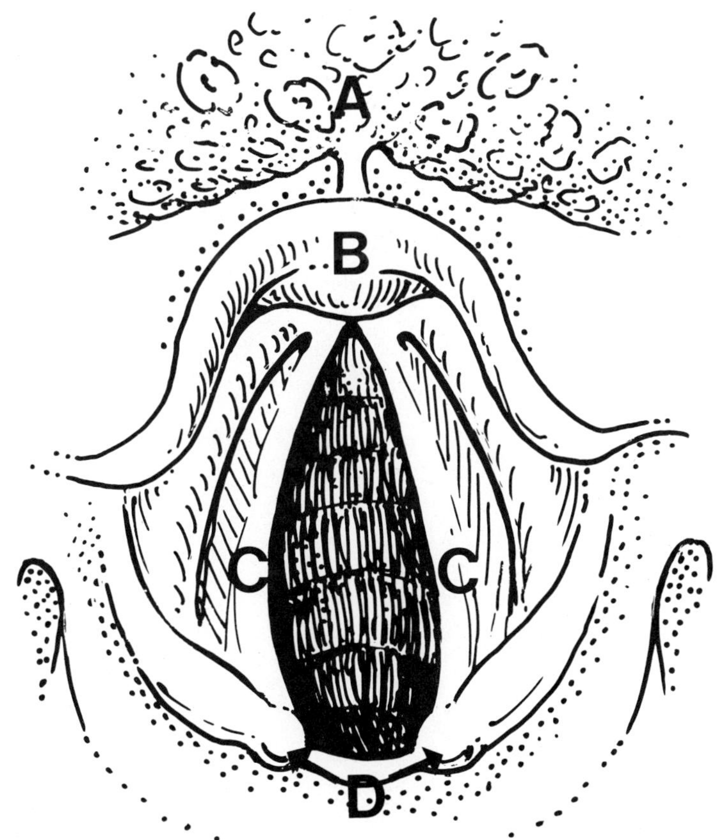

FIGURE 3–9. *A,* Tongue; *B,* epiglottis; *C,* vocal cords; *D,* arytenoids.

into flexion in the supine position. Knowing this, some repositioning and propping with towels under the shoulders will achieve a true "sniffs" position in the small child.

7. Premedication (5 to 7 minutes in advance) with intravenous or aerosolized lidocaine, 2.0 mg/kg, will minimize increases in intracranial pressure that may result from pharyngeal stimulation.

NASOTRACHEAL INTUBATION

Intubation of the trachea through the nasal route offers the following advantages:

Tube can be passed with patient sitting upright (the position naturally assumed by most dyspneic patients).

Tube can be passed without neck manipulation.

Tube fixation is more secure.

Patient cannot bite down on tube.

It is possible to intubate patients with trismus (but if you induce vomiting, you are in trouble).

Contraindications Specific for Nasotracheal Intubation

1. Apneic patient. Since the pure technique (without Magill forceps manipulation) relies on the patient's inspiratory force assisting the tube into the trachea, apnea predisposes to unacceptably high failure rates.
2. Severe facial fractures. Controversy surrounds the potential for "intubating the brain" in the presence of LeFort fractures with potential disruption of the cribriform plate. Cases of intracranial *nasogastric* tube placement have been reported in this setting. Those inexperienced in the technique of nasotracheal intubation should probably avoid it in the presence of severe facial trauma.
3. Blunt laryngeal trauma with suspected tracheal disruption. Blindly passing an endotracheal tube may turn a partial tear into a complete one. Intubation methods using direct vision are preferable.
4. Clinically significant coagulopathy. Epistaxis may be difficult to control in this setting.

Equipment

Mask, eye shield, gloves
Endotracheal tubes
Nasopharyngeal ("trumpet") airways
2% lidocaine jelly
1% phenylephrine spray
10-ml syringe
Laryngoscope handle
Laryngoscope blades—straight and curved, various sizes
Magill forceps
Yankhauer suction apparatus
Benzocaine/tetracaine topical anesthetic spray
Tincture of benzoin
Cloth tape
Pulse oximeter

Technique

1. Adequately prepare for the procedure (see No. 8 in Common Impediments).
2. Briefly explain the procedure to the conscious patient and obtain consent if circumstances allow. Have the conscious, spontaneously breathing patient breathing oxygen through a high FIO_2 mask to begin preoxygenation.
3. Monitor the patient with a pulse oximeter if possible.
4. Place the patient who is neither hypotensive nor spinal-immobilized in the upright position. Gravity will thus assist intubation. Take a position at the side of the bed, facing the patient (right-handed intubator on the right side of the bed).
5. Put on mask, eye shield, and gloves.
6. Determine if one naris is of larger caliber than the other. Use the larger one.
7. Spray benzocaine/tetracaine onto the posterior pharynx, selected naris, and base of the tongue. Spray phenylephrine into the selected naris.
8. Test the integrity of the endotracheal tube balloon by inflating it with 10 ml of air. Deflate the balloon and leave the air-filled syringe attached.
9. Copiously lubricate a flexible nasopharyngeal airway (“nasal trumpet”) with lidocaine jelly, and insert it along the floor of the nasal cavity. Similarly lubricate the balloon end of the selected endotracheal tube.
10. Following some in-and-out manipulation of the nasal trumpet to spread the lubricant, remove it, and insert the endotracheal tube.
11. Advance the tube along the floor of the nasal cavity until the pharynx is reached. (*Do not* direct the tube parallel to the upward slope of the nose (Figure 3–10A, B). With constant, even force, advance the tube through the hypopharynx to the point where the patient’s respirations are maximally audible through the tube and synchronous to-and-fro condensation appears on the tube’s inner surface.

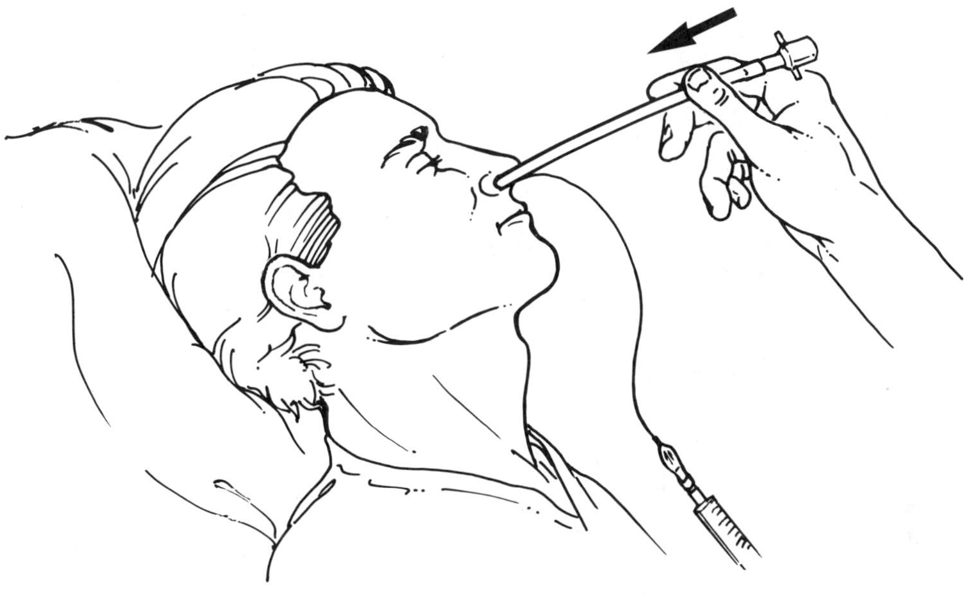

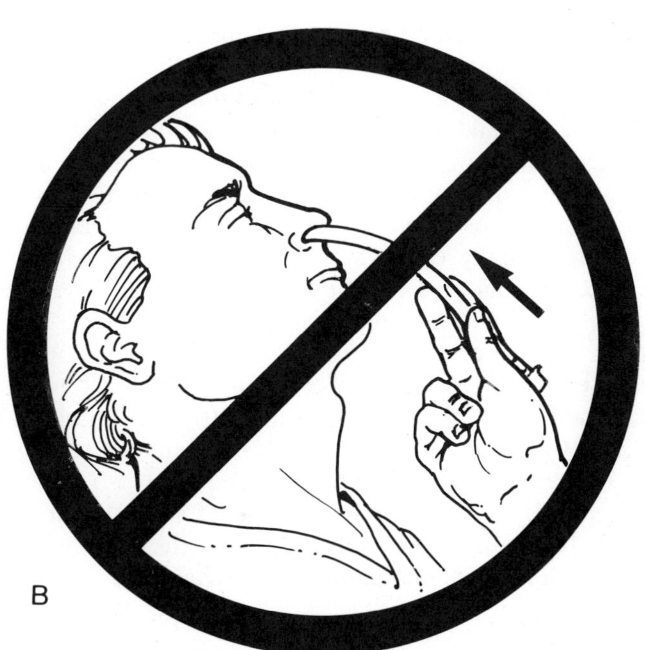

FIGURE 3–10. Nasotracheal intubation.

12. Palpate the cricoid region with the nondominant hand. While observing condensation and listening to respirations, as the patient reaches a point one third of the way into inspiration, quickly advance the tube through the cords into the trachea (Figure 3–11*A, B*). Concurrent mild cricoid pressure (Sellick maneuver) may facilitate passage. Should the tube lodge laterally on this final advancement, withdraw it back to the point of synchronous condensation, rotate it appropriately, and attempt advancement again. Slightly varying the amount of neck flexion/extension in patients without spinal precautions may also improve chances of success.
13. Inflate the balloon with 5 to 10 ml of air, reposition the tube as needed to achieve equal breath sounds over the right and left hemithoraces, and secure the tube with benzoin and tape.
14. Obtain and examine a chest x-ray film to confirm the tube's position.

Specific Potential Complications

Epistaxis
Adenoidectomy (children)
Turbinatectomy
Balloon rupture
Sinusitis

Pearls and Pitfalls

1. A well-lubricated, well-dilated nasal cavity will minimize procedure discomfort and the chance of nasal trauma. The severely dyspneic patient who may be an eventual candidate for nasotracheal intubation should receive topical nasal vasoconstriction and a lubricated nasal trumpet early in his or her emergency department care. This will allow for maximum vasoconstriction and anesthesia by the time of endotracheal tube passage.
2. Avoid the temptation to select too narrow a tube just because the nasal route is attempted. Many experienced intubators believe that excessively small tubes tend to "float around" the hypopharynx and have less chance of finding the larynx. With a well-prepared nasal cavity, tube size should be the same as for the oral route.
3. Do not use an endotracheal tube stylet when intubating through the nose. The procedure succeeds "blind" as a result of the tube's ability to flex as it is aspirated into the larynx. A stylet would prevent this and incur greater risk of trauma on blind advancement.
4. A warm tube is a flexible tube. Wait for 10 to 15 seconds after reaching the pharynx before further advancement. Allowing the tube to be heated to ambient breath temperature will minimize the chance of trauma.

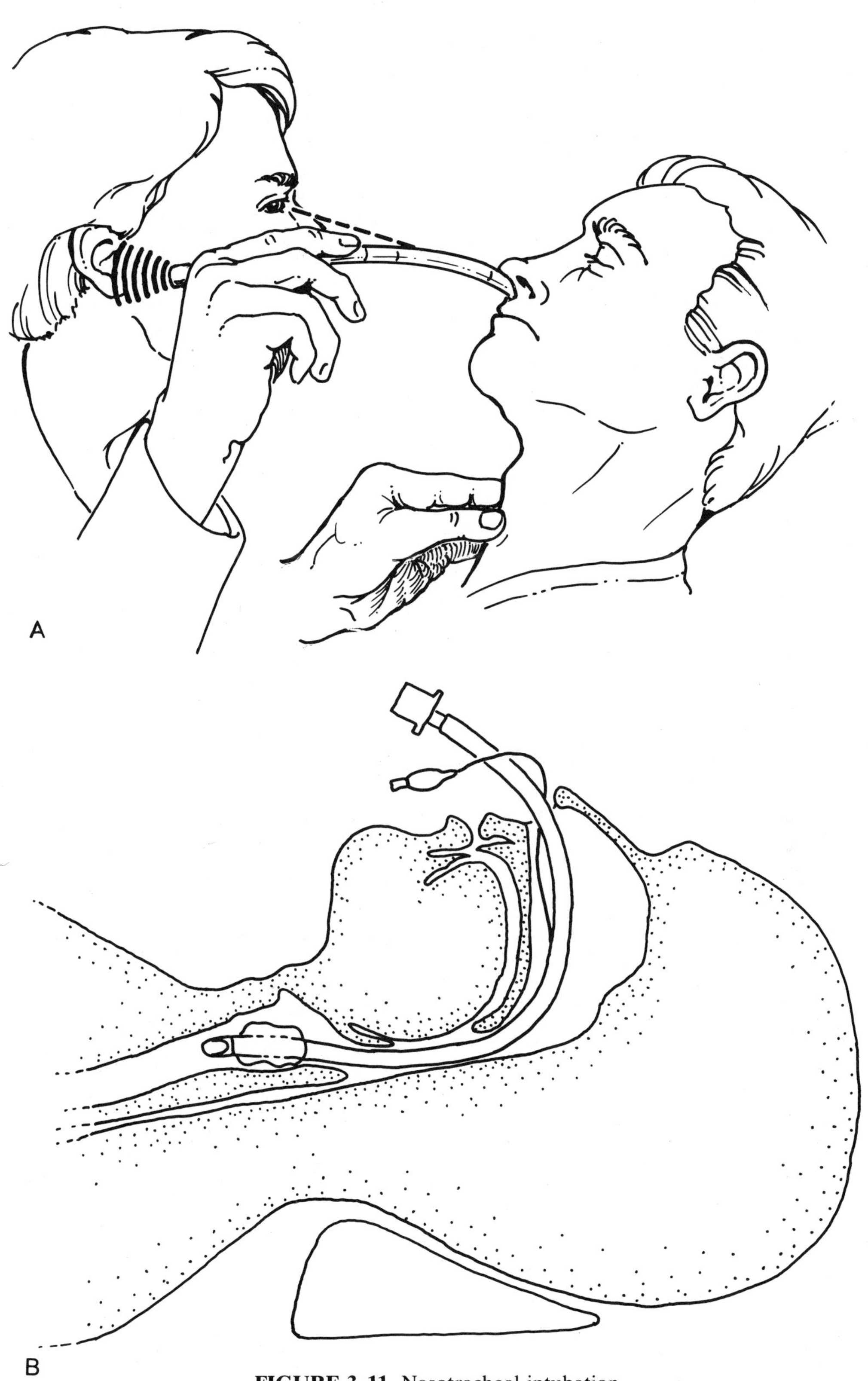

FIGURE 3–11. Nasotracheal intubation.

5. Use of endotracheal tubes whose tips can be directed by traction on a proximal ring (Endotrol, Mallinckrodt Co., St. Louis) (Figure 3–12) greatly increases procedure success rates. Such directable tubes are especially useful for patients with more anteriorly located larynges.
6. In the event of failure of "blind" intubation of the trachea, the tube may still be able to be guided in under direct laryngoscopy with or without use of Magill forceps. Maintain tube advancement in the hypopharynx, and proceed with laryngoscopy with the patient supine as described under Orotracheal Intubation.
7. It is impossible to pass a floppy nasal trumpet through a patient's cribriform plate (fractured or otherwise). Easily passing one through the nasal cavity of a facial trauma victim will, therefore, portend safe nasotracheal intubation in that patient. Even further safety can be achieved with a minor procedure modification: Following trumpet insertion, pass a small-caliber feeding tube through the trumpet and observe it in the pharynx. Remove the trumpet, thread the endotracheal tube over the feeding tube into the pharynx, and remove the feeding tube. Complete the intubation in the usual manner.
8. Nasotracheal intubation takes longer and has a lower success rate than orotracheal intubation, so the nasotracheal route is not the preferred choice when the patient is *in extremis*.

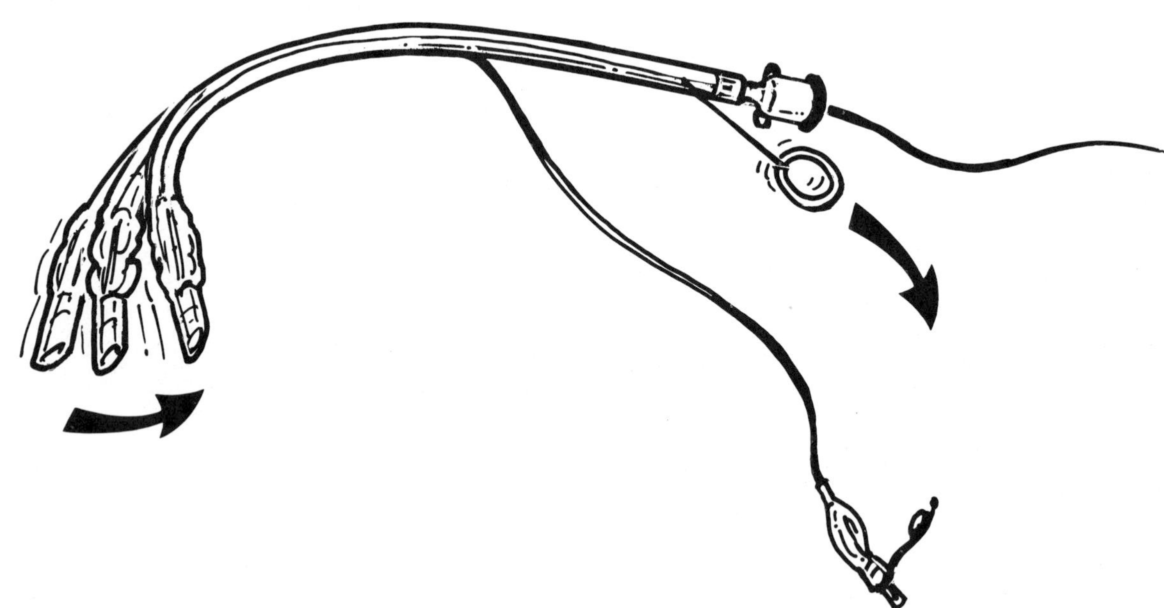

FIGURE 3–12. Directable endotracheal tube.

DIGITAL INTUBATION

Digitally guided intubation may be a viable option when confronted with an apneic, spinally immobilized patient having an anteriorly placed larynx that would prove difficult to intubate safely by other methods. The procedure involves minimal neck manipulation. The problem of visual obscuration of the larynx by vomitus is moot. Digital intubation is easier for the operator with long, thin fingers and more difficult in the patient with a narrow oropharynx.

Contraindications

Patient not deeply obtunded
Patient has intact gag reflex

Equipment

Endotracheal tubes
Stylet
10-ml syringe
Yankhauer suction apparatus
Lidocaine jelly
Bite block or jaw-spreading device
Tincture of benzoin
Cloth tape
Mask
Eye shield
Gloves
Pulse oximeter

Universal Precautions

1. Wear mask.
2. Use an eye shield.
3. Wear gloves.

Technique

1. Adequately prepare for the procedure (see No. 8 in Common Impediments).
2. Monitor the patient with a pulse oximeter if possible.
3. Insert the stylet into the endotracheal tube, making sure no protrusion occurs through the balloon end. Fabricate a gentle curve followed by a "hockey stick" bend to the tube and stylet (Figure 3–13). Test the integrity of the balloon by inflating it with 10 ml of air. Deflate the balloon and leave the air-filled syringe attached.
4. Apply lidocaine jelly to the balloon end of the tube.
5. Put on mask, eye shield, and gloves.
6. Take position at the side of the bed, facing the patient, with your nondominant hand nearest the patient.
7. Vigorously suction the patient's pharynx, ascertaining that no biting down or gag reflex response occurs.
8. Use bag and mask to preoxygenate the patient for at least 30 seconds with 100% FiO_2.
9. Insert the nondominant index and middle fingers into the oropharynx toward the vallecula, depressing the tongue downward and bringing it slightly forward.
10. Grasp the epiglottis between the tips of the fingers, pulling it forward.
11. Pass the endotracheal tube between the fingers through the oropharynx and hypopharynx to a point just past the superior edge of the epiglottis (Figure 3–14).

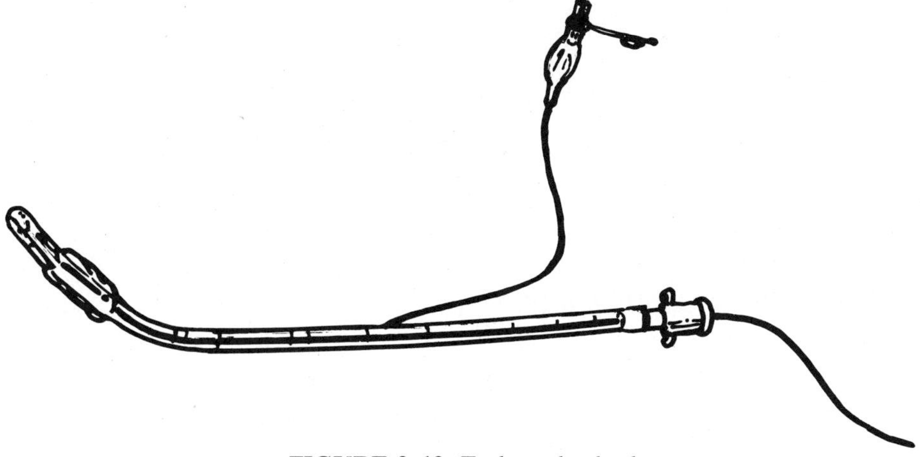

FIGURE 3–13. Endotracheal tube.

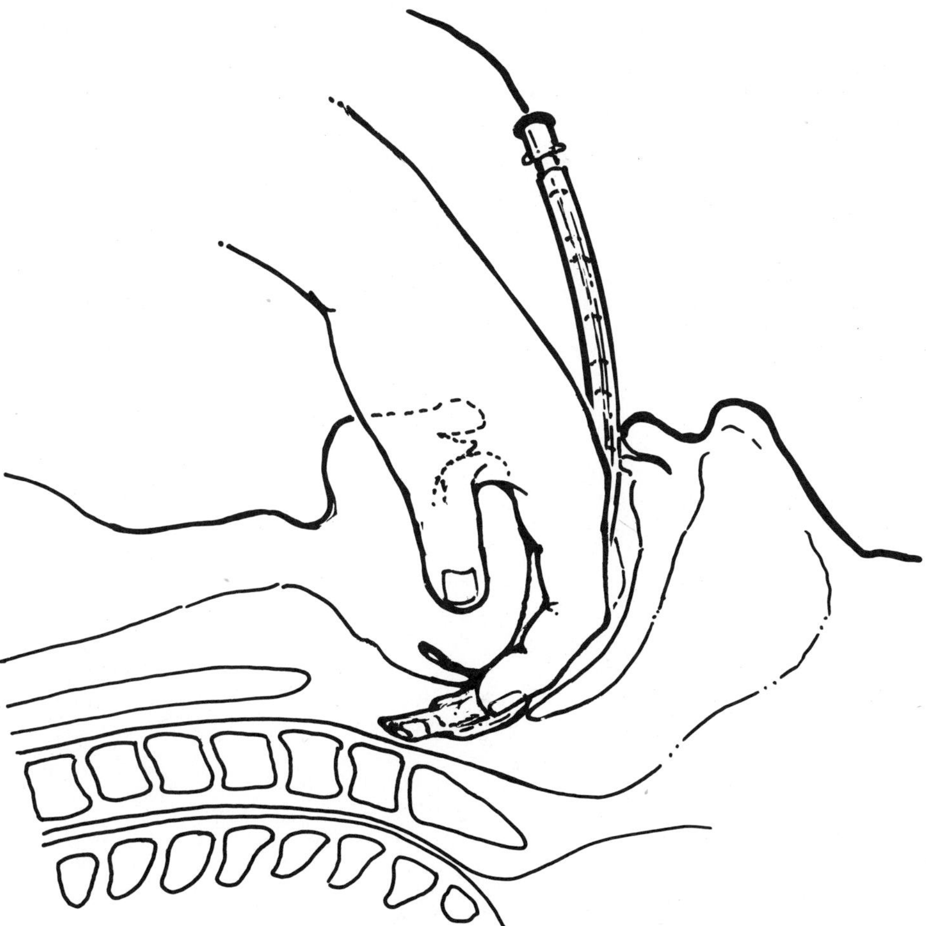

FIGURE 3–14. Digital intubation.

12. Release the epiglottis, grasp the tube between your fingers, and pull it anteriorly against the epiglottis (Figure 3–15).
13. Advance the tube 2 to 4 cm through the cords while maintaining mild anteriorly directed pressure. Remove the stylet, and advance the tube several more centimeters.
14. Inflate the balloon with 5 to 10 ml of air, confirm tube position, reposition as needed, and secure the tube.
15. Obtain a chest x-ray film and examine it.

Specific Potential Complication

Bite injury to the intubator's fingers

Pearls and Pitfalls

1. Should a patient's mouth be too small to accommodate both fingers and the endotracheal tube, it may be possible to pass the tube (without stylet) through the nose into the hypopharynx as in the technique of nasotracheal intubation. It may then be grasped with the fingers, compressed against the epiglottis, and advanced as above.
2. In addition to proper patient selection, the intubator's fingers can be protected further by use of a bite block or oral airway held between the patient's molars by an assistant. Alternately, ratchet-type jaw spreaders may be inserted prior to intubation without much compromise of finger space. With the possible exception of the edentulous patient, the risk to the intubator's fingers will always be finite.

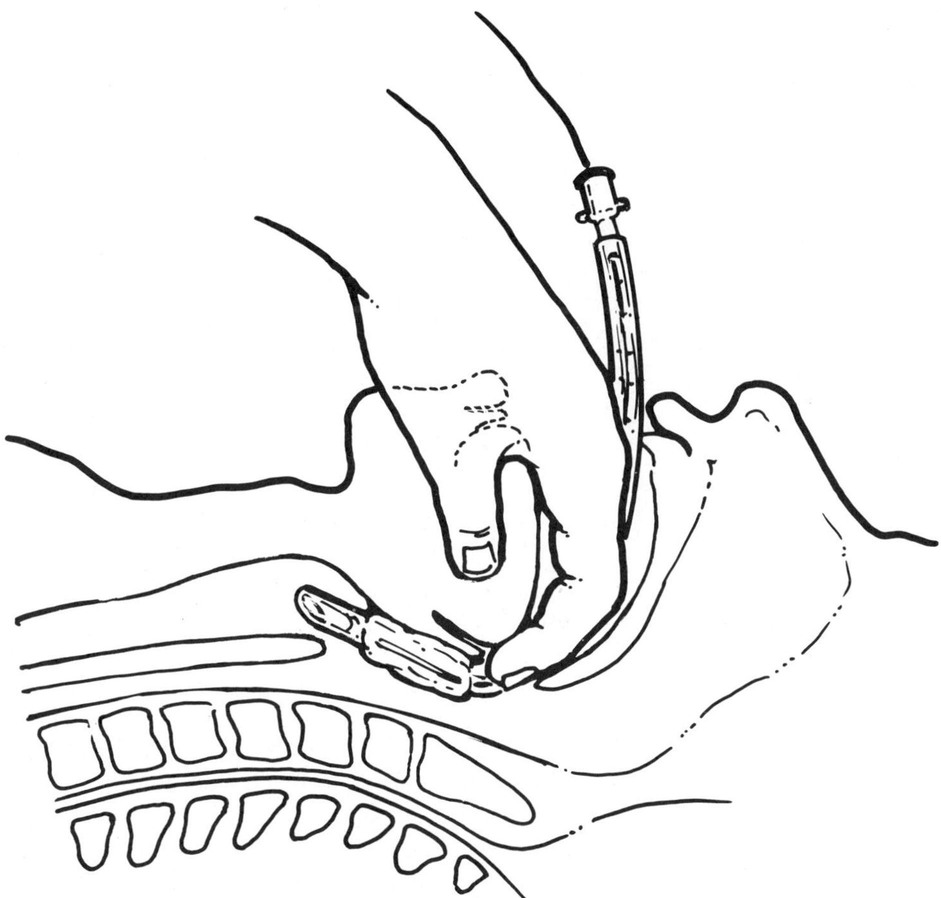

FIGURE 3–15. Digital intubation.

LIGHTED STYLET INTUBATION

The technique of lighted stylet intubation is most applicable in situations in which a digital intubation is applicable. No neck manipulation is required. The risk to the intubator is less, but since a styletted endotracheal tube is advanced through the larynx without direct visualization, the risk to the patient is the same.

Contraindications

Bright ambient light that cannot be eliminated (e.g., prehospital outdoors)
Suspicion of significant anterior neck trauma
Vomitus or foreign body obstruction that cannot be cleared

Equipment

Endotracheal tubes
Lighted stylet
10-ml syringe
Yankhauer suction apparatus
4×4-inch gauze pads
Lidocaine jelly
Tincture of benzoin
Cloth tape
Mask
Gloves
Eye shield
Pulse oximeter

Technique

1. Adequately prepare for the procedure (see No. 8 in Common Impediments). Specifically check for function and attachment of the stylet light.
2. Put on mask, eye shield, and gloves.
3. Insert the stylet into the endotracheal tube to a distance such that the bulb rests 0.5 cm from the end of the tube. Fabricate a 90-degree bend near the end of the tube (Figure 3–16). Test the integrity of the endotracheal tube balloon by inflating it with 10 ml of air. Deflate the balloon and leave the air-filled syringe attached.
4. Apply lidocaine jelly to the balloon end of the endotracheal tube.
5. Take position at the side of the bed, facing the patient.
6. Use bag and mask to preoxygenate the patient for at least 30 seconds with 100% FiO_2.
7. Suction the patient's pharynx.
8. Monitor the patient with pulse oximetry if possible.
9. Turn on the stylet light.
10. With the nondominant hand, grasp the patient's tongue between gauze pads and retract it forward.
11. Insert the tube and stylet along the tongue and down into the hypopharynx.
12. Dim the room lights.
13. Confirming midline transillumination above the laryngeal prominence, advance the tube and stylet inferiorly with mild anterior torque (Figure 3–17).

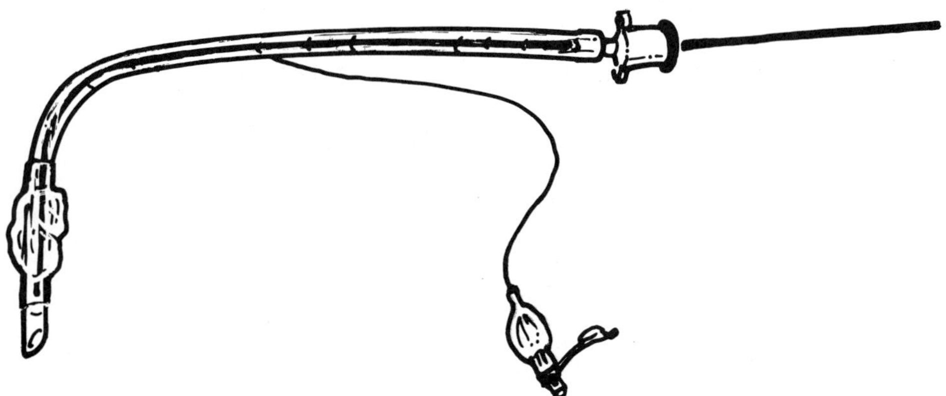

FIGURE 3–16. Lighted stylet endotracheal tube.

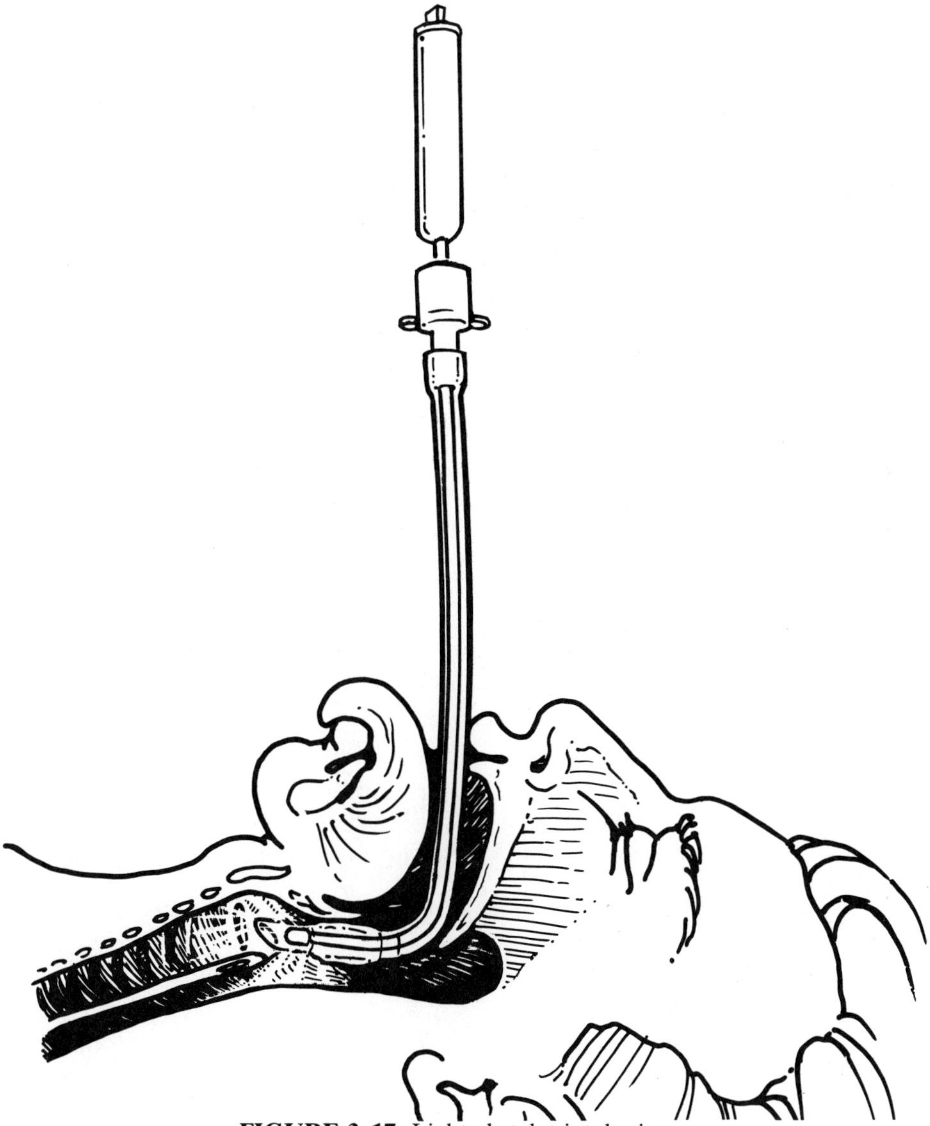

FIGURE 3–17. Lighted stylet intubation.

14. Slide the tube forward a few centimeters off the stylet, and then withdraw the stylet through the tube.
15. Inflate the balloon with 5 to 10 ml of air, confirm tube position, reposition as needed, and secure the tube.
16. Obtain a chest x-ray film and look at it.

Specific Potential Complication

Detachment and loss of stylet bulb into the trachea

Pearls and Pitfalls

1. The dimmer the ambient light, the easier it will be to check for proper tube advancement. A dull subhyoid glow indicates position in the vallecula; bright lateral neck transillumination indicates pyriform recess location. Esophageal location results in subdued, diffuse transillumination or none at all.
2. Patients with anteriorly situated larynges will be more difficult to intubate and will require a greater than 90-degree terminal bend to the stylet.

RETROGRADE TRANSLARYNGEAL INTUBATION

In general, this is an underused technique well worth learning and mastering. In many instances it can supplant cricothyrotomy or translaryngeal jet ventilation. It may be performed in the neck neutral position on the apneic trauma patient without neck manipulation. Anterior vocal cord location does not pose a problem, nor does trismus or facial trauma. The technique is especially well suited to institutions maintaining policy against orotracheal intubation of trauma victims, since both the time required to perform the procedure and the risks of complication are less than with cricothyrotomy. (The relationship between techniques is somewhat analogous to that between Seldinger percutaneous cannulation and peripheral cut down for venous access.)

Contraindications

Massive anterior neck trauma with anatomic distortion
Clinically significant coagulopathy

Equipment

Drapes
Gloves
Mask
Eye shield
Betadine antiseptic solution
1% lidocaine with epinephrine
Syringes
25- to 27-gauge anesthetic needle
1½-inch or greater Seldinger needle accepting guidewire
70-cm angiography guide wire
Hemostat
Magill forceps
Mayo scissors or wire cutter
Endotracheal tubes
Two 10-ml syringes
Yankhauer suction apparatus
Benzocaine/tetracaine topical anesthetic spray
Lidocaine jelly
Tincture of benzoin
Cloth tape
Pulse oximeter

Technique

1. Adequately prepare for the procedure (see No. 8 in Common Impediments). Confirm that the Seldinger needle will accept the guide wire.
2. Explain the procedure to the patient and obtain consent if circumstances allow.
3. Put on mask, eye shield, and sterile gloves.
4. Assume a position at the side of the bed. If necessary, remove the anterior portion of a cervical immobilization collar and substitute sand bag and/or tape immobilization in its place. Palpate the landmarks of the anterior neck.
5. In the conscious patient, spray benzocaine/tetracaine into both nares and into the pharynx. Lubricate the balloon end of the endotracheal tube with lidocaine jelly. Test the integrity of the endotracheal tube balloon by

inflating it with 10 ml of air. Deflate the balloon and leave the air-filled syringe attached.

6. Maintain 100% FiO_2 bag-mask ventilation, and monitor the patient by pulse oximetry if possible.
7. If time permits, prep and drape the area overlying the cricothyroid membrane using sterile technique and infiltrate with anesthetic/vasoconstrictor (1% lidocaine with epinephrine) subcutaneously down to the membrane.
8. With the Seldinger needle on a syringe, perpendicularly pierce the midline skin overlying the inferior portion of the cricothyroid membrane. With retraction on the plunger, advance the needle through the inferior portion of the membrane until air is aspirated back. Advance several millimeters further, and rotate the needle so that the bevel is directed cephalad (Figure 3–18).

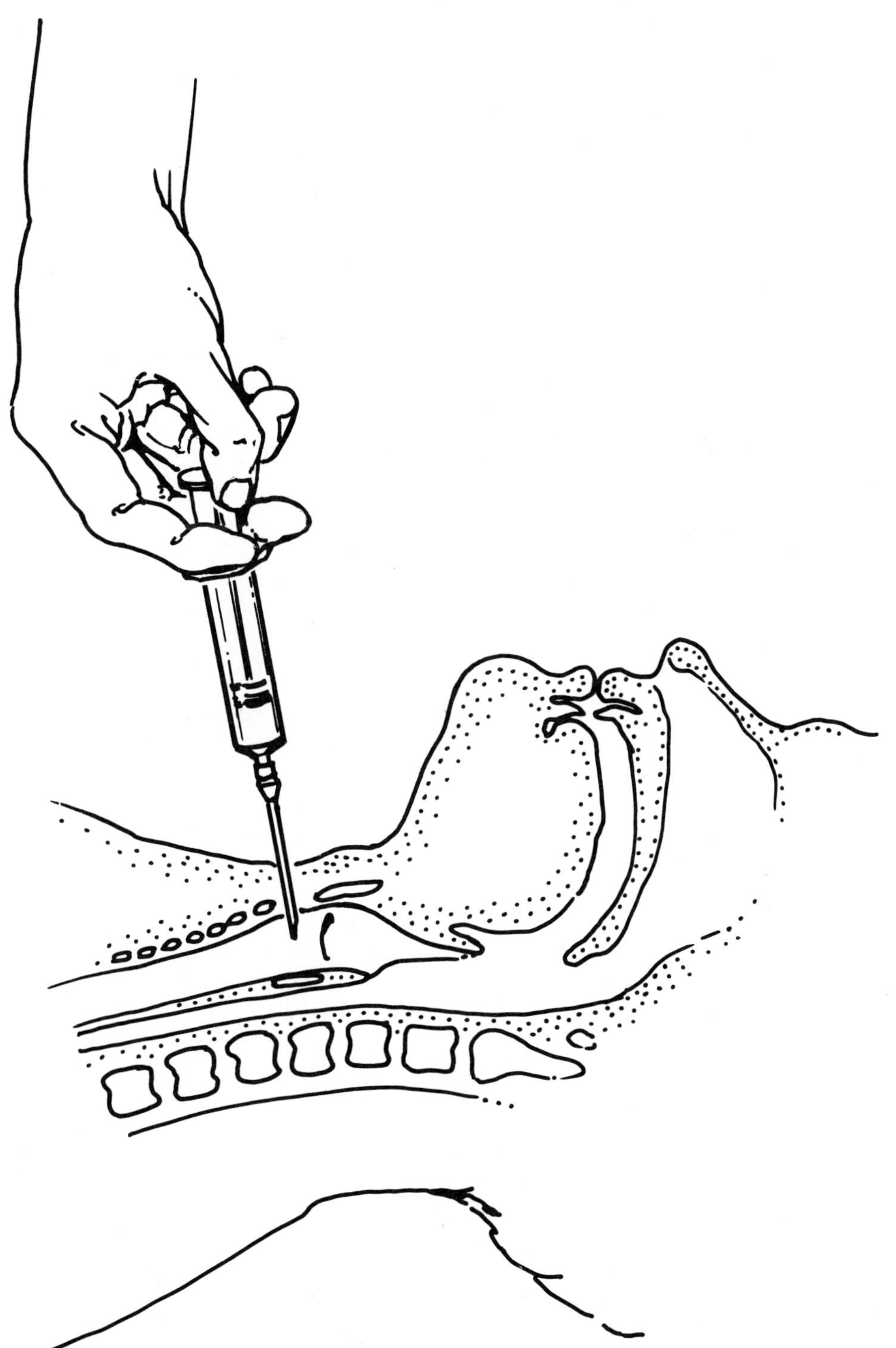

FIGURE 3–18. Retrograde translaryngeal intubation—1.

9. Remove the syringe, angle the needle 30 to 40 degrees cephalad, and thread the guide wire through the needle until a length greater than that of the endotracheal tube protrudes from either the mouth or nose (Figures 3–19 and 3–20). Should no spontaneous exit occur, the wire may be recovered from the pharynx through the mouth with finger or Magill forceps.
10. Remove the needle, and clamp a hemostat on the wire at its entry point into the neck. Excess wire beyond the hemostat can be cut.
11. Thread the superiorly protruding wire into the end hole and through the length of the endotracheal tube (Figure 3–21). Advance the tube over the wire and through the vocal cords.

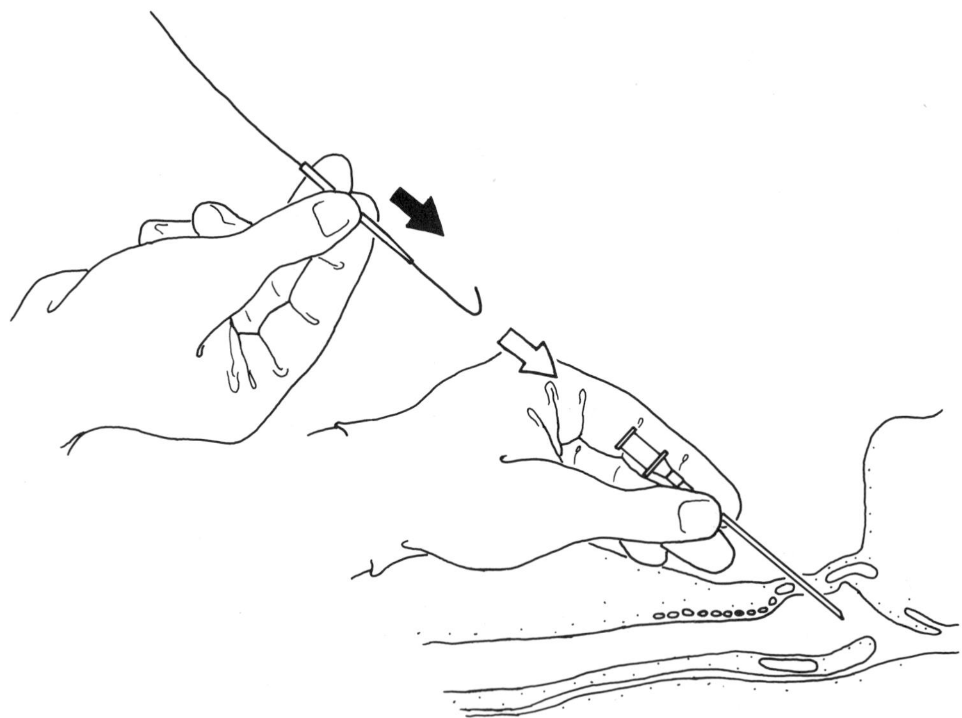

FIGURE 3–19. Retrograde translaryngeal intubation—2.

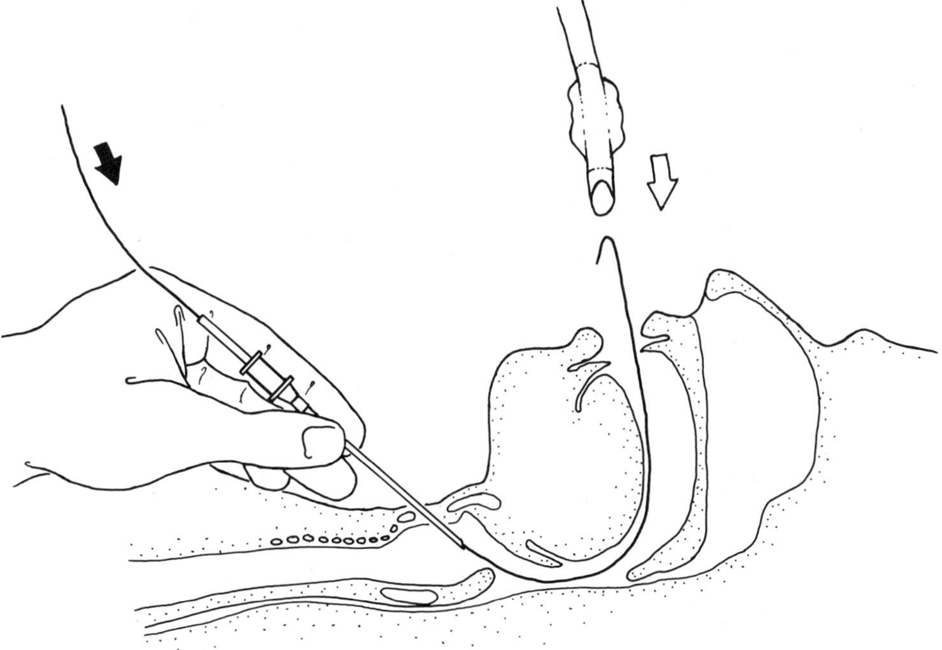

FIGURE 3–20. Retrograde translaryngeal intubation—3.

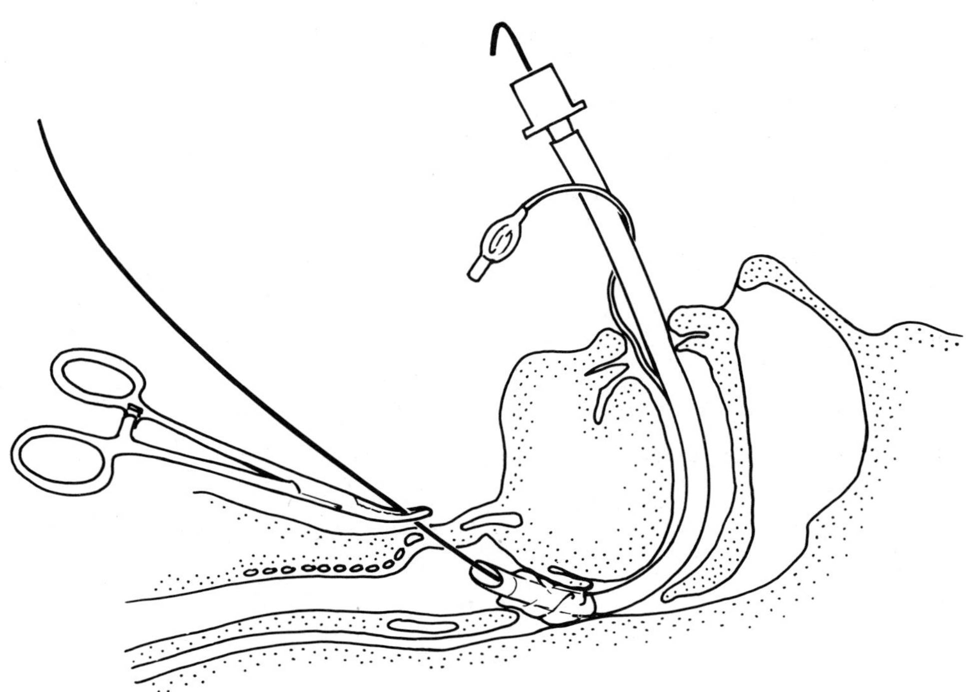

FIGURE 3–21. Retrograde translaryngeal intubation—4.

12. When resistance to further advancement is met on endotracheal tube contact at the wire's entry point inside the larynx, firmly grasp the protruding wire around the fourth and fifth fingers of one hand, and, with the remaining fingers, maintain mild forward force on the tube (Figure 3–22). As the hemostat is released with the other hand, the wire is retracted and the tube moved forward into the trachea.
13. Inflate the balloon with 5 to 10 ml of air, confirm tube position, reposition as needed, and secure the tube.
14. Obtain a chest x-ray film and examine it.

Specific Potential Complications

Bleeding with hemoptysis
Vocal cord damage
Aspiration of broken needle
Wound infection

Pearls and Pitfalls

1. Guide wires provided in standard subclavian vein catheterization kits are *not* long enough to be used in retrograde intubation. Long angiography wires should be part of emergency department standard stock and should be readily accessible.
2. Should it be impossible to recover the wire from the mouth or nose, a standard 14-gauge needle/cannula may be threaded over the wire through the skin and into the trachea, and transtracheal jet ventilation (see page 88) provided as a temporizing measure.
3. Remove the wire in the direction described. Removing it in the opposite direction would bring through the neck wound the length of wire contaminated by the nasopharynx and/or oropharynx and increase the risk of infection.
4. The child in respiratory arrest from epiglottitis may have attempts at standard orotracheal intubation stymied by anatomic distortion of the hypopharynx. The passage of a wire from below will identify the laryngeal opening and facilitate tube passage in this setting.

References

DeGarmo BH, Dronen S: Pharmacology and use of neuromuscular blocking agents. Ann Emerg Med 12:48–55, 1983.
McNamara RM: Retrograde intubation of the trachea. Ann Emerg Med 16:680–682, 1987.
Pointer J: Using nasotracheal intubation to full potential. ER Rep 3:143–148, 1982.
Stewart RD: Tactile orotracheal intubation. Ann Emerg Med 13:175–178, 1984.
Vollmer TP, Stewart RD, Paris PM, et al: Use of a lighted stylet for orotracheal intubation in the prehospital setting. Ann Emerg Med 14:324–327, 1985.

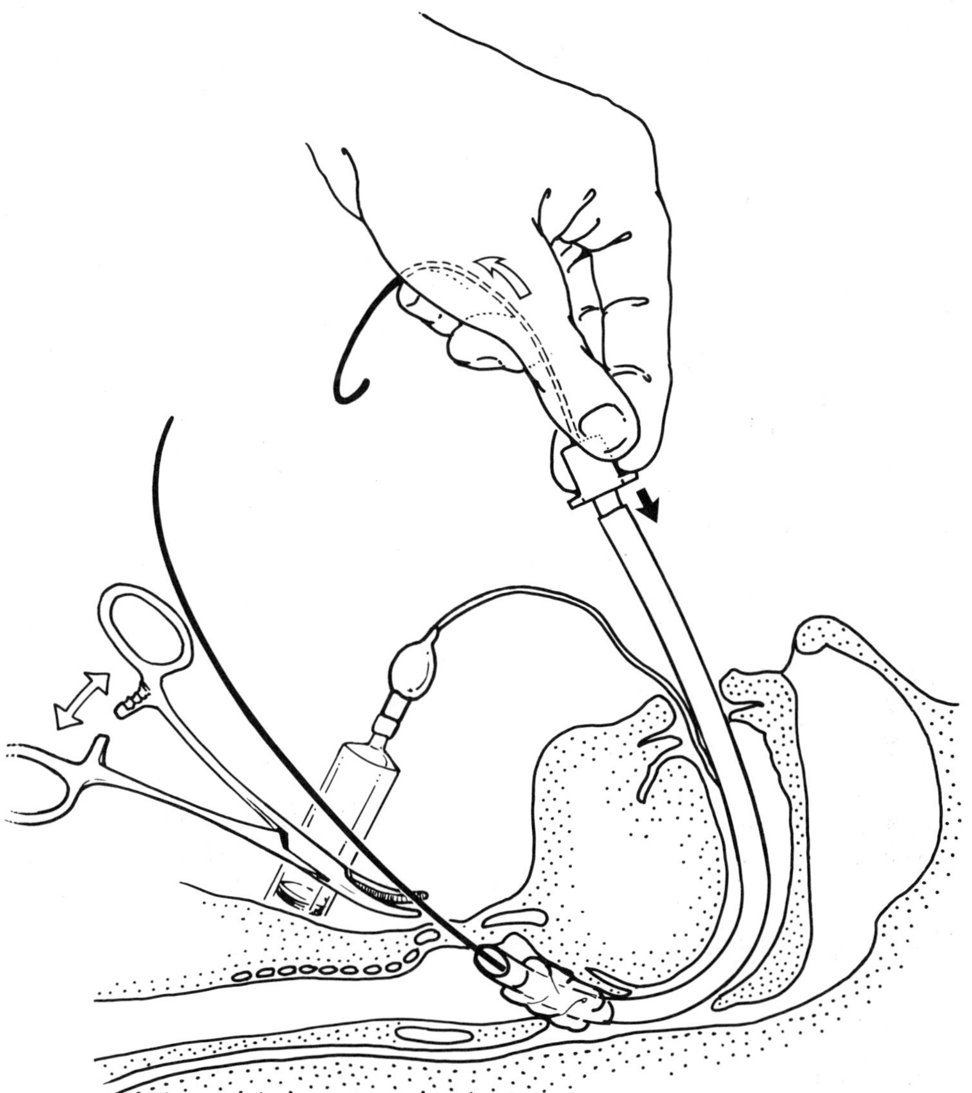

FIGURE 3–22. Retrograde translaryngeal intubation—5.

Needle Cricothyroidotomy

THOMAS TERNDRUP, MD

Indications

When a surgical airway is indicated in a patient younger than 8 years of age

For temporary relief of hypoxemia secondary to airway obstruction

As a temporary guide for standard cricothyroidotomy

When orotracheal or nasotracheal intubation cannot be performed safely and expeditiously

This is a lifesaving procedure for patients *in extremis*

Contraindications

Ability to perform nonsurgical airway management safely and expeditiously

Equipment

Betadine solution, lighting, assistance

Local anesthesia

14-gauge catheter over needle attached to a 10-ml syringe (± filled with sterile saline)

Universal Precautions

1. Wear mask.
2. Use an eye shield.
3. Wear sterile gloves.

Technique

1. If the patient status and circumstances allow (which they almost never do), explain the procedure to the patient and obtain consent.
2. Identify the cricothyroid membrane inferior to the thyroid cartilage and superior to the cricoid rim.
3. Prep for surgery and anesthesia (as time permits).

4. Insert the needle through the skin and then through the inferior part of the cricothyroid membrane, with constant suction and with the needle at a 45-degree angle to the skin, oriented caudad (Figure 3–23).
5. As soon as air bubbles are aspirated, decrease the angle to the skin to about 15 degrees, advance another 1 to 2 mm, and reconfirm aspiration of air into the syringe.

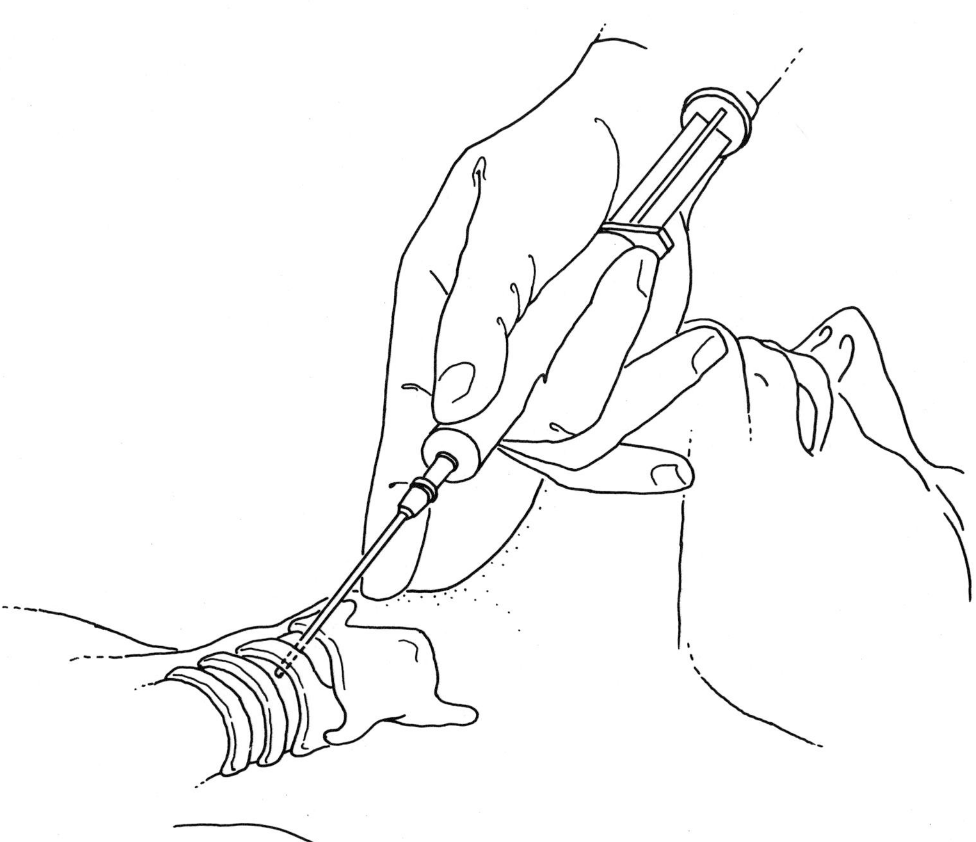

FIGURE 3–23. Needle cricothyroidotomy—1.

6. Rapidly advance the catheter over the needle into the trachea until the hub meets the skin.
7. Reconfirm aspiration of the air with your syringe.
8. Oxygenate and ventilate using one of the following techniques:
   a. Passive apneic diffusion oxygenation: When the airway is totally occluded so no expiration can occur, the Pa_{O_2} can be maintained by flowing 100% oxygen into the lungs at 5 L/min. The Pa_{CO_2} will continue to rise with this technique, usually at a rate of 2 to 3 mm Hg/min, but it can often maintain life for long enough to definitely solve the airway problem.
   b. The adapter from a 3-mm pediatric endotracheal tube fits into the hub of the catheter, allowing ventilation with a self-inflating resuscitation bag device (Figure 3–24). Alternately, the adapter from an 8-mm endotracheal tube can be fitted into the barrel of a 3-ml syringe, the tip of the syringe inserted into the catheter, the hand-held bag-valve device attached to the adapter, and the patient ventilated.
   c. Hand trigger valves are commercially available that allow oxygen from a high-pressure source to be directly insufflated through the catheter. With this technique the valve is opened until adequate chest expansion is observed and then closed to allow exhalation (see Figure 3–25).
9. Ventilate patient for 1 second and allow 2 seconds of exhalation. Exhalation must be through the patient's own airway because of the resistance to air flow through the narrow catheter. Chest compression can be used to increase expiration and flow through a partially obstructed airway.

Complications

Complications of this procedure are basically identical to those of the standard surgical cricothyroidotomy except that no incision is made and the risk for vascular injury is less. There appears to be an increased risk for barotrauma (i.e., subcutaneous emphysema, pneumothorax, and pneumomediastinum) when compared with cricothyroidotomy.

Pearls and Pitfalls

Needle cricothyroidotomy is a temporary measure to create an airway, allowing ventilation and oxygenation. *Adequate* ventilation may be difficult to establish. At best, needle cricothyroidotomy allows for improved oxygenation and ventilation in patients with a complete or nearly complete airway obstruction who would otherwise be unable to be ventilated.

It *may* be the preferred method for surgical airway management in patients younger than 8 years of age.

Immobilization of the proximal trachea by grasping the thyroid cartilage with the nonoperative hand (or by an assistant) improves the success rate.

If the trachea is disrupted below the cricoid or if the cricoid is severely traumatized, the catheter may be inserted lower in the trachea between adjacent tracheal rings, with care taken to avoid the thyroid gland.

References

Extensive experience.

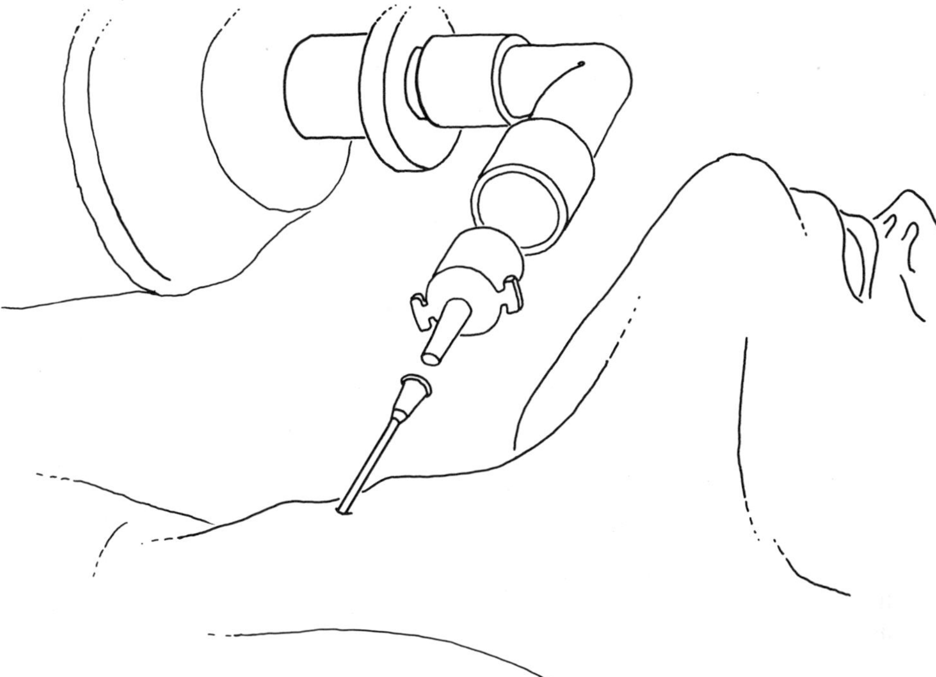

FIGURE 3–24. Needle cricothyroidotomy—2.

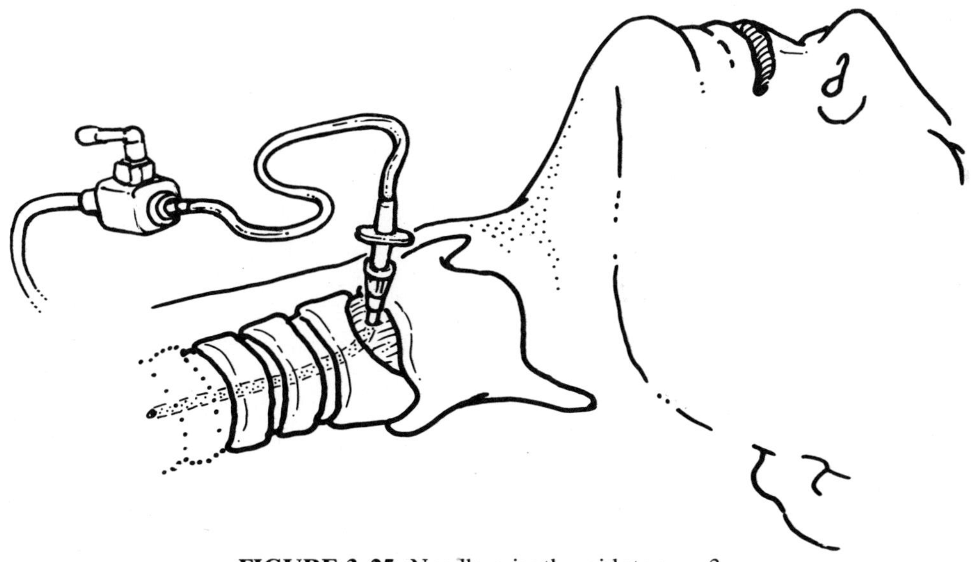

FIGURE 3–25. Needle cricothyroidotomy—3.

4

Bladder Catheterization

DENISE P. GAVULA, DO

INSERTION OF A STRAIGHT OR FOLEY CATHETER

Indications

To obtain an uncontaminated urine specimen for urinalysis and culture
To relieve bladder distention
To drain and measure the volume of residual urine
To monitor urine output
To obtain urine from the unconscious patient

Contraindications

Urethral trauma

Equipment

Bedside collection unit
Betadine ¼ strength
Syringe and sterile water
Sterile gloves
Blue pad or Chux
Sterile sponge forceps
Light source
Straight catheter 16 F (adult)
Foley catheter 16 F (adult)
Straight catheter
- Newborn: 5 and 8 F
- Toddler: 10 F
- Child: 12 F

Foley catheter
- Toddler: 10 F
- Child: 12 F

Universal Precautions

1. Wear gloves.

Technique

Preparation

1. If patient status and circumstances allow, explain the procedure to the patient and obtain consent.
2. Put on sterile gloves using the proper technique.
3. Fill the syringe with the amount of sterile water needed to inflate the balloon.
4. Attach the syringe to the nondraining end of the catheter and gently inflate the balloon to test it and then deflate it completely.
5. Empty the packet of sterile lubricant onto the tray.

Bladder Catheterization of the Female Patient

At each step let the patient know what you will be doing.

---

1. Position the patient supine with knees bent and legs externally rotated and adducted at the hip. (The infant or small child should be placed in the supine frog leg position as shown in Figure 4–1. Two assistants may be needed: one to hold the child and the second to assist with the catheterization.)
2. Place a sterile towel under the hips of the patient, keeping the fingertips sterile by covering them with the folded end of the towel.
3. Place a sterile basin or urine collection cup near the vulva.
4. Stand near the patient's hip facing the patient's head so that your dominant hand is nearest the patient.

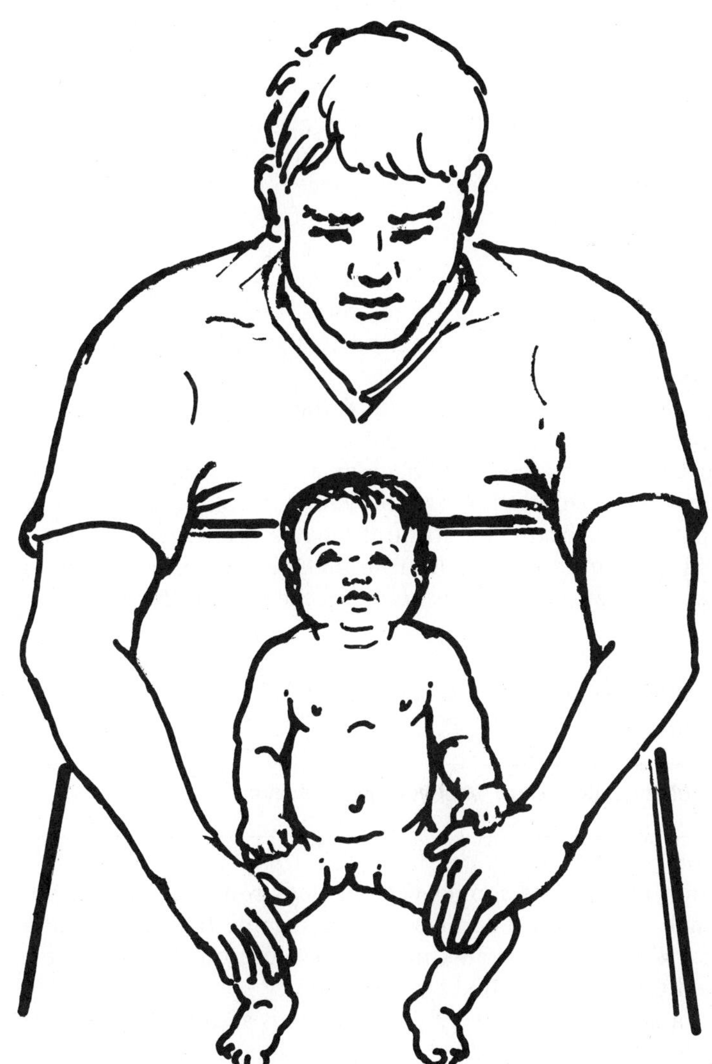

FIGURE 4–1. Position for bladder catheterization—infant.

5. Separate the labia majora and minora with your nondominant hand (Figure 4–2). (Remember, this hand is now contaminated and should not touch the catheter.)
6. Tell the patient that you will be touching her and that it will feel cold. Cleanse the labia minora and urethral opening with your dominant hand using a Betadine-soaked cotton ball held with the sponge forceps or a presoaked Betadine swabstick. The area will be cleansed three times. Each cotton ball or swab should be used only once, wiping with a single downward stroke.
7. Hold the catheter 2 inches from the tip with your dominant hand, and coil the remainder in your hand (see Figure 4–2).
8. Lubricate the catheter tip.
9. Let the patient know that you will be inserting the catheter, and ask her to try to relax.
10. Gently insert the catheter. If you meet resistance, or if the patient appears to be in an unusual amount of discomfort, *stop* and request the assistance of a senior physician.
11. Collect the urine in the sterile container.
12. The straight catheter can be removed when all the urine is drained. The Foley catheter should be inserted to the branching Y if possible and the balloon then inflated.
13. Pull the Foley catheter back until the balloon can be felt to be abutted against the inferior bladder wall.
14. If no urine is obtained, the bladder may be empty or the catheter may be in the vagina. Do not remove this catheter—leave it in place and reexamine the patient to locate the urethral meatus. This first catheter will mark the wrong spot and prevent you from making the same mistake again.
15. Secure a Foley catheter with tape on the skin of the proximal inner thigh.

Bladder Catheterization of the Male Patient

At each step let the patient know what you will be doing.

---

1. Position the patient supine with his legs somewhat adducted. (The infant or small child should be placed in the supine frog leg position as shown in Figure 4–1. Two assistants may be needed: one to hold the child and the second to assist with the catheterization.)
2. Place a sterile towel under the penis and across the thighs of the patient, keeping the fingertips sterile with the folded edges.
3. Place a sterile basin or cup between the patient's thighs.
4. Stand near the patient's hip facing the patient's head so that your dominant hand is nearest the patient.
5. Tell the patient that you will be touching him and that it will feel cold. Grasp the penis with your nondominant hand, and gently retract the foreskin. This may not be possible in some male infants, and the urine sample will need to be obtained by suprapubic aspiration. (Remember, this hand is now contaminated and should not touch the catheter.)
6. Cleanse the urinary meatus with Betadine using a hemostat or sponge

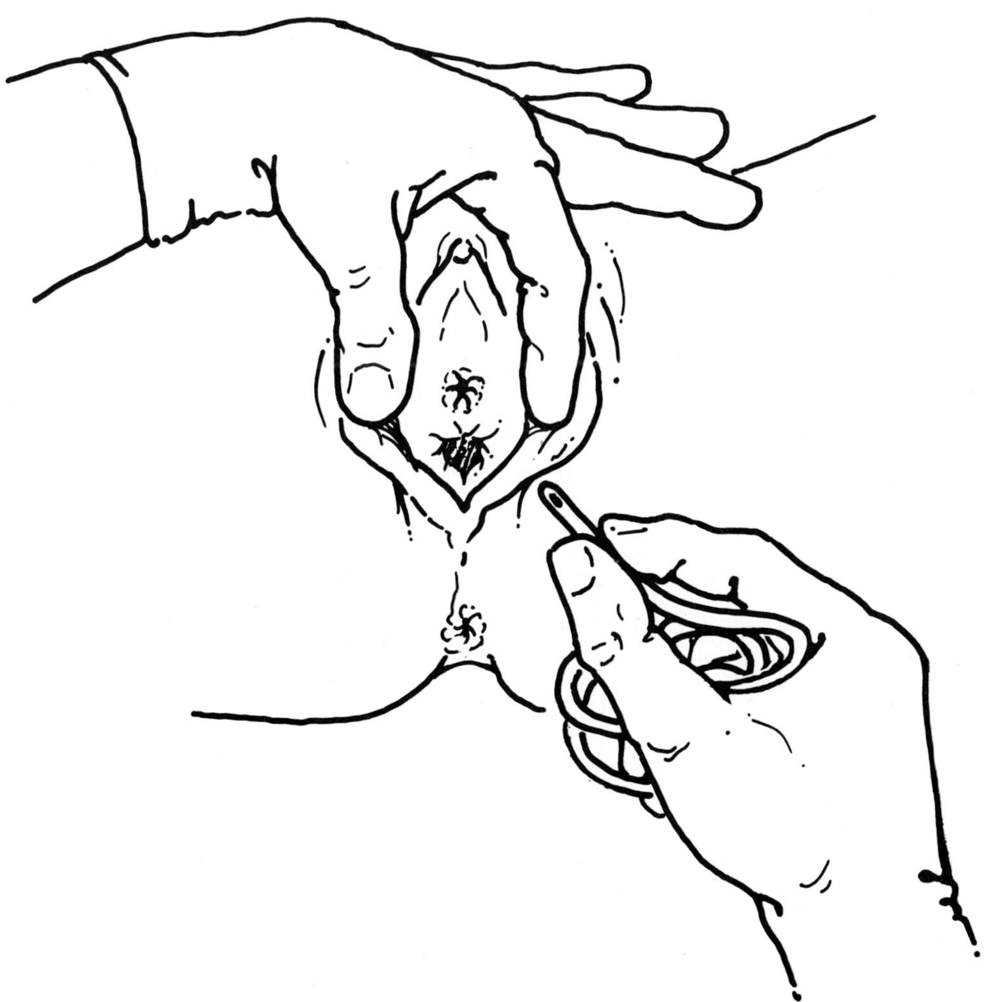

FIGURE 4–2. Bladder catheterization—female.

forceps to grasp the cotton balls or gauze or use prepackaged Betadine swabsticks. Cleanse in a circular pattern from the meatus to the midpoint of the shaft of the penis.

7. Pull the penis gently upward and slightly superiorly to straighten the urethra.
8. Hold the catheter with your dominant hand 2 inches from the tip and coil the remainder in your hand (Figure 4–3).
9. Lubricate the catheter tip.
10. Let the patient know that you will be inserting the catheter, and ask him to try to relax.
11. Gently insert the catheter. If you meet resistance or the patient appears to be in an unusual amount of discomfort, *stop* and request the assistance of a senior physician.
12. Collect the urine in a sterile container.
13. The straight catheter is removed when all the urine is drained. The Foley catheter should be inserted to the branching Y if possible and the balloon then inflated.
14. Pull the Foley catheter back until the balloon can be felt to be abutted against the inferior bladder wall.
15. If no urine is obtained, the bladder may be empty or the catheter may be in the proximal urethra. The balloon should be deflated and the senior physician should be asked for assistance.
16. Secure a Foley catheter with tape on the skin of the proximal thigh.

Complications

Introduction of infection

Pain and injury to the proximal urethra due to inflation of the balloon.

Bruising or irritation of the urethra or bladder wall causing hematuria. Persistent gross hematuria is uncommon.

Vaginal catheterization

Intravesicular knotting

Pearls and Pitfalls

1. Difficult catheterizations in males with enlarged prostates may be facilitated if a coudé catheter is used.
2. It is sometimes helpful (especially in males) to first fill the urethra with lidocaine jelly using a Toomy syringe. This provides some anesthesia (not complete) and better lubrication.
3. Trauma victims should not undergo urethral catheterization until a rectal examination has been performed to rule out urethral disruption or if there is any blood at the urethral meatus or a perineal hematoma. If there is any suspicion of a urethral disruption a retrograde urethrogram should be obtained before any attempt at bladder catheterization is done.

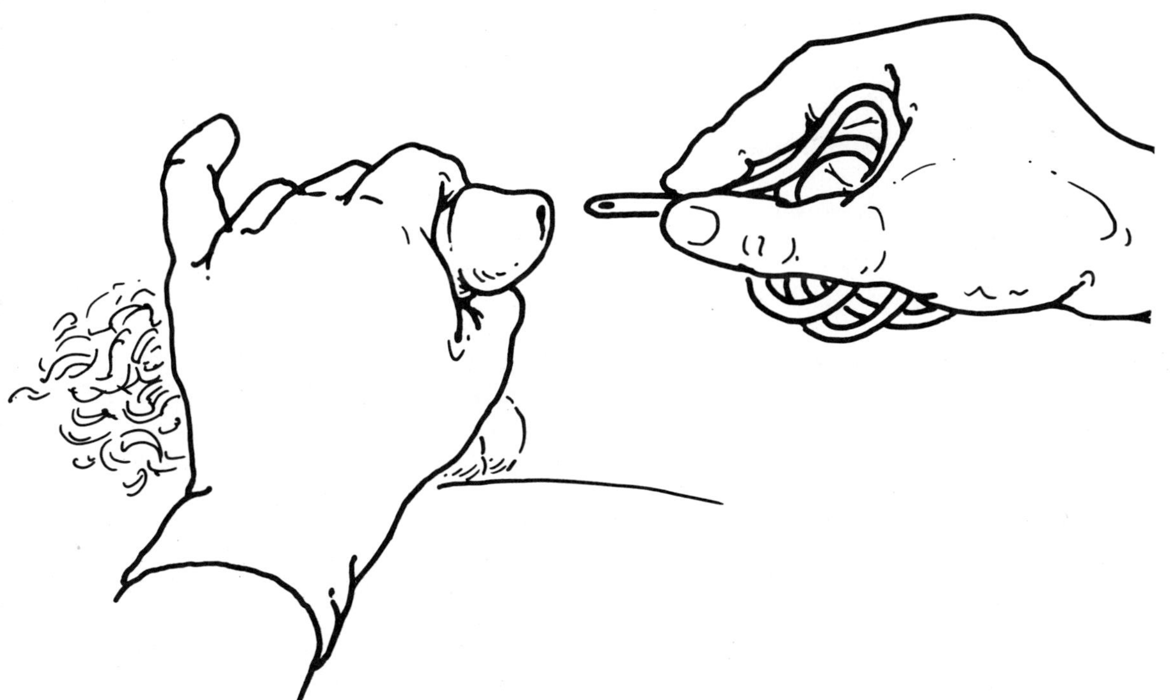

FIGURE 4–3. Bladder catheterization–male.

SUPRAPUBIC BLADDER ASPIRATION

Indication

To obtain a sterile urine specimen for culture in infants and children younger than 2 years of age.

Equipment

Betadine solution or presoaked swabs
Alcohol wipe
Sterile 3-ml syringe with an attached 22-gauge, 1½-inch needle
Sterile gloves

Universal Precautions

1. Wear sterile gloves.

Technique

1. Explain the procedure to the parents, and obtain informed consent.
2. Prior to any attempt you should inquire when the child last voided. If it was within the past hour and a bladder cannot be palpated or percussed, the procedure should not be attempted.
3. Position the child supine.
4. One or two assistants may be needed to hold the child. Gentle occlusion of the tip of the penis of the male infant may prevent him from voiding during preparation for the procedure. If the child voids, wait 1 hour before attempting again.
5. Stand at the side of the child facing the child's head so that your dominant hand is nearest the child.
6. Cleanse the skin with Betadine solution with a circular motion (10 cm diameter) from the center of the pubic bone.
7. The needle should be inserted 2 cm or 2 fingerbreadths above the pubis in the midline at an angle of 10 to 20 degrees (Figure 4–4).
8. Insert the needle and gently aspirate with the syringe while advancing the needle into the bladder.
9. If there is failure to obtain urine, pull the needle back to the level just beneath the abdominal wall and advance it at a different angle (suggested 20 degrees caudad or 20 degrees cephalad to the perpendicular).
10. *The procedure should be attempted only three times.*
11. Urinary catheterization or repeat suprapubic aspiration may be attempted in 1 to 2 hours if there is a failure to obtain urine.

Complications

Microscopic hematuria (gross hematuria uncommon)
Intestinal perforation

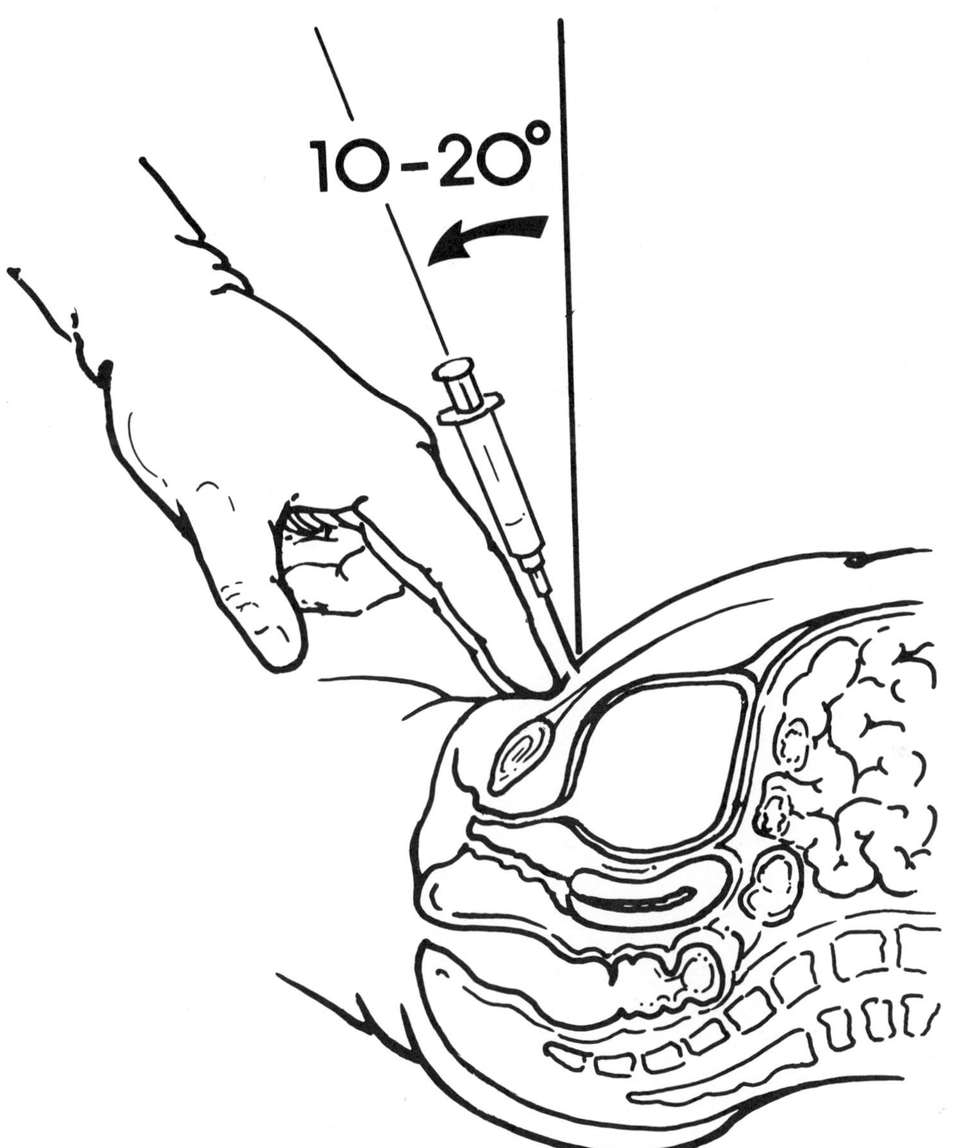

FIGURE 4–4. Suprapubic bladder aspiration.

Infection of the abdominal wall or the urinary tract
Bruising of the abdominal wall

Pearls and Pitfalls

If the infant is dehydrated, wait until intravenous fluid resuscitation has been given before starting the procedure.

References

Nursing Policy and Procedure Manual. Syracuse, NY, State University of New York Health Science Center, 1990.

Ruddy RM: Catheterization of the bladder, suprapubic bladder aspiration. In Fleisher G, Ludwig S (eds): Textbook of Pediatric Emergency Medicine, pp 1306–1309. Baltimore, Williams & Wilkins, 1988.

5

Bone Marrow Aspiration

MARCY LAYTON, MD

Indication

To remove bone marrow for histologic and microbiologic examination

Contraindications

None

Equipment

Sterile gloves
Betadine
Biopsy needle (Jamshidi)
Syringes—20 ml and 5 ml
1% lidocaine
Microscope slides and coverslips
Gauze
Sterile drape
Needles—25-gauge, 1-inch and 20-gauge, 1½-inch
Mask and eye shield

Universal Precautions

1. Wear gloves.
2. Wear a mask.
3. Use an eye shield.

Technique

1. Explain the procedure to the patient and obtain consent.
2. Position the patient in the prone or lateral position.
3. Locate the posterior-superior iliac crest and mark this spot (Figure 5–1).
4. Put on gloves and prep the area with Betadine and drape with a sterile field.
5. Anesthetize the skin and subcutaneous tissue with the 25-gauge, 1-inch needle and 5-ml syringe filled with 1% lidocaine. Anesthetize approximately a dime-sized area of the iliac crest with the longer 20-gauge needle.
6. Place the biopsy needle into its trochanter and enter the bone at the most prominent aspect of the iliac crest.
7. With a twisting motion and continuous downward pressure, advance the needle just through the cortex of bone so the needle is firmly imbedded in bone (Figure 5–2).
8. Remove the trochanter and attach a 20-ml syringe to the needle.
9. Quickly apply negative pressure until several milliliters of fluid have been aspirated.
10. Fluid should be immediately handed to the laboratory technician who will ensure that the specimen is adequate (contains bone spicules) and make smears.
11. Remove the needle from the biopsy site and apply a pressure bandage.

Complications

Excess bleeding
Infection if improper sterile technique

Pearls and Pitfalls

1. Bone marrow aspiration can be extremely painful. Prior administration of a narcotic and/or sedative will increase the patient's comfort.
2. In patients with myelofibrosis, aspiration will be difficult and you may need to proceed to a biopsy alone.
3. In osteoporotic women, you must be careful not to insert the needle entirely through bone.

Reference

Extensive experience.

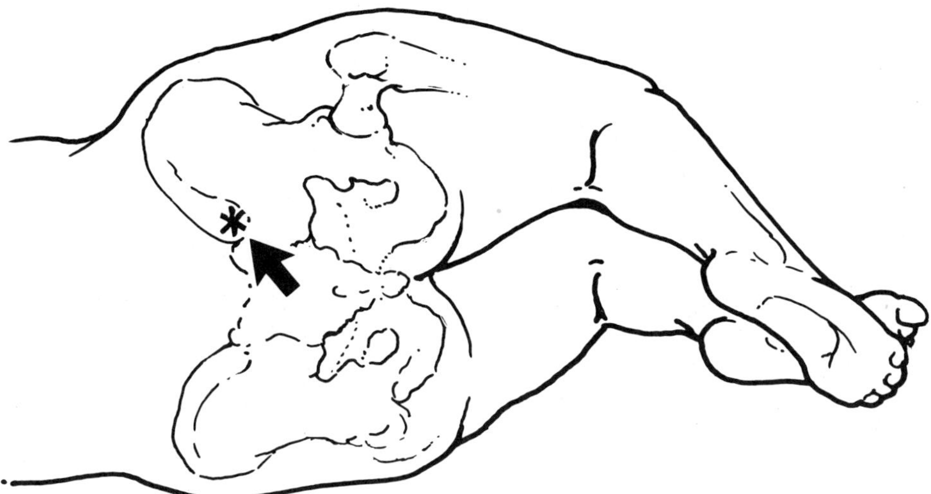

FIGURE 5–1. Position for bone marrow aspiration.

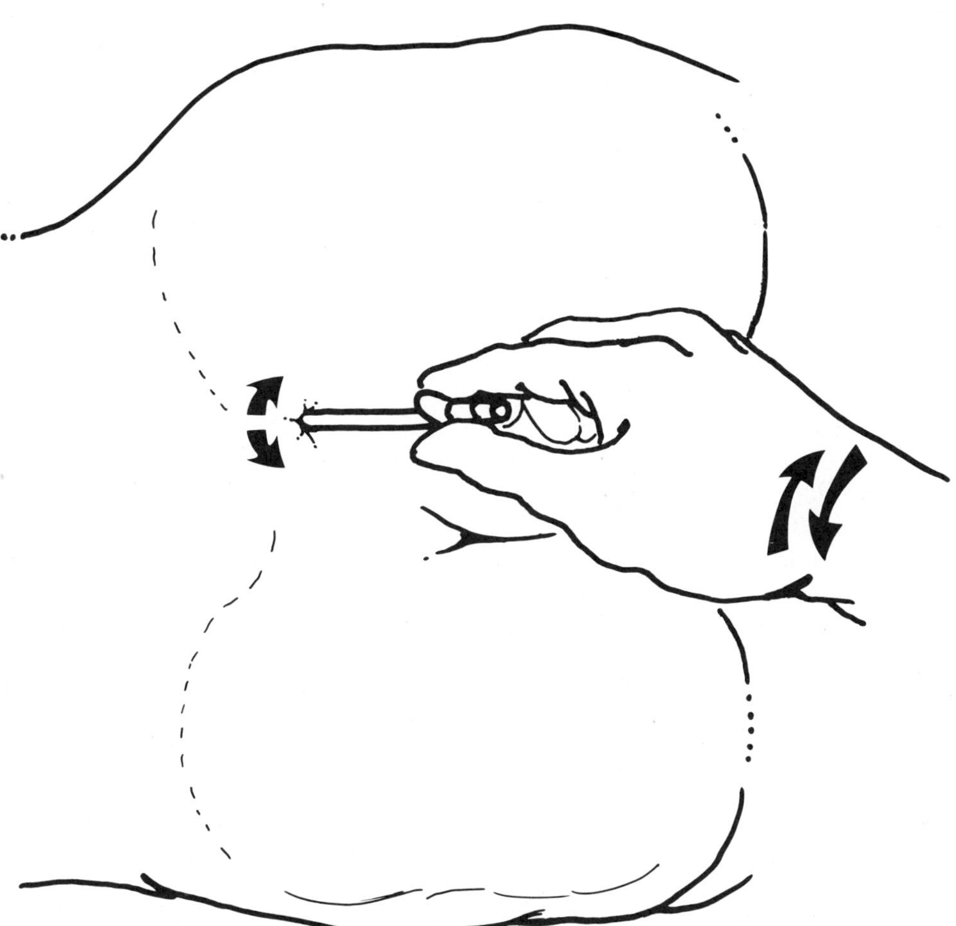

FIGURE 5–2. Bone marrow aspiration.

6 Culdocentesis

LUKE YIP, MD

Indications

When suspicious of a rupturing, ruptured, or chronic ectopic pregnancy when a sonogram is not readily available and the patient is hemodynamically stable

As a confirmatory (diagnostic) procedure when an ultrasound shows fluid in the pelvis and the patient is hemodynamically stable

In a patient with multiple trauma when diagnostic peritoneal lavage is absolutely contraindicated

The hemodynamically unstable patient is best managed by an emergency laparoscopy and/or an exploratory laparotomy.

Contraindications

When laparoscopy and or exploratory laparotomy is clearly indicated

Suspicion of a rupturing, ruptured, or chronic ectopic pregnancy when a sonogram is readily available and the patient is hemodynamically stable

A pelvic mass and or a nonmobile retroverted uterus diagnosed on a bimanual pelvic examination

Coagulopathy

Equipment

Pelvic examination table and setup
Vaginal (bivalve) speculum
Uterine cervical tenaculum
Two ringed forceps
No. 19-gauge butterfly needle (≥ 2½-cm needle length) with attached tubing
10-ml syringe
20-ml syringe
20-gauge, 1-inch needle
1% lidocaine with epinephrine
Cotton balls
4×4-inch gauze pads
Betadine solution
Mask
Eye shield
Sterile gloves

Universal Precautions

1. Wear sterile gloves.
2. Wear a mask.
3. Use an eye shield.

Technique

1. Explain the procedure to the patient and obtain consent.
2. Place the patient in the usual lithotomy position for a pelvic examination.
3. Put on mask, eye shield, and sterile gloves.
4. Prepare the needed equipment by filling the 20-ml syringe with 5 ml of anesthetic solution. This syringe is then attached to the female end of the butterfly tubing. The needle end of the butterfly is then securely held with the ring forceps (Figure 6–1).
5. After you have performed a careful bimanual pelvic examination to exclude a pelvic mass or a nonmobile retroverted uterus, introduce the vaginal speculum into the vaginal orifice in the usual manner.
6. Open the height and angle adjustment of the speculum wide.
7. After the cervix is well visualized, grasp its lower lip with the tenaculum held in your nondominant hand (Figure 6–2).

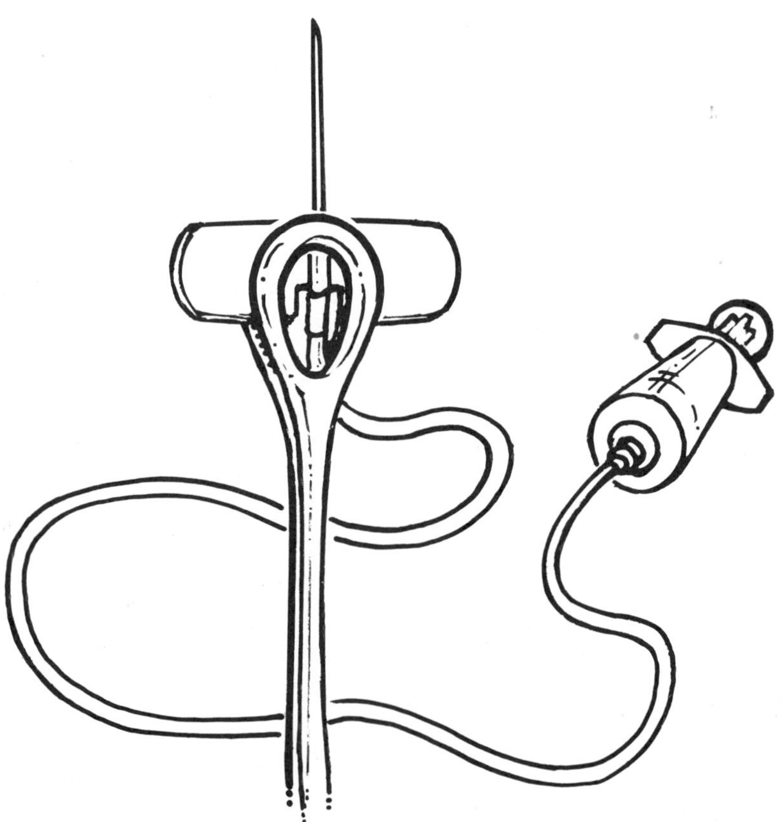

FIGURE 6–1. Culdocentesis needle.

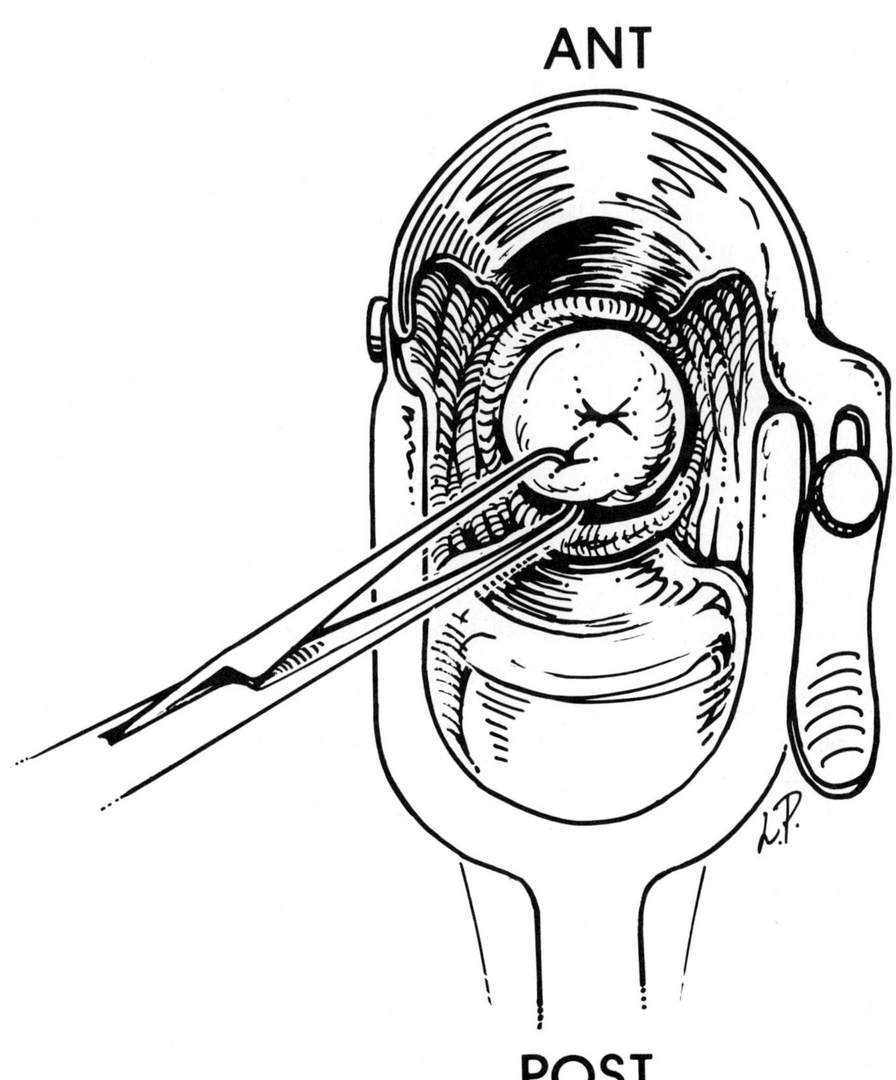

FIGURE 6–2. Culdocentesis: visualization.

8. Using your nondominant hand, apply gentle continuous traction and elevate the cervix at the same time to expose the rectouterine pouch (pouch of Douglas; posterior fornix).
9. Wash the vaginal wall of the rectouterine pouch with cotton balls soaked in Betadine solution (use the second ring forceps to hold them).
10. With your dominant hand, direct the butterfly needle held in the ring forceps into the midpoint of the rectouterine pouch approximately 1 cm inferior to where the vaginal wall joins the cervix (Figure 6–3).
11. Inject 1 to 2 ml of the anesthetic into the local area under the mucosa.
12. Now advance the needle completely into the pouch of Douglas while your assistant maintains a gradual, continued aspiration of the tubing with the 20-ml syringe.
13. Free flow of fluid into the syringe confirms the correct location of the needle tip.
14. If *no* fluid is aspirated, withdraw the needle and reintroduce it, directing it slightly lateral to the midline on either side. The procedure is repeated two times, once to the right and once to the left of the midline.
15. When fluid returns, change to the 10-ml syringe and withdraw a sample of fluid to send for hematocrit determination.
16. Remove the needle, tenaculum, and speculum.

Interpretation

Nondiagnostic: dry tap or less than 2 ml of clotted blood is aspirated.

More than 2 ml of free-flowing, nonclotting blood is suggestive of a hemoperitoneum.

Active intraperitoneal bleeding will result in a hematocrit greater than 10.

More than 10 ml of clear fluid is suggestive of a ruptured ovarian cyst, ascites, carcinoma, etc.

Ectopic pregnancy is highly favored if the culdocentesis sample has a hematocrit greater than 15.

Chronic ectopic pregnancy is favored if the sample has a hematocrit greater than 60.

Hematocrit less than 10 is suggestive of a nonectopic cause (e.g., corpus luteal cyst).

Complications

Perforation of hollow viscus, vein, artery, unsuspected tubo-ovarian abscess, or unsuspected pelvic kidney

Inadvertent puncture of the rectum

Pyosalpinx

Bleeding

Pearls and Pitfalls

1. Prudence dictates that a patient who is hemodynamically unstable or seriously suspected of having an ectopic pregnancy should have intravenous access

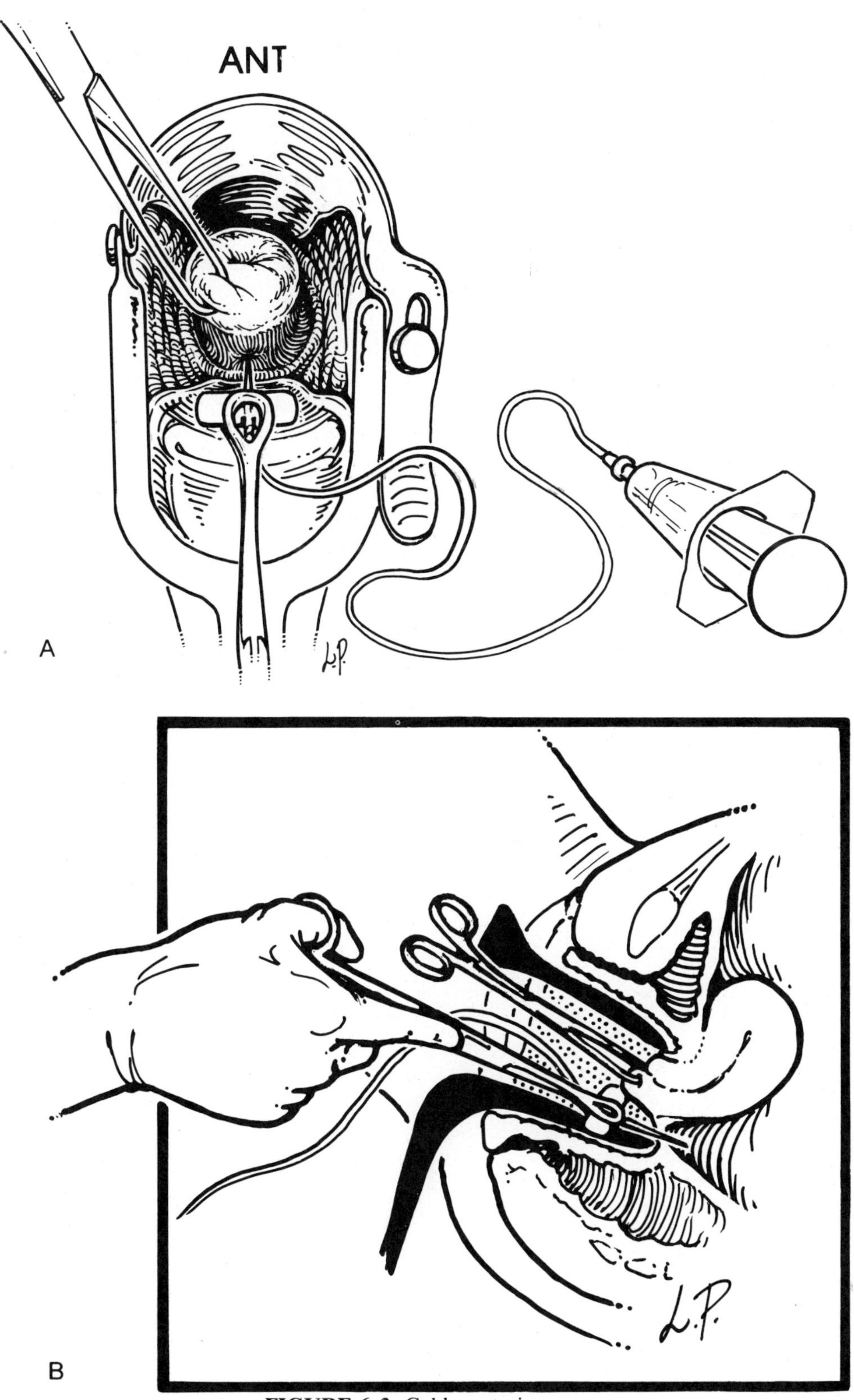

FIGURE 6–3. Culdocentesis.

and a blood sample drawn for a complete blood cell count, coagulation profile, and type and cross-match before attempting any diagnostic procedures.

2. A *positive* culdocentesis (tap) is the *only* diagnostic result (e.g., a negative or "dry" tap is nondiagnostic).
3. A positive tap only indicates the presence of intraperitoneal blood, which in the proper clinical setting is highly suggestive of a rupturing, ruptured, or chronic ectopic pregnancy or disruption of a solid viscus (e.g., spleen, liver).
4. A *true* negative tap will at best rule out a ruptured ectopic pregnancy; it *will not* rule out an unruptured ectopic pregnancy.
5. Fresh vascular blood should clot in 5 minutes; true peritoneal blood should *not* clot unless there is very active fresh bleeding.

7

Emergency Childbirth

MICHAEL S. JASTREMSKI, MD

Indication

Active labor with imminent delivery likely

Contraindications

You've got no choice!

Equipment

Mask, cap, gown
Goggles
Sterile gloves
Two clamps
Scissors
Bulb syringe
Blanket or warm towels
Sterile towel
Betadine
Sterile drapes

Universal Precautions

1. Wear mask and goggles.
2. Wear a gown and gloves.

Technique

1. If time allows, explain the procedure to the mother and father. If the father is present, assess his level of anxiety and ability to contribute in a positive way before deciding if he may stay.
2. Position the mother supine with legs bent at knees, flexed and maximally abducted at the hips.
3. Wash your hands.
4. Put on cap, mask, goggles, gown, and gloves.
5. Stand or sit between the mother's legs facing her head.
6. Prep the perineum with Betadine.
7. Assess the frequency and duration of contractions and observe associated cervical dilatation, crowning, and bulging of the perineum.

Delivery **is imminent when the contractions last 1 to 2 minutes and occur at intervals of 2 to 3 minutes and there is crowning with contractions or cervical effacement with the infant's head visible between contractions.**

---

8. Drape.
9. Normal vertex deliveries proceed naturally and spontaneously. Your function is to ensure that the delivery proceeds gradually and in a controlled manner, since a rapid, explosive delivery can be damaging to both mother and child. Place your left hand on the infant's head (Figure 7–1). This hand gently controls the delivery of the head. Your right hand, covered by a sterile towel, exerts forward pressure on the chin through the perineum, which will extend the infant's neck to facilitate delivery of the face and chin (Figure 7–1).

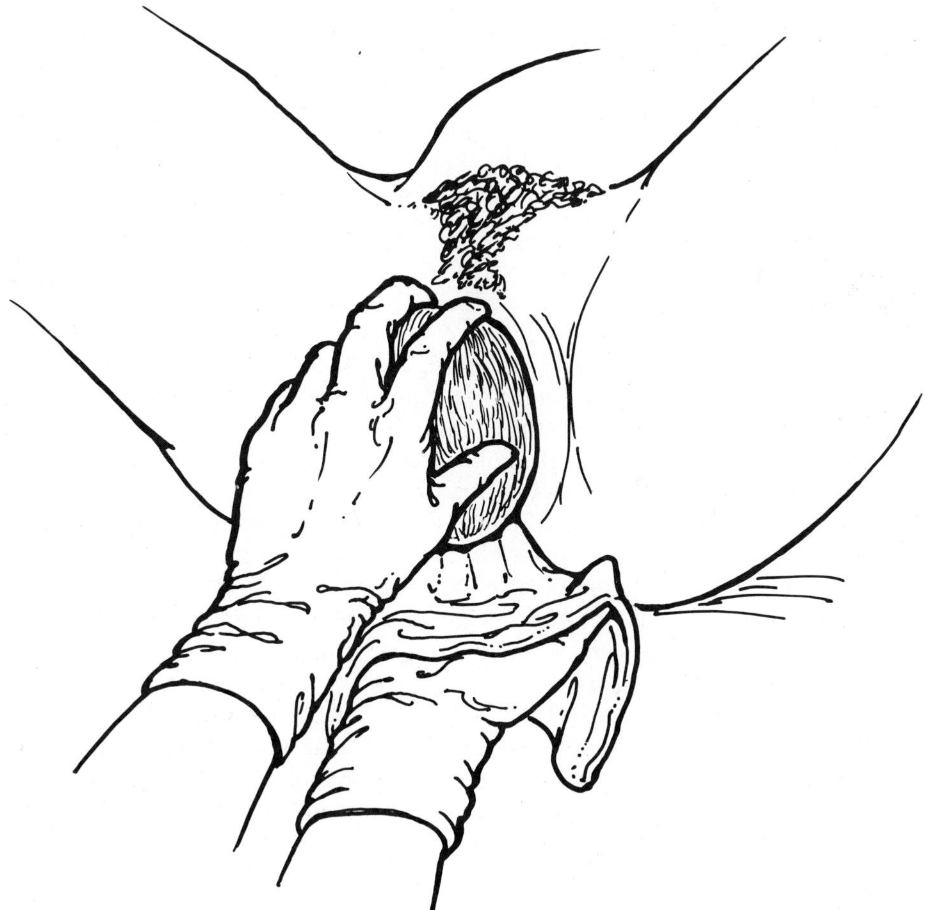

FIGURE 7–1. Delivery of the head.

10. After the head is delivered, continue to support it with your left hand (Figure 7–2), while using your right hand to feel for the umbilical cord around the infant's neck. If the cord is around the infant's neck, as occurs in approximately 20% of deliveries, carefully loosen it and pass it over the infant's head. If the cord is too tight to be freed from the infant's neck, immediately clamp it with two clamps and cut it between the clamps.
11. After the head has been delivered and the umbilical cord managed if necessary, suction the infant's mouth and nose with a bulb syringe (Figure 7–3).
12. Deliver the shoulders and then the rest of the body. Delivery of the shoulders may be facilitated by first downward traction on the head to deliver the anterior shoulder, followed by upward traction to deliver the posterior shoulder. Traction should be gentle and not rotary.
13. After the infant is completely delivered, hold the body and head down at an angle of 10 to 15 degrees to aid drainage of airway secretions and below the vagina to allow drainage of blood from the placenta into the infant.
14. Clamp the umbilical cord in two places and cut it within a minute of delivery, if it did not have to be cut when the neck was delivered.

Keep the infant warm.

---

15. Suction the infant's mouth and nose again, and determine the infant's status. Spontaneous breathing, a vigorous cry, and a pulse greater than 100 beats per minute indicate the infant is well. If these are not present, stimulate the infant with back rubbing or snapping the bottom of the infant's foot. If this fails, begin resuscitation of the infant.
16. Deliver the placenta. Signs of placental separation include a gush of blood, further extrusion of the cut umbilical cord, and an elevation of the uterus in the abdomen. Often the placenta will be completely expelled spontaneously. If not, place one hand on the abdomen above the pubic symphysis and push downward with the fingers pushing the placenta toward the vagina while the other hand is used to keep the cord taut with very gentle pressure. Do not attempt to remove the placenta by pulling on the cord.
17. Palpate and elevate the uterus after the placenta is delivered. Massage the uterus through the abdominal wall to stimulate contractions if there is persistent bleeding. Continued bleeding after massage has been tried may be treated with oxytocin, 5 to 10 IU (0.5 to 1 ml), given intravenously.

Complications

Atypical presentations
Infant distress
Persistent maternal bleeding
Incomplete delivery of the placenta

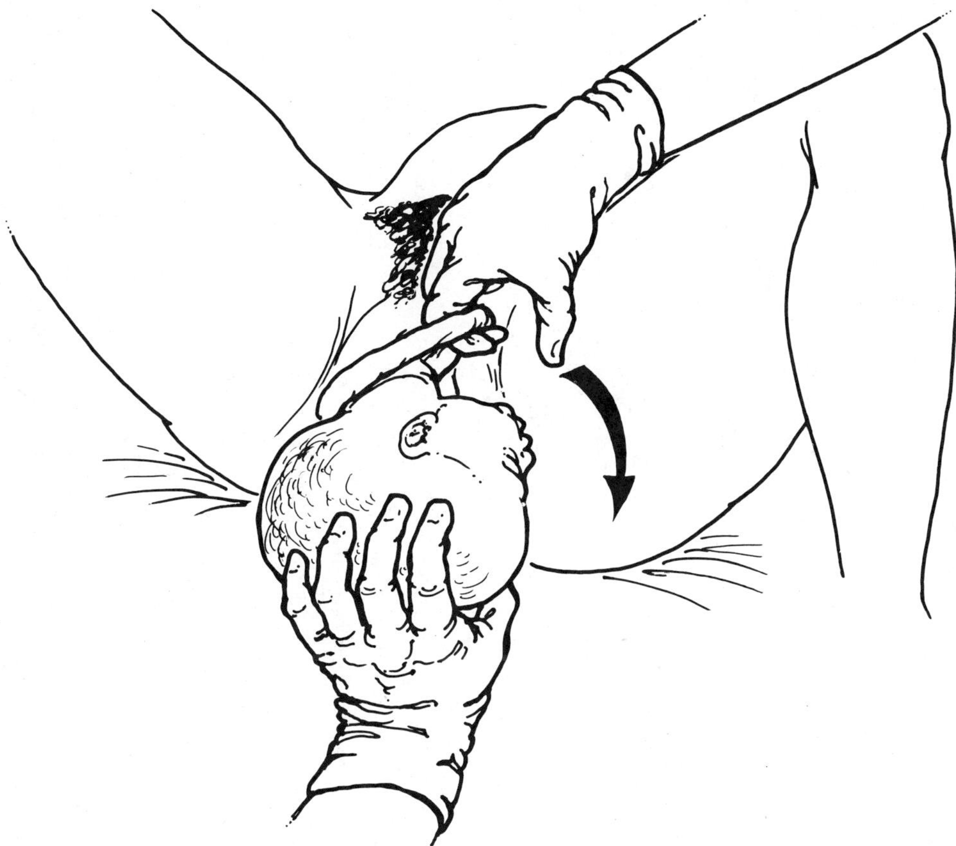

FIGURE 7–2. Management of the umbilical cord.

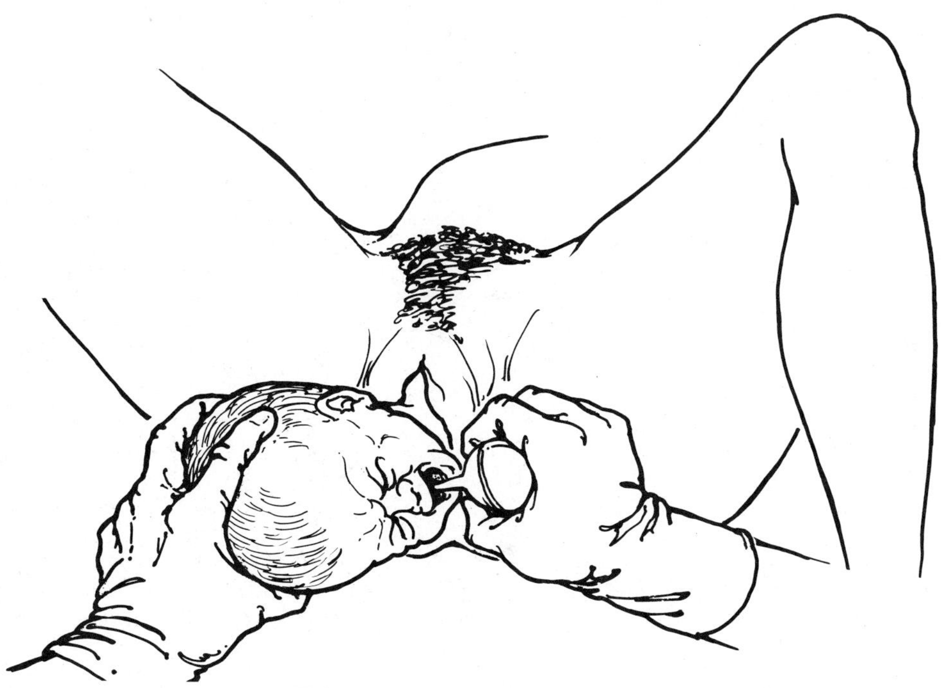

FIGURE 7–3. Clearing the airway.

Pearls and Pitfalls

1. Do not panic; almost all births proceed normally.
2. Do not let the mother use the toilet.
3. Save the placenta for subsequent examination by the obstetrician to ensure it has been completely delivered.
4. Make sure you keep the infant warm.

Reference

Doan LA: Emergency childbirth. In Roberts JR, Hedges JR (eds): Clinical Procedures in Emergency Medicine, pp 708–731. Philadelphia, WB Saunders, 1985.

8

Foreign Body Removal

Removal of Foreign Bodies from the Ear

LEO ROTELLO, MD

Indication

If it is in there, it needs to come out.

Contraindications

Avoid the use of magnets in patients who have metal tympanotomy tubes in place.

Avoid instillation of solution in the external auditory canal if perforation is suspected. If irrigation becomes necessary in a patient with suspected perforation, it should be done with a sterile solution.

Common Types of Foreign Bodies Encountered

Small batteries
Insects
Small toys
Food
Paper

Equipment

Otoscope
Headlight mirror
Straight, alligator, or mosquito forceps
Suction device or Barron suction catheter
Wire loops
Mineral oil, 2% lidocaine solution, or alcohol solution
Magnet
20-ml syringe
Flexible 18-gauge angiocath
Ear curette
Hooked probe

Universal Precautions

None

Technique

1. Explain procedure to patient and/or parents.
2. Stand on the affected side of the patient, with the patient seated in an examining chair with a headrest.
3. Perform a thorough otoscopic evaluation of both ears.
4. Visually identify the object to be removed, if possible.
5. Typically these patients are children, and reassurance and/or mild sedation is the key to successful examination and removal of the object.
6. Attempt removal first with the use of a straight mosquito or alligator forceps under direct visualization (Figure 8–1).
7. If the above attempt is unsuccessful, an attempt may be made to irrigate the object out with any form of sterile solution. To irrigate, fill a 20-ml syringe with room temperature saline or sterile water and direct a forceful stream against the wall of the canal. The stream should not be directed against the object since this may further imbed it.
8. If unsuccessful with attempt at removal by irrigation, an attempt at removal may be made with suction, using a soft pliable Frazier suction tube. Magnets may also be used to attempt to remove metallic objects.
9. For insects, instillation of mineral oil, 2% lidocaine, or alcohol solution into the external auditory canal should be first done to kill the insect. The insect can then be gently grasped with alligator forceps and removed. Often this is unsuccessful, and I have found the use of a small suction catheter with the suction setting at 120 to 180 mm Hg to be quite successful and effective in the removal of insects from the external auditory canal.
10. Another method that may be helpful is the application of cyanoacrylate adhesive (Super Glue) to a small metal or plastic stick that is then carefully attached to the object in the canal. Wait for it to set and then remove the stick with the object attached.
11. An attempt may also be made to pass an ear curette, wire loop, or hooked probe beyond the object to draw it out.
12. After removal, instill corticosporin otic suspension into the canal and have the patient continue this for several days.
13. If the above attempts are unsuccessful, consultation with an otolaryngologist should be obtained.

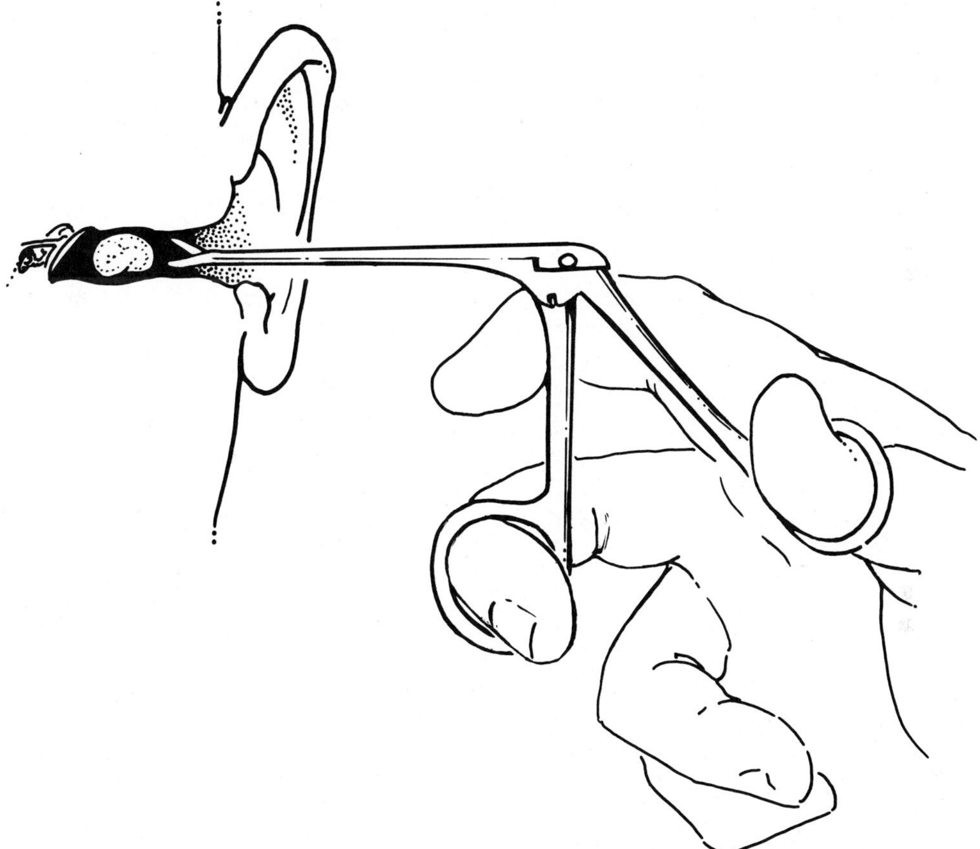

FIGURE 8–1. Removal of foreign body from the ear.

Complications

Tympanic membrane rupture
Auditory canal laceration
Subsequent infection
Bleeding

Pearls and Pitfalls

1. Reassurance and mild sedation are the best anesthetics. Anesthesia of the external auditory canal can be obtained only through local subcutaneous injection and is extremely painful for the patient.
2. The first attempt at removal is the one most often successful.
3. Smooth, round objects are best removed with a soft, pliable suction catheter.
4. Removal of metal objects should be attempted with the use of a magnetic device.
5. Avoid irrigation of objects that will absorb liquid and swell (e.g., paper, insects).
6. Do not persist with your attempts if the patient cannot cooperate. These patients may require general anesthesia to avoid trauma to the ear and to successfully accomplish the procedure.

If all of the above methods are attempted, 90% of foreign objects in the external auditory canal should be successfully removed without the necessity for consultation with an otolaryngologist.

References

Baker MD: Foreign bodies of the ears and nose in childhood. Pediatr Emerg. Care 3:67, 1987.

Brownstein DR, Hodge D: Foreign bodies of the eye, ear, and nose. Pediatr Emerg Care 4:215, 1988.

Pride H, Schwab R: A new technique for removing foreign bodies of the external auditory canal. Pediatr Emerg Care 5:135, 1989.

Votey S, Dudley JP: Emergency ear, nose, and throat procedures. Emerg Med Clin North Am 7(1):117, 1989.

Warren J, Rotello LC: Removing cockroaches from the auditory canal: A direct method. N Engl J Med 320:322, 1989.

Removal of Foreign Bodies from the Eye

LEO ROTELLO, MD

Indication

To remove any superficial ocular foreign body

Contraindication

Intraocular foreign body

Equipment

- Ophthalmoscope
- Local anesthetic (e.g., proparacaine HCl 0.5%)
- Topical antibiotic (e.g., sulfacetamide drops or ointment)
- Cycloplegic (e.g., homatropine 5%)
- Fluorescein strips
- Wood's lamp
- Cotton-tipped applicators
- 25-gauge needle or foreign body spud
- Sterile irrigation fluid
- Eye patches with tape
- Visual acuity chart
- Slit lamp

Universal Precautions

None

Technique

1. Explain the procedure to the patient in a reassuring manner and obtain consent.
2. Document visual acuity.
3. Position the patient sitting in an examination chair with headrest.
4. Stand at the side of the chair facing the patient on the side of the involved eye.

5. Instillation of topical anesthetic will facilitate examination and treatment.
6. Carefully examine the eye, including inversion of the upper lid. The ophthalmoscope makes a handy bright light source and magnifying glass. Visualize the inner aspects of the lids as well as the cornea.
   a. Lower lid: pull down lid and ask the patient to look up and visualize for complete examination.
   b. Upper lid: eversion of an upper lid is accomplished by placing a tongue blade on the upper lid and pulling the lid upward by the lashes. You can then examine the underside of the lid as the patient looks down.
7. Identify location of foreign body:
   a. Corneal—should be removed with sterile irrigation from the squeeze bottle only. Corneal foreign bodies should not be removed with a cotton-tipped applicator since extensive corneal damage may occur.
   b. Conjunctival—may be dislodged with irrigation or with the use of a moistened cotton-tipped applicator, brushing lightly to dislodge the foreign object.
   c. Imbedded foreign body—may require the use of a sharp instrument (e.g., 25-gauge needle or foreign body spud). Introduce needle or spud tangential to the globe, and ask patient to focus in the distance. Attempt to remove the foreign body with the needle or spud. This procedure is greatly facilitated with the use of a slit lamp to identify and assist in removal of the foreign object (Figure 8–2).
8. After foreign body removal:
   a. Determine if there is a corneal abrasion:
      1) Touch moistened fluorescein strip to the lower conjunctival sac and ask patient to blink.
      2) Examine cornea with a Wood's lamp. Corneal abrasion stains bright yellow.

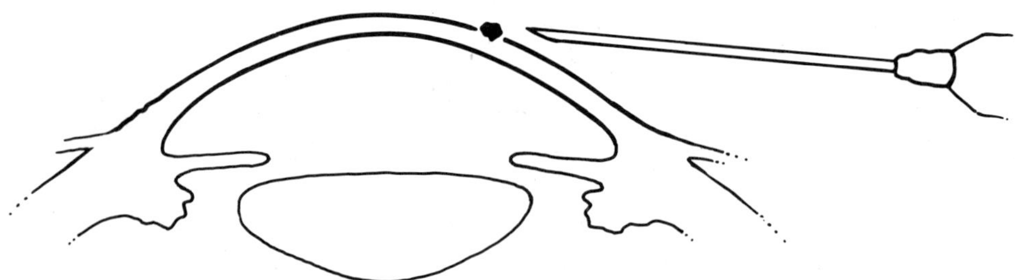

FIGURE 8–2. Removal of corneal foreign body.

   b. Apply topical antibiotic ointment and patch eye securely.
   c. Refer patient to an ophthalmologist within 24 hours for reevaluation and reexamination.
9. Difficulty in removing a foreign object requires immediate ophthalmologic consultation.
10. All patients with corneal abrasions or ocular foreign body removal should receive a tetanus toxoid immunization if required.

Complications

Infection
Globe perforation
Bleeding
Allergic reactions to anesthetics or antibiotics

Pearls and Pitfalls

1. Topical corticosteroids should not be administered for abrasions or foreign bodies.
2. Patients should never be prescribed topical anesthetics on leaving the emergency department.
3. Refer all patients with corneal abrasions or foreign body removal for follow-up ophthalmologic examination within 24 hours.
4. If topical anesthesia was used, do not discharge the patient until the anesthesia effect has worn off so it can be determined if the patient still perceives the presence of a foreign body.
5. A corneal abrasion often gives the sensation of a foreign body under the upper lid after the foreign body is gone.
6. Patients with large corneal abrasions often have considerable ciliary spasm and will have great symptomatic relief from the application of a topical cycloplegic.
7. Systemic analgesia is often necessary for the first 24 to 48 hours after a corneal abrasion.

Situations for Immediate Ophthalmologic Consultation

Penetrating ocular injury
Globe injury
Injury associated with a full-thickness laceration of the eyelid
Evidence of rust ring after the removal of a metallic foreign object
Inability to remove the foreign body

References

Brownstein DR, Hodge D: Foreign bodies of the eye, ear, and nose. Pediatr Emerg Care 4:215, 1988.
Clark RB, et al: Optimizing visual outcome in ocular emergencies: I. Nontraumatic Lesions. Pract J Primary Care Physician 7:105–112, 1986.
Clark RB, et al: Optimizing visual outcome in ocular emergencies: II. Ocular trauma. Pract J Primary Care Physician 7:113, 1986.

Fishhook Removal

MICHAEL S. JASTREMSKI, MD

Indication

People just do not take you seriously when there is a Hula Popper hanging from your nose.

Contraindications

None, since the hook has to come out. However, specialty consultation should be obtained if the hook is in a critical area such as the eye.

Universal Precautions

1. Wear gloves.
2. Take care not to hook yourself, especially if it is a lure with multiple triple hooks.

Equipment

Gloves
5-ml and 20-ml syringes
25-gauge, 1-inch needle
18-gauge, 1 1/2-inch needle
Local anesthetic
Betadine skin prep
Scalpel with No. 11 blade
Hemostat
Wire cutters
Saline for irrigation
4 × 4-inch gauze pads
Antibiotic ointment
Band-Aid

Technique

Note: There are a variety of methods for removing fishhooks, which means that the infallible method has yet to be discovered. I will present several options in the order I usually try them.

1. Explain the procedure to the patient and obtain consent.
2. Have the patient lie comfortably on a stretcher with the hooked part up and stand next to the impaled area.
3. Prep the area around the hook with Betadine.
4. Put on gloves.
5. Use the 25-gauge needle and 5-ml syringe to infiltrate the area with local anesthetic.
6. Many fishing lures have multiple triple hooks. When there are multiple hooks it is a good idea to cut the shaft of the offending hook with the wire cutters so the rest of the hooks can be removed from the work area. It is quite embarrassing if you hook the patient or yourself with a second hook while attempting to remove the first one.

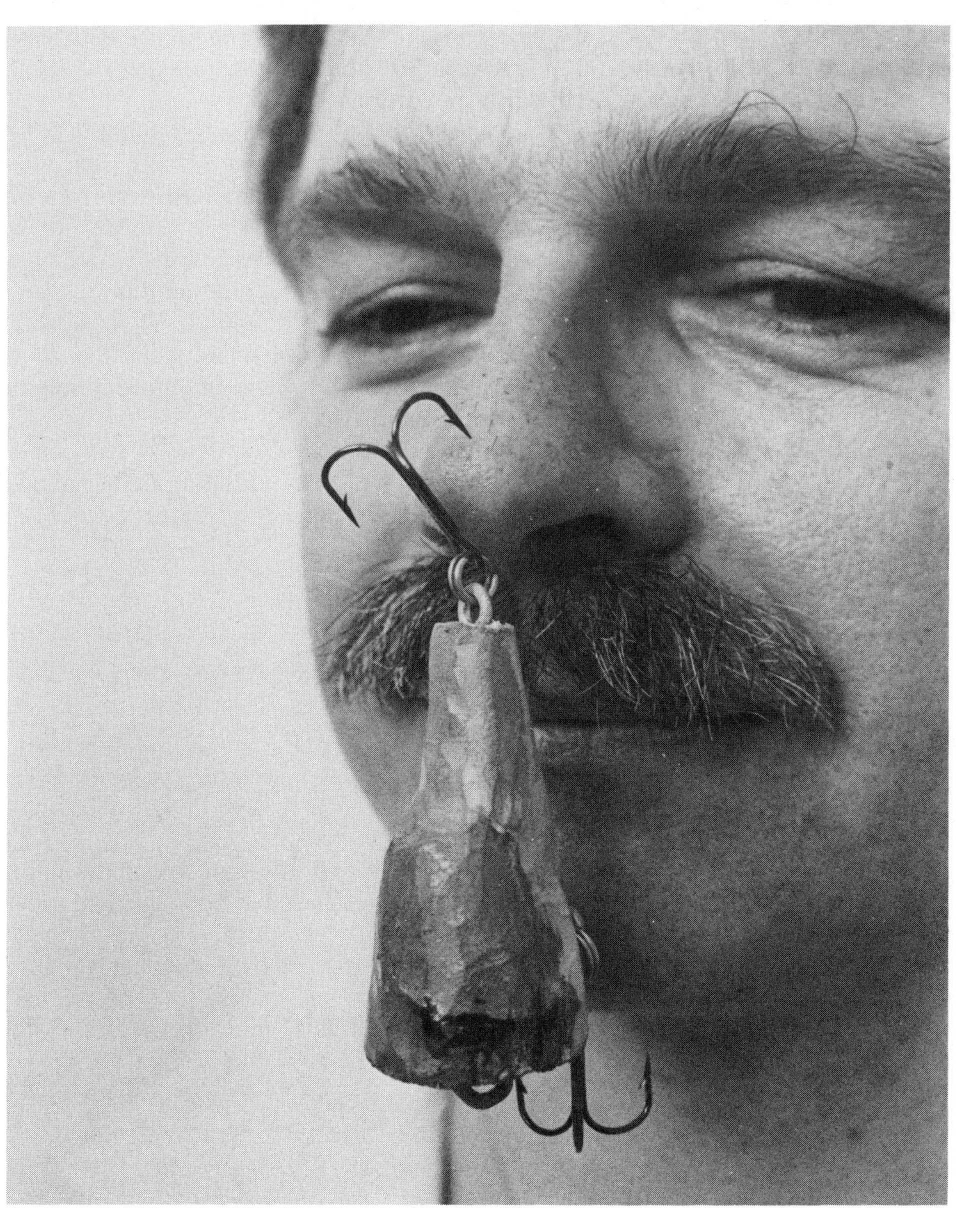

7. Option 1: The streamside technique (Figure 8–3).
   a. Use the index finger of your nondominant hand to depress the tip of the hook, thus disengaging the barb. A slight inward pressure applied to the curve of the hook may facilitate this.
   b. While keeping the tip of the hook depressed with your index finger, grasp the curve of the hook with the thumb and index finger of your dominant hand and pull it out (actually it is more like ripping). Some experts suggest that several feet of string (or fishing line) be looped around the curve of the hook, then wrapped around the dominant hand to provide greater traction.

   Note: Beware of flying hooks if you use the string technique.
8. Option 2: Push it out (Figure 8–4)
   a. Grasp the shank of the hook with the index finger and thumb of your dominant hand.
   b. Rotate the hook so the tip and barb exit the skin. This may not be possible if there is a solid structure (bone or fingernail) or a vital structure (e.g., eye) in the path the tip would follow to exit.
   c. Cut off the tip and barb with wire cutters.
   d. Pull the rest of the hook back out through the entrance wound.
9. Option 3: Cut it out
   a. Use the scalpel with a No. 11 blade to extend a small incision from the entrance wound to the barb.
   b. Grasp the tip of the hook with the hemostat and lift it out.
10. Cleanse the wound (or wounds); apply an antibiotic ointment and cover it with a Band-Aid.
11. If you used the incision technique, irrigate it with saline using the 20-ml syringe and 18-gauge needle, close it with a Steri-Strip or suture, apply an antibiotic ointment, and cover with a Band-Aid.
12. Determine if tetanus immunization is required.
13. Advise the patient of the risk of and signs of infection and instruct him or her to return if there is any suspicion of infection.

Complications

Infection
Hooking yourself

Pearls and Pitfalls

If the offending lure was the fisherman's favorite and you had to cut the hook, advise him or her that replacement hooks can be purchased at finer sporting goods stores and the lure repaired.

I personally have not had great success with option 1; I may not rip hard enough.

Option 3 allows for thorough irrigation of the tract, which should lessen the incidence of infection.

Reference

Extensive experience

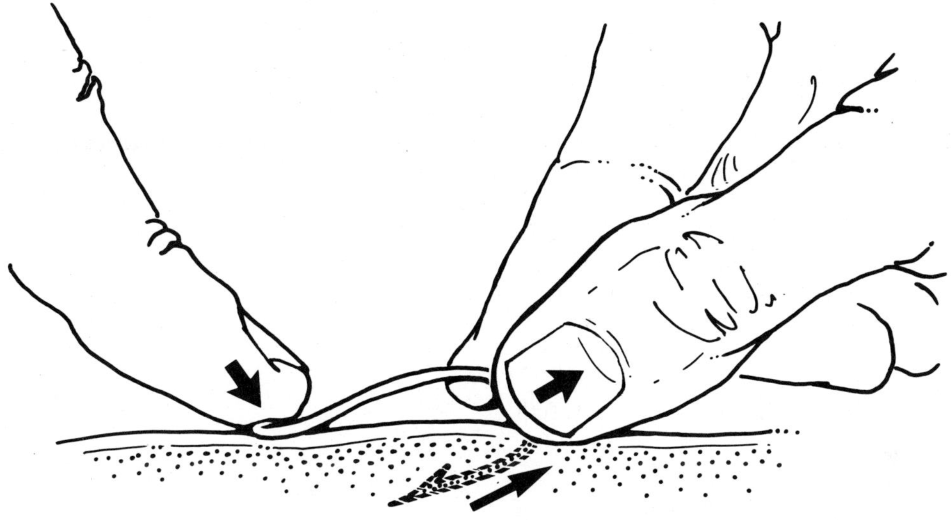

FIGURE 8–3. Fishhook removal: streamside technique.

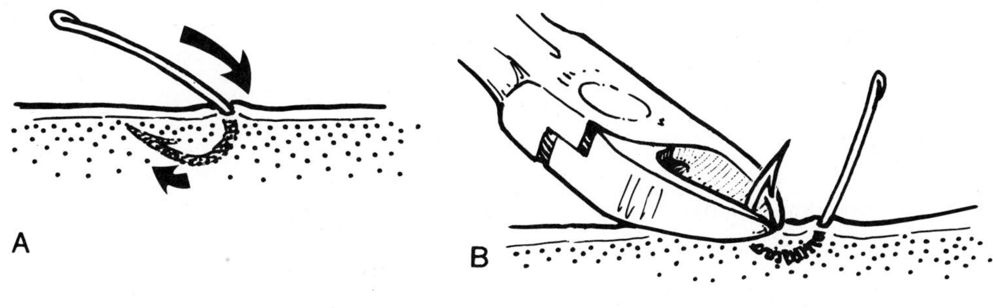

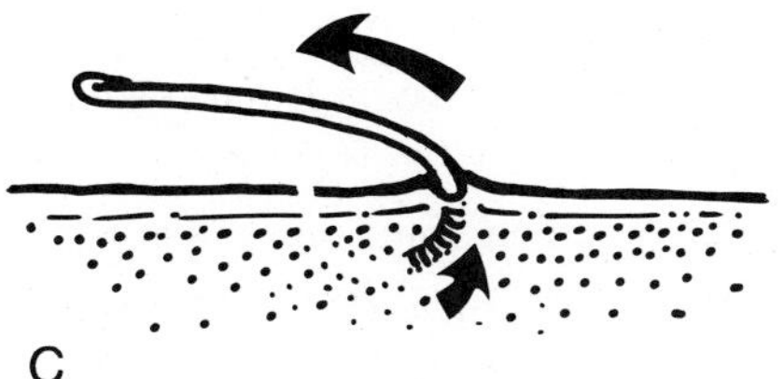

FIGURE 8–4. Fishhook removal.

Removal of Foreign Bodies from the Nose

LEO ROTELLO, MD

Indication

If it is there, it needs to come out.

Contraindications

None; however, general anesthesia may be necessary for an uncooperative child.

Common Types of Foreign Bodies Encountered

Beads
Toy parts
Paper
Food particles
Crayons

Equipment

Mask, eye shield, gloves
Nasal speculum or diagnostic otoscope
Headlight mirror
Right angle hooks
Wire loop
Alligator and bayonet forceps
Frazier pliable suction catheters and No. 5 Barron suction catheter
No. 8 F Fogarty catheter
Topical anesthetic (i.e., 4% cocaine solution or 4% topical lidocaine)
Topical vasoconstrictor (0.25% to 0.5% phenylephrine)
Nasal speculum

Universal Precautions

1. Wear gloves.
2. Wear a mask.
3. Use an eye shield.

Technique

1. Explain the procedure to the patient and parents (since the patient will probably be a child) and obtain consent.
2. Put on mask, eye shield, and gloves.
3. Position the patient sitting in examination chair with headrest.
4. Stand at the side of the chair facing the patient on the side of the nare containing the foreign body.
5. Perform a complete visual examination of the nasal passage.
6. Local mucosal anesthesia should be applied. This may be done with the use of a 4% solution of cocaine to a maximum dose of 3 mg/kg. Also topical 4% lidocaine with 1/1000 epinephrine or 0.25% to 0.5% phenylephrine solution can be used as an alternative to cocaine. The total dose of lidocaine that should be administered is also 3 mg/kg. The anesthetic can be dripped into the nose by use of a dropper, or anesthetic-soaked cotton pledgets can be placed in the nose. For complete nasal anesthesia, three pledgets must be placed: one on the floor of the nose, the second in the middle meatus, and the third in the roof of the nasal cavity. Pledgets should be left in place for 10 to 15 minutes.
7. In cooperative patients, before instrumentation, an attempt should be made to have the patient expel the foreign body by forcefully blowing the nose while occluding the opposite nare. This may be met with some success after the local vasoconstrictor is applied.

8. If the previous fails, one or more of the following instrumentation techniques should be attempted:
   a. Blunt hook, ear curette, or wire loop may be passed beyond the object and attempts made at extraction.
   b. An alligator, bayonet, or other such forceps may be used to grasp the object and remove it under direct visualization, especially irregularly shaped foreign objects.
   c. Hard, round, smooth objects may be further impacted using hooks or forceps, so sharp instrumentation should not be used with such objects. In this situation, first try suction applied to the foreign object using a soft, pliable Frazier suction catheter with the suction set at approximately 180 mm Hg.
   d. If this is unsuccessful, a No. 4 to No. 8 F Fogarty vascular catheter may be passed *above* the foreign body; the balloon is inflated once beyond the foreign body and then withdrawn until resistance is met. At this point, gentle traction should be applied until the object is removed (Figure 8–5).
9. If these attempts fail, consultation with an otolaryngologist should be obtained.

Complications

Epistaxis
Aspiration of the foreign body (potentially lethal)
Subsequent infection

Pearls and Pitfalls

1. Irrigation is inappropriate with nasal foreign bodies since the irrigant, along with the foreign body, may be aspirated into the airway.
2. A unilateral purulent nasal discharge in a child is due to a foreign body until proven otherwise.

References

Brownstein DR, Hodge D: Foreign bodies of the eye, ear, and nose. Pediatr Emerg Care 4:215, 1988.
Fox JR: Fogarty catheter removal of nasal foreign bodies. Ann Emerg Med 9:37, 1980.
Votey S, Dudley JP: Emergency ear, nose, and throat procedures. Emerg Med Clin North Am 7:117, 1989.

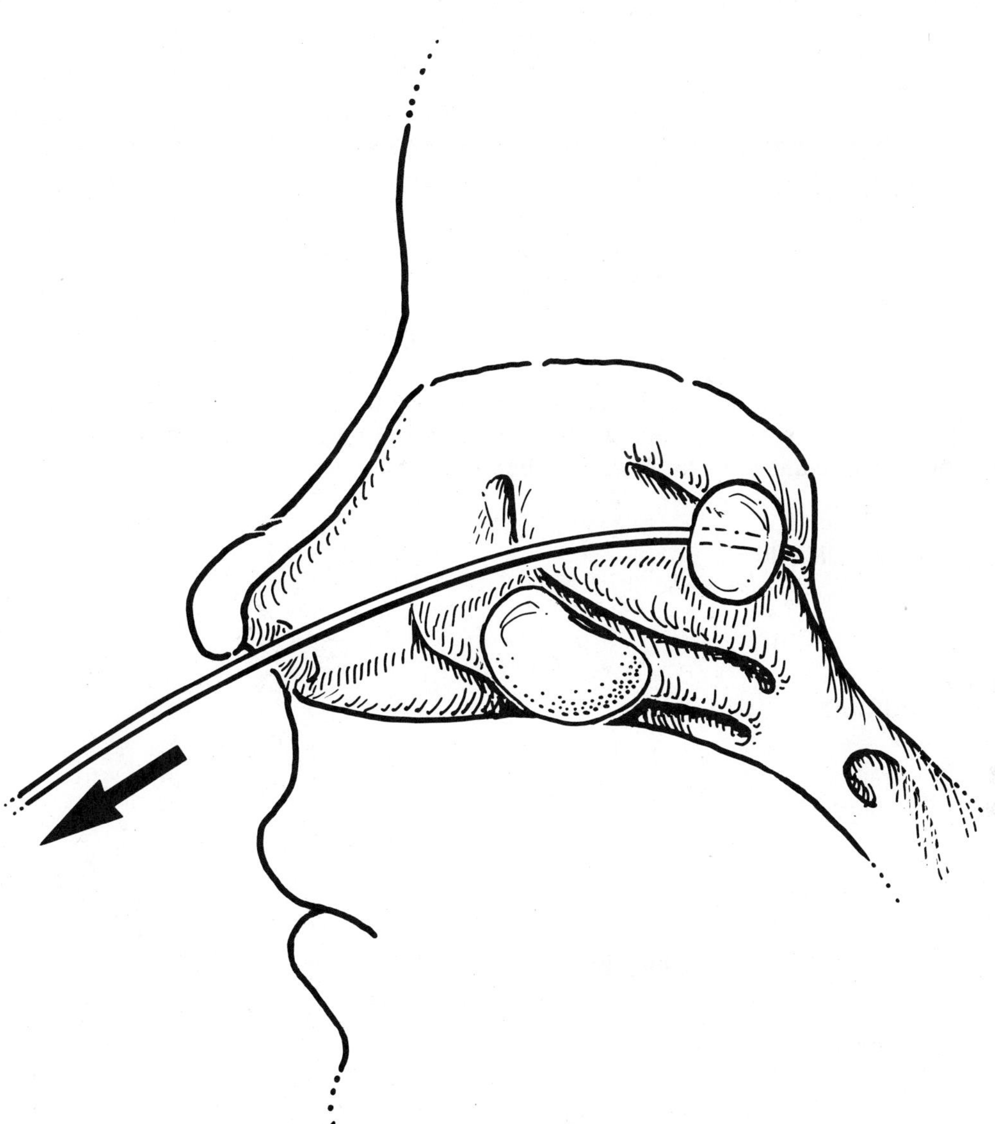

FIGURE 8–5. Removal of nasal foreign body.

Removal of Protective Headgear

MICHAEL S. JASTREMSKI, MD

Indication

When an injured patient is wearing a protective helmet (e.g., football, motorcycle), it must be removed so treatment can proceed. However, these helmets provide little protection to the cervical spine and their improper removal may worsen spinal cord damage if the neck has been fractured.

Contraindications

None

Equipment

Gloves
Bandage scissors

Universal Precautions

1. Wear gloves (there may be blood under the helmet).

Technique

1. Explain the procedure to the patient.
2. Remove glasses if the patient is wearing them.
3. Kneel (if patient is on the ground) or stand (if patient is on a stretcher) at the patient's head facing his or her feet.
4. Supply in-line stabilization by placing your hands on each side of the helmet with your fingers on the mandible. Gently pull the patient's head toward you, exerting enough force to keep the neck immobile without producing vigorous traction (Figure 8–6).
5. While you maintain in-line stabilization, have your assistant stand or kneel at the patient's side.
6. If the helmet has a chin strap, have the assistant cut it (Figure 8–7).

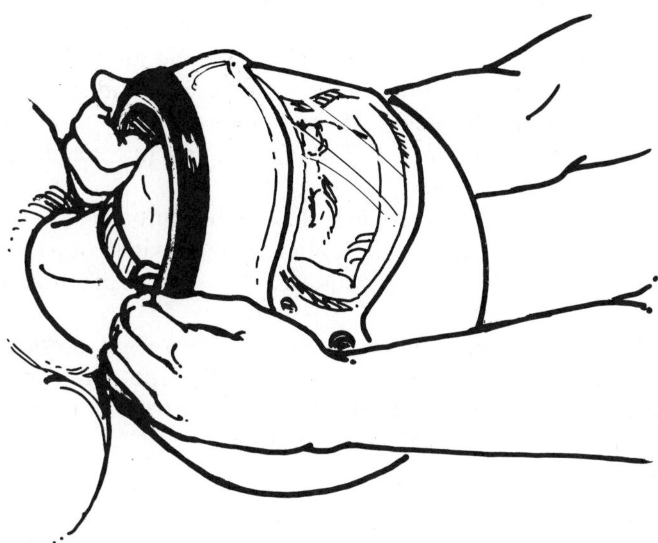

FIGURE 8–6. Helmet removal: Step 1.

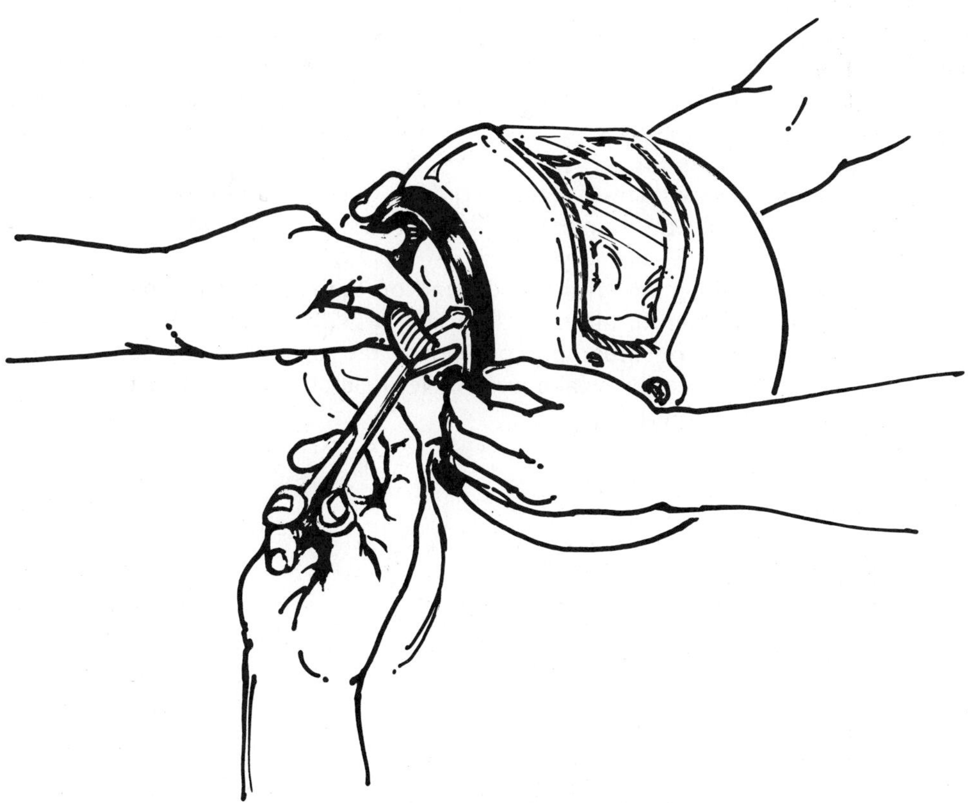

FIGURE 8–7. Helmet removal: Step 2.

7. Without removing your hands, have the assistant cup the mandible with one hand and place his or her other hand to the back of the neck. The assistant then maintains continuous cervical spine stabilization by applying caudally directed pressure, but not vigorous traction (Figure 8–8).
8. Remove your fingers from the patient's mandible and grasp the lower edge of the helmet. Pull the edges of the helmet laterally to clear the ears and then gently pull the helmet off. Full face helmets may need a little backward tilt to clear the nose (Figure 8–8).
9. When the helmet is off, resume in-line stabilization from above by placing your hands on each side of the patient's head with your fingers under the mandible. Remember, use adequate, but gentle pressure, not vigorous traction (Figure 8–9).
10. Have the assistant immobilize the spine with a rigid cervical collar, backboard or Kendrick extrication device (KED), tape, and sandbags.
11. Resuscitate the patient following the ABCs of trauma resuscitation.
12. Obtain and look at cervical spine x-ray films.

Complication

Exacerbation of cervical spine injury

Pearls and Pitfalls

When the patient is unconscious or under the influence of mind-altering drugs, awake and complaining of neck pain, or has neurologic deficits or the helmet shows evidence of trauma, you should presume the neck is fractured until proved otherwise by a complete x-ray series (lateral, anteroposterior, odontoid, obliques, and flexion extension views).

Vigorous traction may distract certain types of fractures and further injure the spinal cord. Thus, only the minimal pressure necessary to immobilize the neck should be applied.

The urgency of helmet removal will depend on the status of the patient. It is very difficult to maintain an airway or ventilation with a helmet in place, so if there are any airway or breathing problems, the helmet must be removed immediately. If the patient is awake and stable, helmet removal may be delayed until after the primary survey.

Reference

McSwain NE: To doff a helmet. Emerg Med, August: 104–105, 1982.

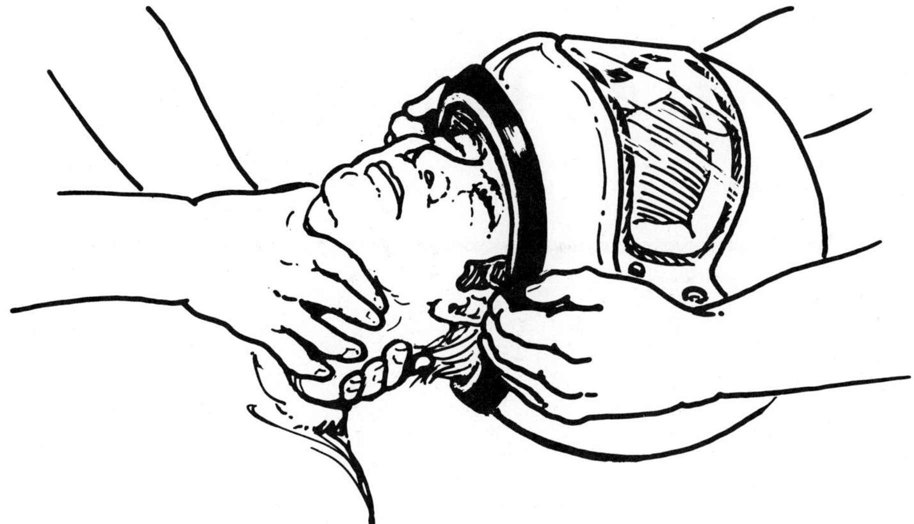

FIGURE 8–8. Helmet removal: Step 3.

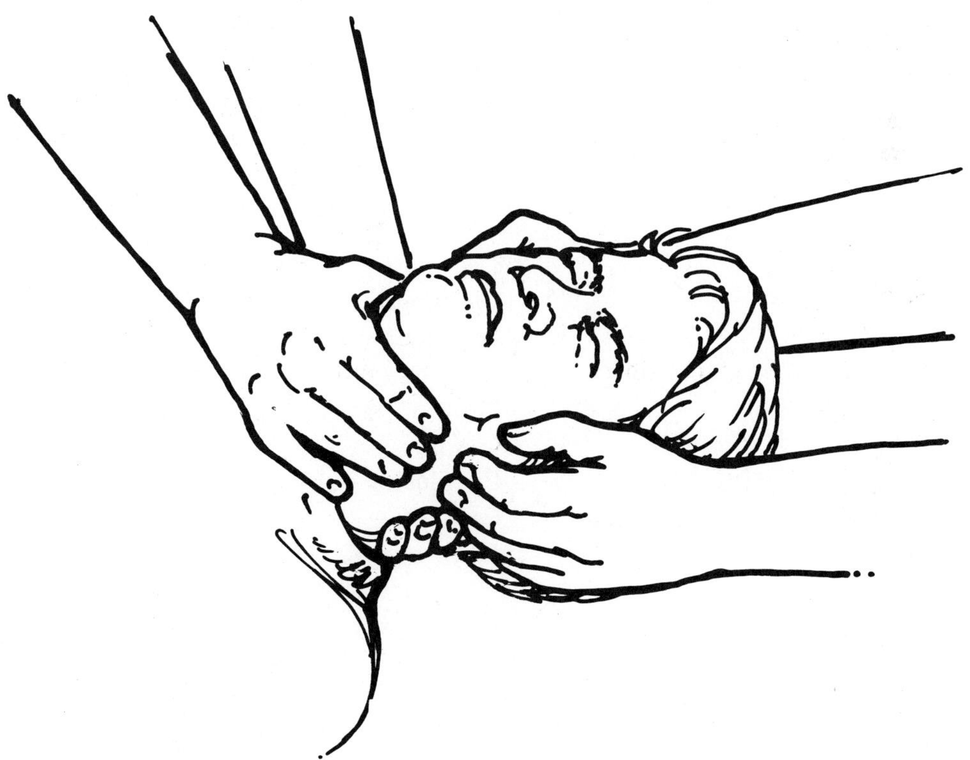

FIGURE 8–9. Helmet removal: Step 4.

Removal of Rectal Foreign Bodies

LEO ROTELLO, MD

Indications

To remove any visually identified rectal foreign body in a patient without evidence of perforation. Suspicion of perforation requires immediate surgical consultation.

Contraindications

Uncooperative patient (to emergency department removal)
Suspected perforation
High-lying foreign bodies that cannot be visualized directly
Fragile foreign body (e.g., light bulb) with a high risk of breakage and subsequent bowel damage

Equipment

Rubber gloves
Light source
Rigid anoscope and flexible sigmoidoscope
No. 24 F Foley catheter
No. 6 endotracheal tube
Lubricant
20-ml syringe
1% lidocaine solution
Assorted forceps: sponge, Kelly, straight
Mask
Gown
Eye shield
Cap

Universal Precautions

1. Wear gloves, gown, cap, and mask.
2. Use an eye shield.

Technique

1. Explain the procedure to the patient and obtain informed consent.
2. Perform a digital rectal examination.
3. Obtain biplanar abdominal films for localization and identification of the object and to look for extraluminal air.
4. Position patient in lithotomy position or, if available, on a sigmoidoscopy table.
5. Local anesthesia may be given by means of perineal injections of 1% lidocaine solution to both anesthetize and relax the anal sphincter. Mild systemic sedation may be given if the patient is significantly uncomfortable or anxious.
6. Attempt gentle manual digital removal.
7. If manual digital removal fails, lubricate anoscope and insert it after telling patient what you are about to do (Figure 8–10).

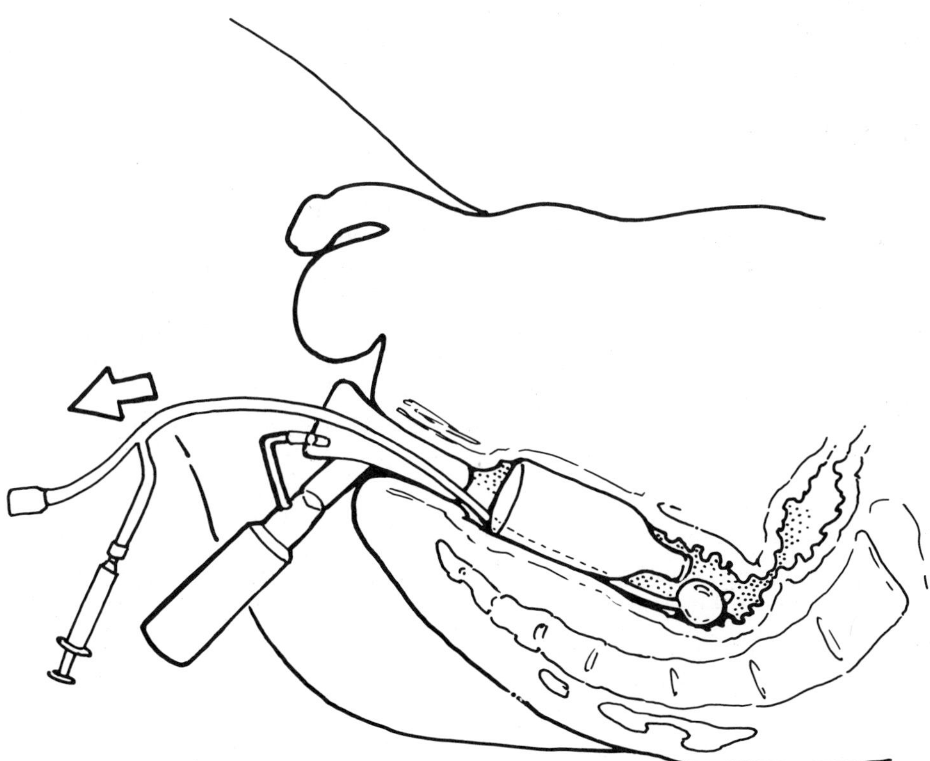

FIGURE 8–10. Removal of rectal foreign body.

a. Solid objects: If the object is easily visualized, you can also try to grasp it with a small forceps or other clamping device. If this is met with difficulty, attempt to pass a No. 24 F Foley catheter above the object, inflate the balloon, and try to draw it manually down with gentle traction.

b. Hollow objects: Hollow objects are difficult in that they may cause a suction injury to the colon. If the hollow object is inverted with the opening facing up, it may be beneficial to pass a small endotracheal tube (No. 6) or large No. 24 F Foley catheter above the object and insufflate air to break the vacuum seal and facilitate removal. Attempts should then be made to gently withdraw the object.

8. If the object is larger than the orifice of the anoscope, pull it tight against the anoscope with the Foley catheter, being careful not to trap any mucosa between the object and anoscope. Then gently withdraw the anoscope and object as a unit.
9. If these attempts fail, surgical consultation should be attained.
10. After removal of the object, perform follow-up sigmoidoscopy to look for perforation or hemorrhage.

Complication

Perforation with sepsis
Bleeding
Vagal stimulation with bradycardia and hypotension

Pearls and Pitfalls

1. Always obtain a complete history and perform a physical examination.
2. If object is above the rectum, the patient should be admitted.
3. General sedation may be very helpful in relaxing the anal sphincter.
4. If after approximately 30 minutes of attempts at removal you are unsuccessful, surgical consultation should be requested for evaluation of the situation.
5. Abdominal films should always be taken to localize as well as identify more than one foreign body in the rectum.
6. Ingenuity is the most useful tool in removal of some rectal foreign bodies.

References

Brenner BE, Simon RR: Anorectal emergencies. Ann Emerg Med 12:367–376, 1983
Garber HI, Rubin RJ, Eisenstat TE: Removal of a glass foreign body from the rectum. Dis Colon Rectum 24(4):323, 1981.
Wigle RL: Emergency department management of retained rectal foreign bodies. Am J Emerg Med 6:385–389, 1988.

Ring Removal

MICHAEL S. JASTREMSKI, MD

Indication

To remove and preserve a ring that may cause vascular compromise of a finger

Contraindications

Digit that is already ischemic
Displaced fracture or dislocation distal to the ring

Equipment

Petroleum jelly, Surgilube, or soap
Ice
Curved mosquito clamp
2-0 silk suture or umbilical tape or string

Universal Precautions

1. Wear gloves if the patient has any lacerations.

Technique

1. Explain the problem to the patient and obtain his or her agreement to proceed.
2. Elevate the hand and ice pack the involved digit for 10 to 15 minutes.
3. While keeping the hand elevated, slather up the finger with a lubricant (e.g., petroleum jelly, soap) and attempt to work the ring off.
4. If this fails, proceed to the wrapping technique:
   a. Use the mosquito clamp to slip an end of the umbilical tape or suture material under the ring (Figure 8–11, step 1).*
   b. Take the long end of the tape or suture that is distal to the ring, lubricate it with petroleum jelly, and then use it to tightly wrap the finger starting at the ring. Make sure each successive loop touches the previous one so no skin bulges out between loops. The proximal interphalangeal joint is usually the major problem area, so wrap this area tightly and carefully (Figure 8–11, step 2).
   c. Grasp the short end of the tape or suture that is on the proximal side of the ring with four fingers or the mosquito clamp. Pull this end toward the fingertip and then unwind the tape. This should progressively advance the ring off the finger (Figure 8–11, step 3).
   d. It may be necessary to repeat this process several times.
5. If the wrapping technique fails, use a ring cutter to remove the ring.

Complications

Ischemia of the digit
Unsuccessful removal

Pearls and Pitfalls

Do not save the ring and lose the finger. If the digit is truly ischemic (pale, mottled, no capillary refill), immediately cut the ring off.

This condition may be very painful so a digital block may be necessary for the patient's comfort.

If you are unsure about the perfusion status of the finger, attach a pulse oximeter to the tip. If you can obtain a pulse oximeter reading from that finger, the perfusion is still adequate.

Reference

Smith R: Emergency ring removal. In Jastremski M, Cantor R, Olson C, Smith R, Tyndall G (eds): The Whole Emergency Medicine Catalog. Philadelphia, WB Saunders, 1985.

---

* The figure is from Smith R: Emergency ring removal. In Jastremski M, Cantor R, Olson C, Smith R, Tyndall G (eds): The Whole Emergency Medicine Catalog, p 365. Philadelphia, WB Saunders, 1985.

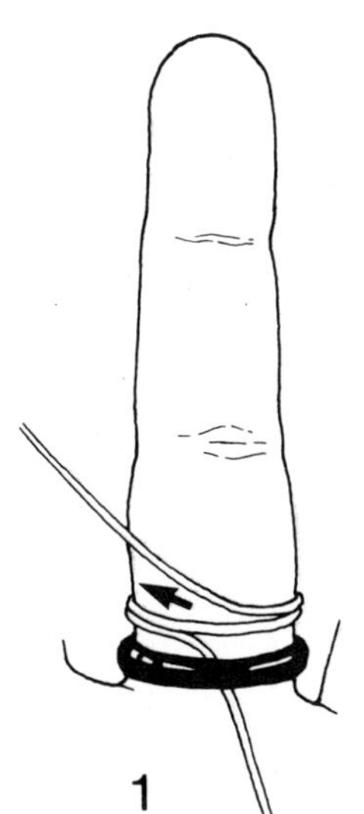

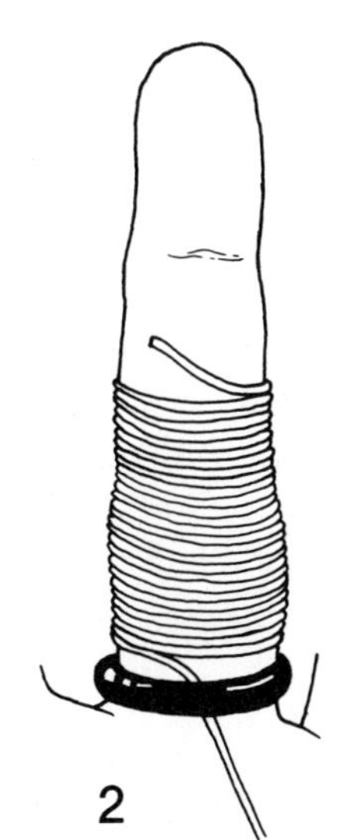

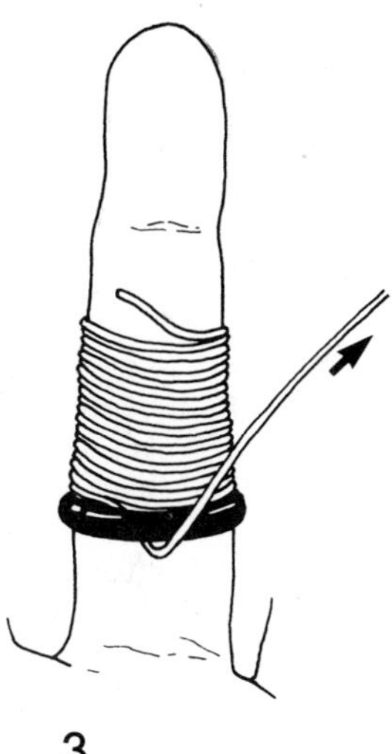

FIGURE 8–11. Ring removal.

Tooth Reimplantation

MICHAEL S. JASTREMSKI, MD

Indication

To preserve a normal tooth that has been traumatically dislodged

Contraindications

Replacement of a primary tooth may lead to facial deformity or hinder the eruption of the permanent tooth.

A badly damaged or carious tooth should be removed.

Life-threatening injuries that require immediate attention should be managed and stabilized first.

Equipment

Gloves
Face shield
Suction
Tools for dental anesthesia (see Chapter 2)
20-ml syringe
19-gauge needle
Saline solution
Coe-Pak dental splint
Tongue blade
Headlight

Technique

1. Immediately place the dislodged tooth in saline or, better yet, the tooth-preserving solution system. Do not touch the root!
2. Explain the procedure to the patient and obtain consent. Carefully and clearly emphasize that the tooth may not reattach, with the probability of successful reattachment decreasing about 1% per minute since it was dislodged. Also advise the patient that replanted teeth almost always require a root canal procedure within a few weeks.
3. Position the patient sitting in an examining chair and stand facing the patient.
4. Prepare the Coe-Pak splint material following the directions included with it.

5. Inspect the socket and gently irrigate it with saline solution using the 20-ml syringe and the 19-gauge needle to remove any clot or debris. *Do not* scrape the socket.
6. If the irrigation is too painful, administer a dental block (see Chapter 2).
7. Holding the dislodged tooth by the crown only, gently rinse it with saline or running water. *Do not* scrub or wipe it in any manner since this may remove any remaining fibers of the periodontal ligament that play a crucial role in reattachment.
8. Insert the tooth back into its socket, being very careful to maintain normal anatomic alignment. This is done by holding the crown of the tooth between the thumb and index finger of your dominant hand while grasping the alveolar ridge on each side of the socket with the thumb and index finger of your other hand (Figure 8–12).

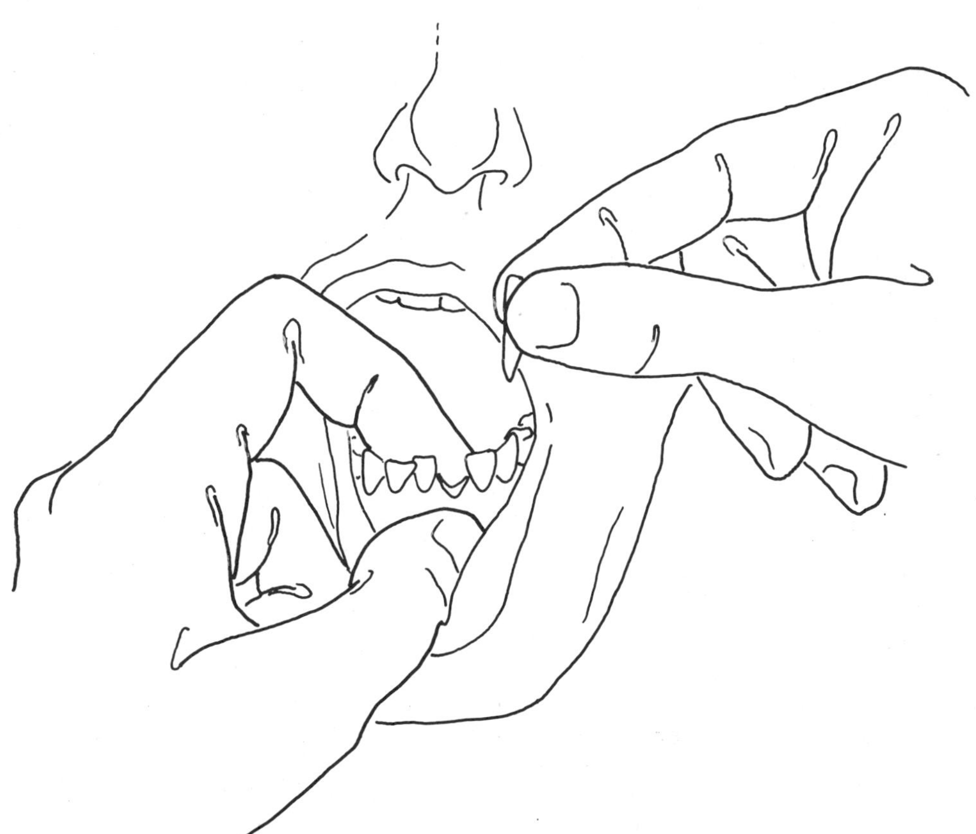

FIGURE 8–12. Tooth reimplantation.

9. If the tooth will not completely return to the socket or if the alignment is unsatisfactory, as often happens with molars (test this by having the patient gently approximate his upper and lower teeth), an immediate dental or maxillofacial surgical consultation is needed. Have the patient keep the tooth in its socket by softly biting on a piece of gauze until the consultant arrives.
10. Repair any gingival lacerations that require suturing.
11. If you achieve good alignment, the next step is to stabilize the tooth. The easiest way for the nondentist to accomplish this is with a periodontal splint fashioned from Coe-Pak. Coe-Pak is made by mixing a base and a catalyst into a material that is initially plastic and malleable but subsequently hardens to anchor the tooth. Roll the Coe-Pak into a rope and apply it for a distance of three teeth on either side of the replanted tooth on both sides of the teeth. Mold the splint over the gum line and between the teeth using your fingers or a blunt instrument (Figure 8–13).
12. Follow-up care includes
    a. Referral to a dentist within 24 to 48 hours
    b. Liquid diet
    c. Prophylactic antibiotics—penicillin VK 500 mg four times a day unless the patient is allergic to penicillin
    d. Consideration of the need for tetanus immunization

Complications

Unsuccessful replantation
Malalignment
Infection

Pearls and Pitfalls

1. Do not replant primary teeth.
2. Do not be overly optimistic about the tooth surviving, especially if more than 30 minutes has elapsed since it was dislodged.
3. The Coe-Pak splint is also very good for stabilizing teeth that are loosened but not dislodged.
4. If you are called for advice about managing a dislodged tooth before the patient comes to the hospital, prearrival instructions should be as follows:
    a. Rinse the tooth in water, but do not scrub it. Then try to put it back in its socket. If the patient can do this, then he or she should gently bite on a piece of cloth and immediately come to the hospital.
    b. If the patient or a bystander cannot get the tooth back into its socket, instruct him or her to keep the tooth moist in a cup of water or milk or by holding the tooth under the patient's tongue and bring the tooth and the patient to the hospital as quickly (but safely) as possible.

Reference

Medford HM: Temporary stabilization of avulsed or luxated teeth. Ann Emerg Med 11:490, 1982.

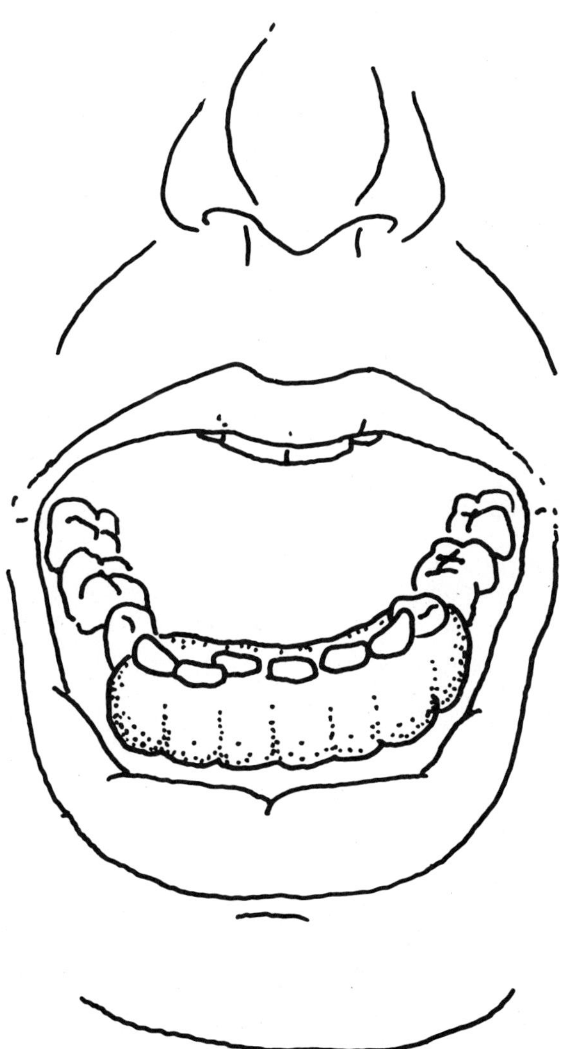

FIGURE 8–13. Dental splint.

Removal of Vaginal Foreign Bodies

LEO ROTELLO, MD

Indication

If it is there, it needs to come out.

Contraindication

Suspected perforation

Equipment

Rubber gloves
Vaginal speculum
Nasal speculum
Sponge forceps
1% lidocaine jelly

Universal Precautions

1. Wear gloves and mask.
2. Use an eye shield.
3. Wear a gown or plastic apron.
4. Use a noseplug (optional).

Technique

1. Obtain a history.
2. Explain the procedure to the patient and obtain consent.
3. Perform an abdominal examination, including a rectal examination.
4. Place the patient in the lithotomy or knee-chest position or use a gynecologic examination table.
5. Perform direct visual inspection of the vaginal vault using a lighted speculum (a nasal speculum is often effective in children). Carefully look for evidence of trauma in addition to the foreign body.

6. Grasp the object with a sponge forceps (other forms of clamps will also suffice).
7. Remove the object slowly.
8. Obtain cultures (gonococcus, *Chlamydia,* bacteria) and smears (Gram stain, potassium hydroxide, hanging drop).
9. If the procedure is painful for the patient, the vaginal vault can be anesthesized with 1% lidocaine jelly or systemic sedation and analgesia may be used.
10. If the object cannot be visualized, perform a bimanual examination to localize the object and manipulate it into view so it can then be grasped and removed with a repeat speculum examination.
11. If the object still cannot be visualized, a pelvic x-ray or ultrasound may be helpful for localization, although this is infrequently necessary.
12. Advise the patient to douche with dilute vinegar or a commercially available product when she gets home.
13. After the foreign body is removed, perform a bimanual examination looking for clinical signs of perforation or infection.

Complications

Perforation
Bleeding
Local infection, salpingitis
Systemic infection
Toxic shock syndrome

Pearls and Pitfalls

1. Rubber objects usually cause an irritant effect.
2. Cottons and wools usually cause an odorous discharge.
3. Plastics, glass, and ceramic foreign bodies are usually asymptomatic.
4. The most common vaginal foreign body is the tampon.
5. An accurate history may be difficult to obtain in a child.
6. Any patient with an unexplained vaginal discharge should be examined for the presence of a foreign body (especially children).

Indications for Admission or Urgent Gynecologic Consultation

Perforation with or without peritonitis or sepsis
Difficult-to-remove or nonvisualized foreign bodies
Intrauterine foreign bodies
Toxic shock syndrome

References

Chapman GW Jr: An unusual intravaginal foreign body. Natl Med Assoc 76:811, 1984.
Parsons L, Somers SC: Gynecology. Philadelphia: WB Saunders, 1978.

Zipper Removal

MICHAEL S. JASTREMSKI, MD

Indication

To release penile or labial skin caught in a zipper

Contraindications

None

Equipment

Gloves
Bone cutter

Universal Precautions

Wear gloves

Technique

1. Explain the procedure to the patient and obtain consent.
2. Determine the need for local or intravenous anesthesia depending on the patient's degree of pain and anxiety.
3. Put on gloves.
4. Locate (Figure 8–14) and squeeze the median bar of the zipper with the bone cutter (Figure 8–15). This will cause the zipper guides to spread open so the two sides of the zipper may be pulled apart and the entrapped skin freed.
5. Cleanse the abraded skin and apply a topical antibiotic ointment.

Complications

Bleeding (usually can be controlled with pressure)
Infection
Embarrassment

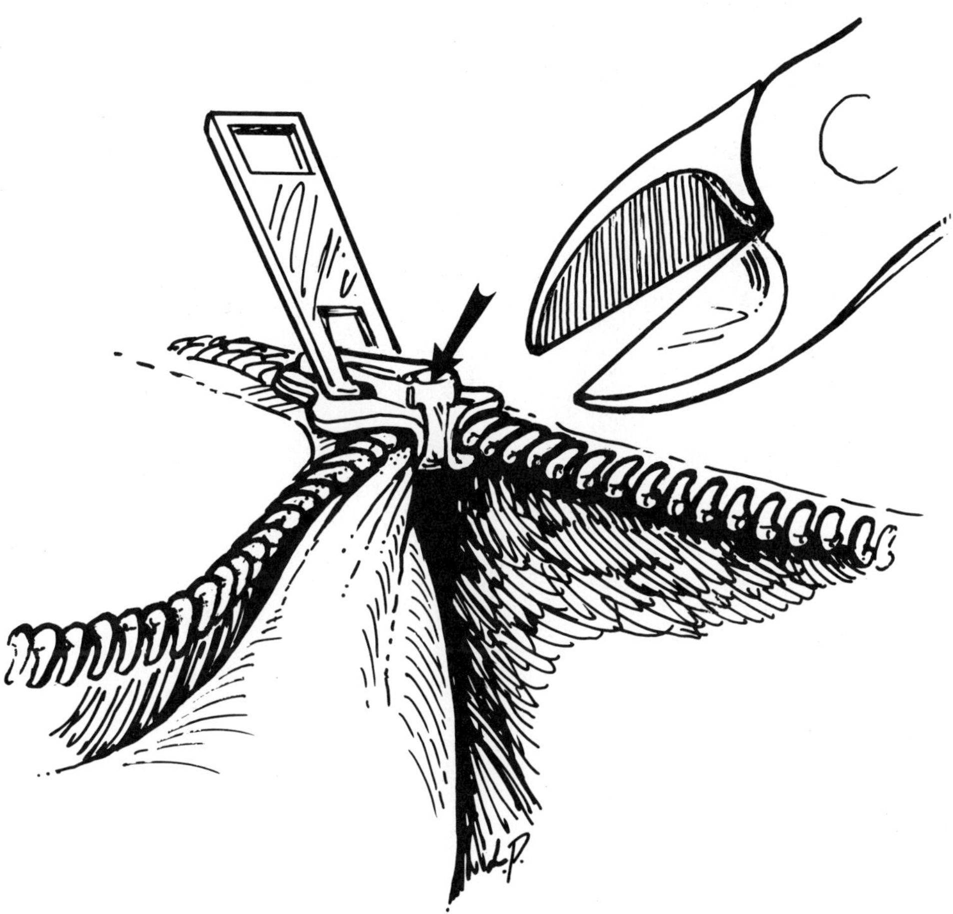

FIGURE 8–14. Location of median bar. (→)

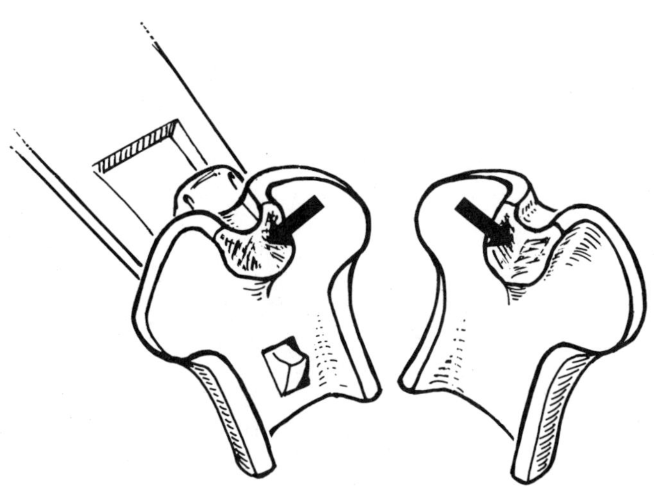

FIGURE 8–15. Cut median bar. (→)

Pearls and Pitfalls

Minor degrees of entrapment may be freed by a quick manipulation of the zipper without the need for anesthesia or tools.

Reference

Flowerdew R, Fishman IJ, Churchill BM: Management of penile zipper injury. J Urol 117:671, 1977.

Gastrointestinal 9

Anoscopy

DAVID G. HEISIG, MD

Indications

Visual examination of the anal canal and distal rectum in patients with lower gastrointestinal tract bleeding, rectal foreign bodies, or other rectal pathology

Contraindications

Granulocytopenia (strong relative)

Extremely painful local pathologic process. It may be prudent to delay this examination under these circumstances.

Equipment

Anoscope (preferably beveled) with obturator

Light source compatible with anoscope

Face shield

Nonsterile gloves

Lubricating jelly

Universal Precautions

1. Wear gloves.
2. Face shield
3. Gown (optional, but wise)

Technique

1. Explain the procedure to the patient and obtain consent.
2. Place patient in the left lateral (Sims') position with his or her knees tucked up against the chest.
3. Drape the patient to preserve modesty.
4. Perform a careful digital rectal examination.
5. Test the light source. Lubricate the anoscope.
6. Holding the obturator in place with your thumb or thenar eminence, gently advance the anoscope through the anal aperture in line with the anal canal (Figure 9–1).
7. Once the anoscope has entered the anal canal, angle it toward the sacrum to negotiate the anorectal junction and advance it to the handle.
8. Remove the obturator (standing clear of involuntarily expelled gas or liquid stool).
9. Straighten the scope and carefully examine the anorectal mucosa while you slowly withdraw the anoscope. Obtain specimens for ova and parasites, culture, Wright stain, and pathology as indicated by visual finding.
10. The beveled end usually allows optimum evaluation of a quadrant per pass, thus at times necessitating four passes to complete a full circumferential evaluation.

Complication

Trauma to the anorectal mucosa may occur rarely if excessive force is applied.

Pearls and Pitfalls

1. Lidocaine jelly may make the examination more tolerable, especially if a painful pathologic condition is present.
2. Hold the obturator firmly in place while advancing the anoscope. If it slips, remove the scope rather than attempting to reinsert it since this may cause sensitive anorectal mucosa to be pinched (thus likely ending your chance of completing the examination).
3. If a painful pathologic condition will allow only one pass, line the beveled tip up with the quadrant your digital examination identified as most problematic.
4. If the anoscopy is being performed for possible *Neisseria,* use water as the lubricant. Lubricating gels may prevent the *Neisseria* from growing in culture.

Reference

Extensive experience

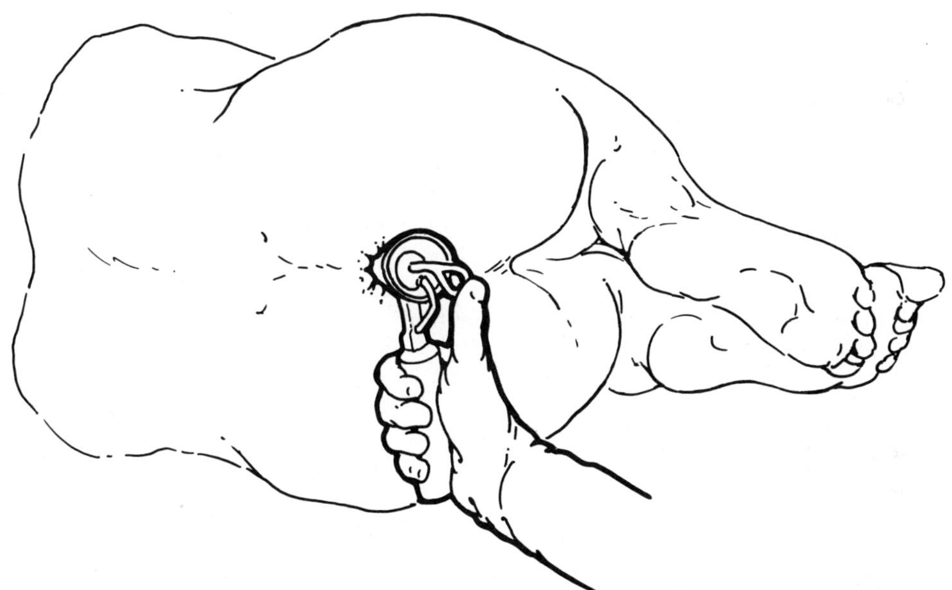

FIGURE 9–1. Anoscopy.

Balloon Tamponade of Bleeding Gastroesophageal Varices

DAVID G. HEISIG, MD

Indications

Acutely bleeding gastroesophageal varices

Although endoscopic sclerotherapy is often used first, balloon tamponade is still useful when endoscopic sclerotherapy fails or is unavailable. Parenteral administration of vasopressin and transcutaneous or parenteral administration of nitroglycerin should be used in conjunction with balloon tamponade in the presence of an acute hemorrhage.

Contraindications

There are no true contraindications to this procedure in a patient with a life-threatening gastroesophageal hemorrhage, but if endoscopic sclerotherapy is readily available it should be attempted first. Sclerotherapy may be more acutely definitive and is often better tolerated.

Equipment

Sengstaken-Blakemore tube or a Linton-Nachlas tube (or another similar brand of tube) with the manufacturer's instructions (Figure 9–2)
Stethoscope
Large-volume syringe (50 or 60 ml) with a tip compatible with the tube balloon ports
Lubricating jelly
Traction frame bed
Suction apparatus
Nasogastric tube (12 F, 14 F)
Scissors
Mask

Eye shield
Gown or plastic apron
Gloves

Universal Precautions

1. Wear mask, gown or plastic apron, and gloves.
2. Use an eye shield.

Technique

1. Explain procedure to the patient and obtain consent if circumstances permit (many of these patients will be *in extremis).*
2. Remove the tube from the package and test its balloons for air leaks. Read the manufacturer's recommendations!
3. Lavage the patient as best possible and suction the orohypopharynx thoroughly.
4. Lubricate the tube generously and pass it through either the nose or the mouth into the esophagus.
5. Advance the tip of the tube into the stomach. (*Note:* The gastroesophageal junction lies approximately 40 cm below the incisors of the average adult.)
6. Inflate the gastric balloon about 50 ml (using air).
7. Inject air through the port leading to the gastric cavity and listen for it with the stethoscope over the left upper quadrant and epigastrium. An x-ray film may also be used to ensure the location of the gastric balloon within the stomach.

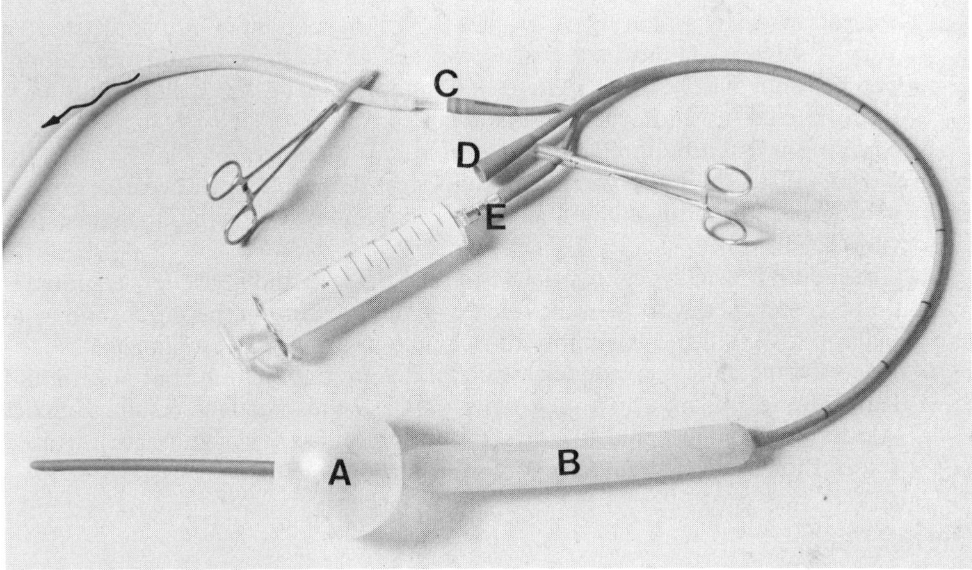

FIGURE 9–2. Sengstaken-Blakemore tube. *A,* gastric balloon; *B,* esophageal balloon; *C,* port to esophageal balloon; *D,* port to gastric tube; *E,* port to gastric balloon. Arrow points to pressure manometer.

8. Inflate the gastric balloon slowly to its maximum capacity, which is specified by the manufacturer (often 250 to 275 ml).
9. Apply moderate traction (3–5 lb) on the tube, which can be maintained using the traction frame. The patient's head should be held steady with the applied traction.
10. Inflate the esophageal portion of the tube if bleeding has not been controlled thus far.
11. If the particular tube you have chosen does not have an intraesophageal port allowing suctioning of the portion of the esophagus above the balloon, then pass a small nasogastric tube into the midesophagus.
12. Attach the ports draining the gastric cavity and the portion of the esophagus above the balloon to intermittent suction.
13. Obtain and look at chest and abdominal x-ray films to confirm correct placement (Figure 9–3).

Note: The Linton-Nachlas tube has a larger gastric balloon and no esophageal balloon, so minor adjustments in the above technique are necessary. Use the manufacturer's recommendation regarding the amount of air to be used in the balloon.

Complications

Aspiration
Migration of the balloon/tube into the hypopharynx with asphyxiation
Esophageal perforation

Pearls and Pitfalls

1. It is probably wise to insert an endotracheal tube in all patients before placing a Sengstaken-Blakemore (or similar) tube to minimize the chance of aspiration or hypopharyngeal occlusion. If the patient is not intubated, a pair of scissors should be taped to the bed so the balloon inflation tubing can be immediately cut to deflate the balloons should the balloon pull back into the pharynx and occlude the airway.
2. Sedation is often required to increase patient tolerance.
3. Never inflate the balloons quickly and stop if the patient develops sudden chest pain during insufflation since this may indicate impending esophageal rupture.
4. The mouth is usually less restrictive to tube passage and hence less traumatic.
5. Some clinicians advise periodic release of the pressure in the intraesophageal balloon to lessen the possibility of ischemic injury to the esophagus.
6. Once the bleeding has stopped, you can deflate the balloons but you should leave the tube in place for 24 hours in case the bleeding resumes. Strict attention should be paid to correcting any coexistent coagulopathy. Rapid referral for more definitive treatment is appropriate.

References

Bayless TM: Current Therapy in Gastroenterology and Liver Disease 1984–1985. Toronto, BC Decker, 1984.

Sleisenger MH, Fordtran JS: Gastrointestinal Disease: Pathophysiology, Diagnosis, and Management, 4th ed. Philadelphia, WB Saunders, 1989.

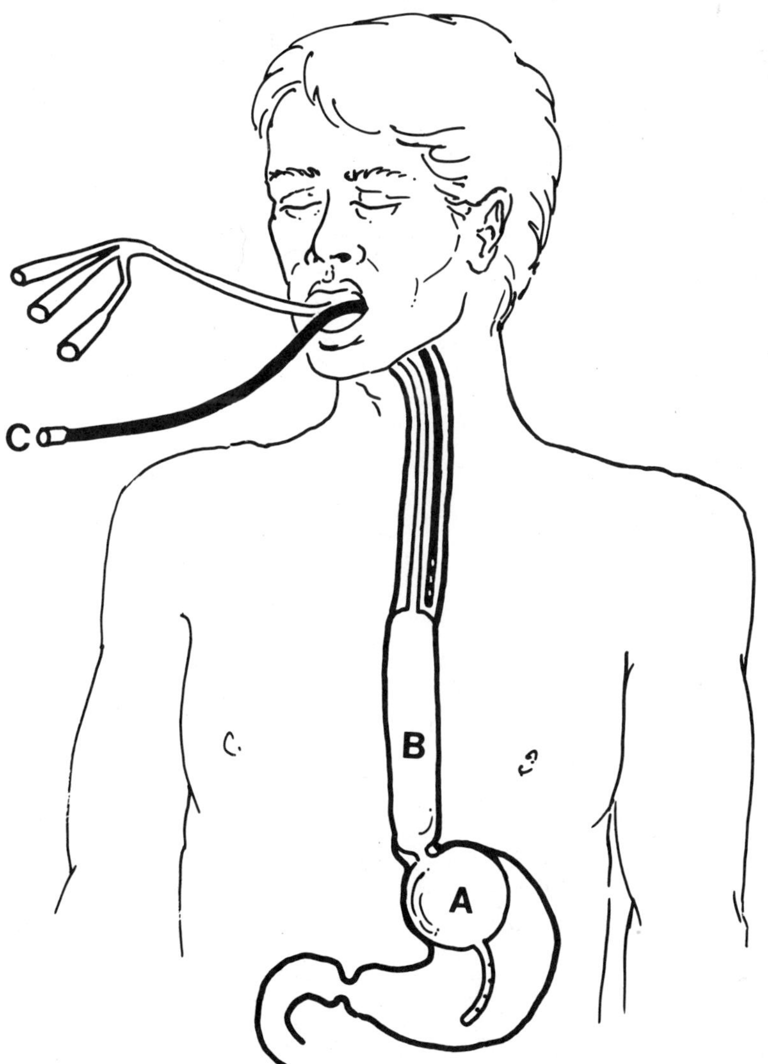

FIGURE 9–3. *A,* gastric balloon; *B,* esophageal balloon; *C,* esophageal tube.

Gastric Lavage

CONNIE WALLECK, RN

Indications

Upper gastrointestinal tract bleeding
Ingestion of poisons or toxins
Life-threatening overdose of drugs
Control of temperature extremes

Contraindications

Suspected rupture of esophagus
Ingestion of caustic substances
Ingestion of petroleum distillates (relative)

Equipment

Large-bore (32 F) Ewald tube or 18 F Salem sump tube
Large 2- to 3-L inflow bottle (bag)
Large-bore inflow and outflow tubing
Y connector
Outflow bottle
50-ml Toomey syringe
Lubricant
Hemostats (for clamping tubing)
Gown
Gloves
4 × 4-inch gauze pads
Face shield

Universal Precautions

1. Wear gloves.
2. Wear gown or plastic apron.
3. Use a face shield.

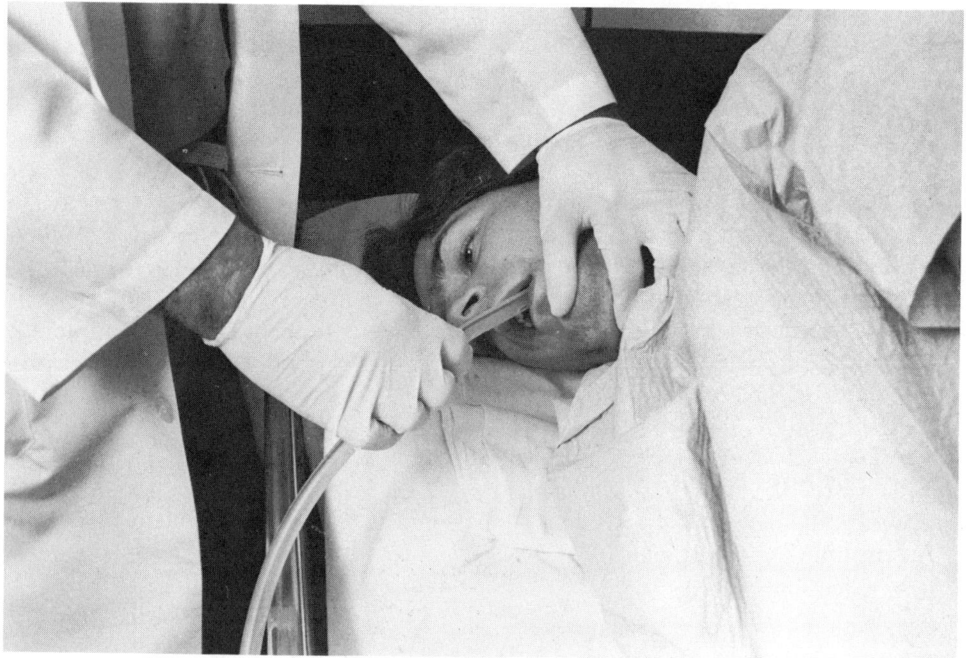

FIGURE 9–4. Ewald tube insertion.

Technique

1. Explain the procedure to the patient and obtain consent if circumstances permit.
2. Lubricate the Ewald tube.
3. Put on gloves and gown.
4. Ensure that the patient is conscious with an intact gag reflex. If this is not the case, the trachea must be intubated with a cuffed endotracheal tube (see Chapter 3) before beginning gastric lavage.
5. Position the patient lying on the stretcher with the patient's left side up and the feet higher than the head (so the mouth is lower than the larynx to lessen the possibility of aspiration) (Figure 9–4).
6. Flex the patient's head.
7. Stand at the patient's anterior side facing the patient.
8. Insert the Ewald tube through the mouth and advance it into the stomach using gentle pressure. This may be facilitated by grasping the tongue with a 4 × 4-inch gauze pad and pulling it out of the way. (If you choose to use a Salem sump tube see page 164 for the technique of nasogastric tube insertion) (see Figure 9–4).
9. Confirm correct tube placement by return of gastric contents and/or auscultation of injected air over the stomach.
10. Send a sample of gastric contents to the toxicology laboratory in cases of ingestion.
11. Drain all gastric contents.

12. Hook up the lavage system (Figure 9–5).
13. Fill inflow bottle (bag) with iced normal saline or regular normal saline with inflow tubing clamped.
14. Clamp outflow tubing, open inflow tubing, and infuse 250 ml of solution initially. The volume of each infusion may be increased to 500 ml as tolerated by the patient.
15. Clamp the inflow tubing and open the outflow tubing allowing the lavage solution to drain by gravity to a container on the floor or a low stool. When most of the lavage fluid has returned, repeat the process.
16. Infuse and drain solution until return fluid is clear.
17. In overdose cases, administer the following after lavage is completed: activated charcoal, 50 to 100 g, and a cathartic such as magnesium citrate or sorbitol.

Complications

Aspiration
Electrolyte imbalances
Perforation of the esophagus or stomach
Trauma to gastric mucosa
Reflux esophagitis
Cardiac dysrhythmias
Hypothermia (if iced saline used in large amounts)
Acidosis

Pearls and Pitfalls

1. Suction oral cavity frequently during procedure to prevent possible aspiration.
2. Assess for tube patency.
3. Assess for tube placement before beginning the lavage since it may have coiled in the oral pharynx or esophagus or may have entered the lungs. If there is any question about tube placement obtain an x-ray film before starting the lavage. Lung lavage can be fatal.
4. Maintain airway.
5. Keep accurate inflow and outflow record to prevent distention.
6. Drainage may be facilitated by rolling the patient from side to side.
7. Restrain patient as needed to prevent removal of tube.
8. If a Salem sump is used, draining will need to be done by aspirating with a Toomey syringe. Syringe aspiration should be avoided if at all possible when an Ewald tube is used since this may cause severe suction damage to the gastric mucosa.
9. When using gastric lavage to treat hypothermia, warm the lavage fluids with a blood warmer or in a microwave oven.

Reference

Extensive experience

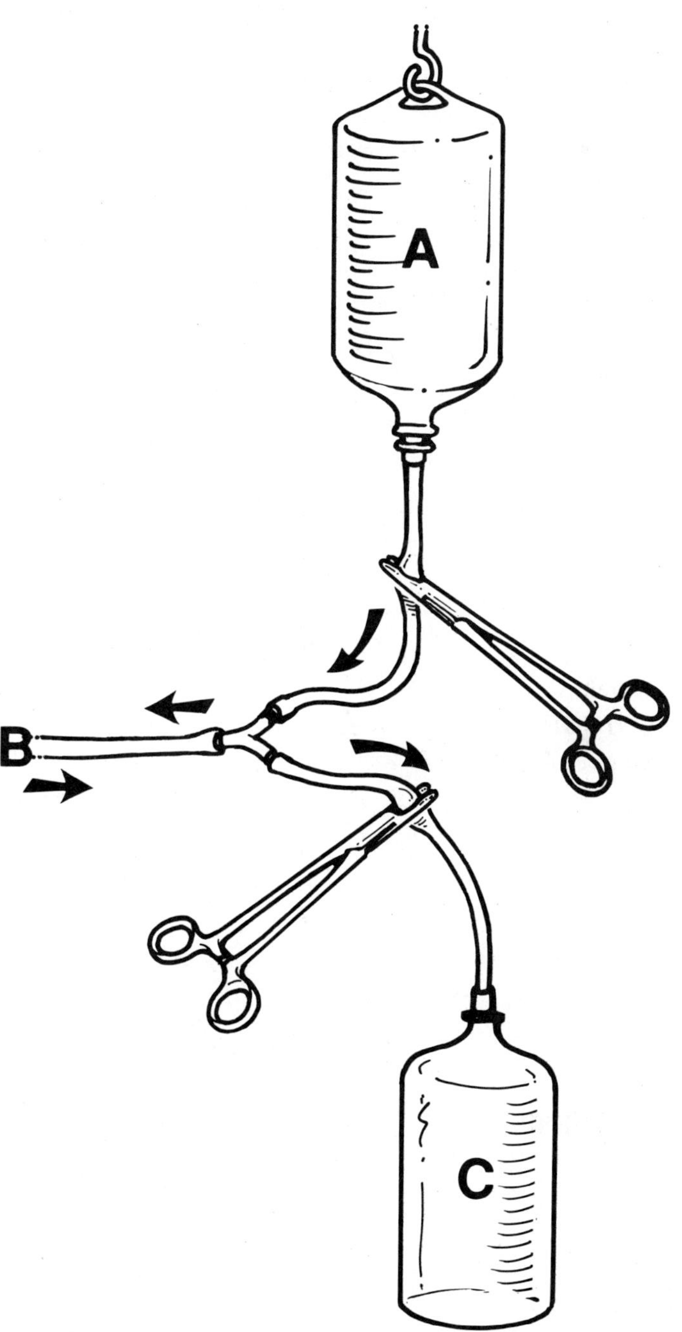

FIGURE 9–5. *A,* Inflow bottle; *B,* lavage tube; *C,* outflow collection bottle.

Nasogastric Tube Insertion

MARCY LAYTON, MD

Indications

Relief of ileus
Gastric lavage—gastrointestinal bleeding, overdosed patients
Medicating comatose and/or intubated patients
Enteral feeding

Contraindications

Recent esophageal surgery
Coagulopathy (relative)
Recent nasal surgery or trauma

Equipment

Nasogastric tube, Nos. 14 to 18 F
Petrolatum or lidocaine jelly
Gloves
Toomey syringe
Tape
Glass of water
Mask and eye shield

Universal Precautions

1. Wear mask and gloves.
2. Use an eye shield.

Technique

1. If the patient's condition allows, explain the procedure to the patient and obtain consent.
2. Ideal positioning is with patient sitting at 90 degrees with neck flexed forward (to compress the trachea).
3. Determine which nasal passage is widest.
4. Put on gloves, mask, and eye shield.

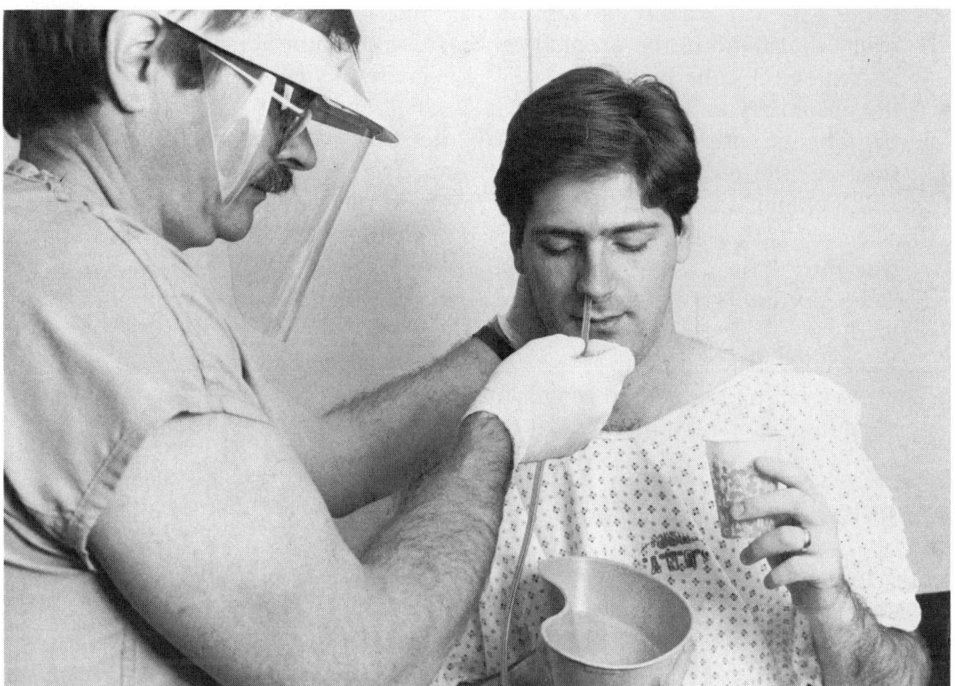

FIGURE 9–6. Nasogastric tube insertion.

5. Apply lubricant to the distal end of the nasogastric tube.
6. Insert nasogastric tube into nares just to nasopharynx (Figure 9–6).
7. If patient is able to cooperate, have him or her swallow sips of water as nasogastric tube is advanced into the stomach.
8. To ascertain if position is correct, aspirate stomach contents with Toomey syringe and auscultate over stomach as air is injected through the syringe.
9. Tape tube in position, out of reach of patient.

Complications

Local trauma due to tube irritation

Endobronchial placement (if unsure of position, check with an x-ray film)

Continual twisting of tube in nasopharynx

Sinusitis

Otitis media

Epistaxis

Perforation of cribriform plate, nasopharynx, or esophagus

Pearls and Pitfalls

1. If the patient is uncooperative, mild sedation and restraint may be needed.
2. If the patient has a pronounced gag reflex, anesthetize the nasopharynx with a short-acting anesthetic spray (e.g., Cetacaine) or use lidocaine jelly as the lubricant.

3. If the patient is edentulous, insertion of the tube can be facilitated by using your other hand in the oropharynx to guide the tube down the esophagus.
4. Stiffening the tube by placing it in an icebath may ease insertion if it coils in the nasopharynx.
5. In patients with head and/or facial injuries who may have a basilar skull fracture, the orogastric route is recommended to lessen the risk of sinusitis and meningitis and to avoid insertion of the tube into the brain.
6. The orogastric route may also be used in a patient with a severe coagulopathy who must have a gastric tube.
7. Tube position should be confirmed by x-ray film before beginning enteral feedings.
8. Very difficult intubations may be facilitated by placement under direct vision using a laryngoscope and Magill forceps.
9. As a last resort, endoscopy can be used.

Reference

Broughton WA, Green AE, Hall MW, Bass JB: The technique of placing a nasoenteric tube. J Crit Illness 5:1101, 1990.

Paracentesis

GARY A. JOHNSON, MD

Indications

Diagnostic

Suspected infectious peritonitis (especially spontaneous bacterial peritonitis or tuberculous peritonitis)
Ascites of uncertain origin (e.g., malignant, chylous, or pancreatic)

Therapeutic

Respiratory distress secondary to ascites

Contraindications

Large or small bowel obstruction (relative)
Multiple, previous abdominal procedures (relative)
Coagulopathy (relative)
Pregnancy (relative; if necessary, use supraumbilical site)

Equipment

Note: It is convenient to use a prepared kit that contains all the necessary items.

18- or 16-gauge needle with wire and catheter (for Seldinger technique) or 16-gauge needle with catheter that passes through needle
5-ml syringe
25-gauge, 1-inch needle
Antiseptic solution (e.g., Betadine)
Local anesthetic
Sterile 4 × 4-inch gauze pads
Sterile drapes
Intravenous tubing
Collection bag or bottle
Stopcock

Universal Precautions

1. Wear gown, mask, and sterile gloves.
2. Use an eye shield.

Technique

1. If ileus or obstruction is clinically possible, get a flat and upright abdominal x-ray film before proceeding.
2. Explain the procedure to the patient and obtain consent.
3. Have the patient void or insert a Foley catheter to decompress the bladder.
4. Position the patient supine on a stretcher and stand at the side you will puncture (either side is acceptable if using the infraumbilical approach).
5. Select the puncture site (midline infraumbilical or either lower quadrant just lateral to the anterior rectus muscle). In general, avoid previous surgical sites and do not go lateral enough to hit retroperitoneal structures (e.g., ascending or descending colon). The midline infraumbilical approach is preferable because of the relative absence of vascular structures in the anterior abdominal wall (Figure 9–7).
6. Put on mask, eye shield, gown, and sterile gloves.
7. Prep the area with Betadine and drape with sterile towels.
8. Infiltrate the skin and subcutaneous tissues with 1% lidocaine using the 5-ml syringe and 25-gauge, 1-inch needle.
9. Place an 18- or 16-gauge needle through the skin 2 or 3 cm lateral to the planned puncture site of the anterior fascia. With the needle in the subcutaneous tissue, move the needle and syringe as a unit over to the site of fascial puncture (Figure 9–8). (This provides a "Z" pathway for the needle and will make leakage of peritoneal fluid unlikely after the needle and catheter are removed [Figure 9–9]).

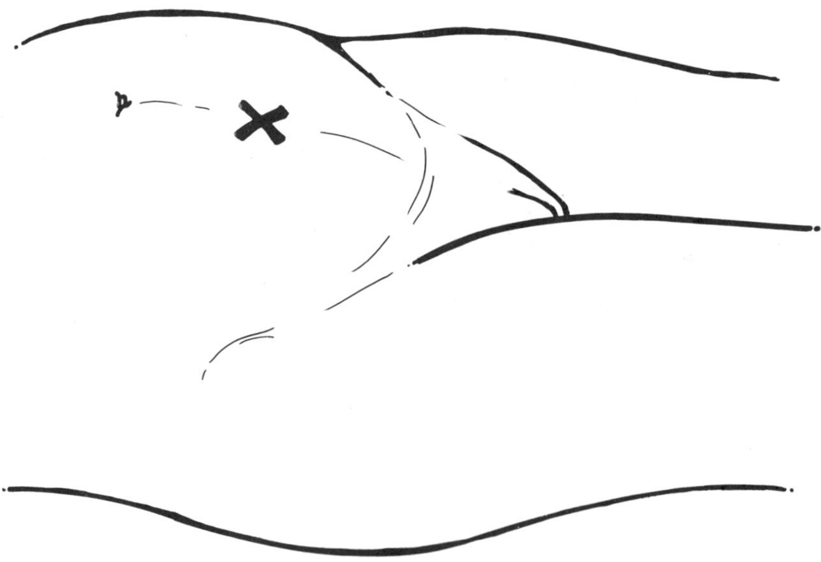

FIGURE 9–7. Site for paracentesis.

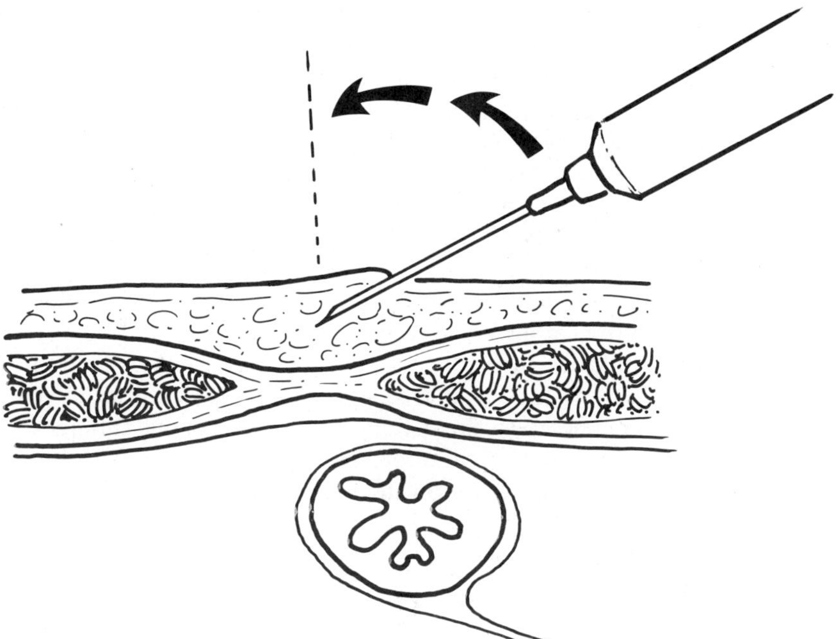

FIGURE 9–8. Needle path for paracentesis.

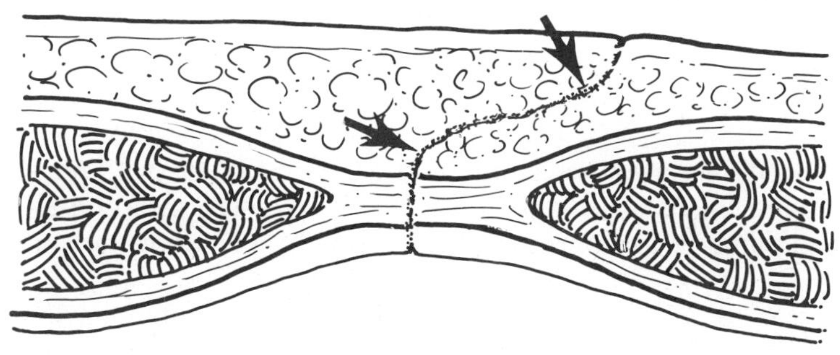

FIGURE 9–9. Arrows indicate Z tract.

10. Enter the peritoneal cavity with negative pressure applied to the needle through the syringe. Resistance will decrease when the anterior wall is penetrated. Do not advance the needle more than 1 cm past the abdominal wall. Peritoneal fluid will be easily aspirated when the needle is in the appropriate position.
11. Use one of three methods:
    a. Obtain peritoneal fluid through the needle (this is not recommended unless 30 ml or less of fluid is to be obtained).
    b. Use the Seldinger technique and place a wire through the needle. Allow enough length of wire to pass through the needle to ensure the wire is in the peritoneal cavity. Remove the needle while securing the wire with your hand. Place a catheter over the wire and slide the catheter into the peritoneal cavity. (A dilator may be needed to pass the catheter through the abdominal wall.) Hold the catheter in place while removing the wire (Figures 9–10 and 9–11).
    c. Pass a catheter through the needle and then remove the needle. Secure the needle on the catheter with a guard.
12. Fluid may be withdrawn through a stopcock, syringe, and collection bag or directly into a sterile 1-L vacuum bottle (allowing the vacuum to pull fluid into the bottle) connected to the catheter with intravenous tubing.
13. When finished, remove the catheter, place a bandage over the needle insertion site, and hold pressure on the wound site.

Complications

Pain

Infection (either introduced from skin or from bowel perforation)

Bowel puncture

Bladder puncture

Bleeding

Failure to obtain fluid

Persistent leakage of peritoneal fluid from puncture site

Pearls and Pitfalls

1. The "Z" needle insertion technique is crucial for patients with tense ascites since they are likely to leak peritoneal fluid from the insertion site if the needle and catheter are introduced in a straight line from the skin to the fascia.
2. Patients who have spontaneous bacterial peritonitis often have minimal tenderness. Therefore, paracentesis needs to be performed on most patients with known ascites and either unexplained fever or increased white blood cell counts.
3. Spring-loaded stopcocks are available that will help you to withdraw peritoneal fluid into a syringe and then push the fluid back into the stopcock and into a collection container without having to either remove the syringe or turn a valve on the stopcock.
4. Catheter manipulation (turning or withdrawing) is often repeatedly necessary to continue the flow of peritoneal fluid.

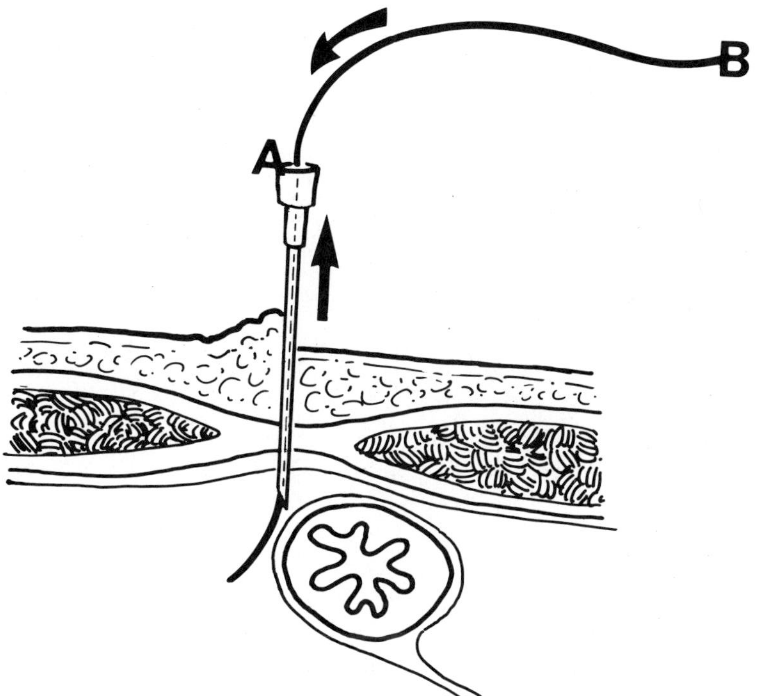

FIGURE 9–10. *A,* Needle; *B,* guidewire.

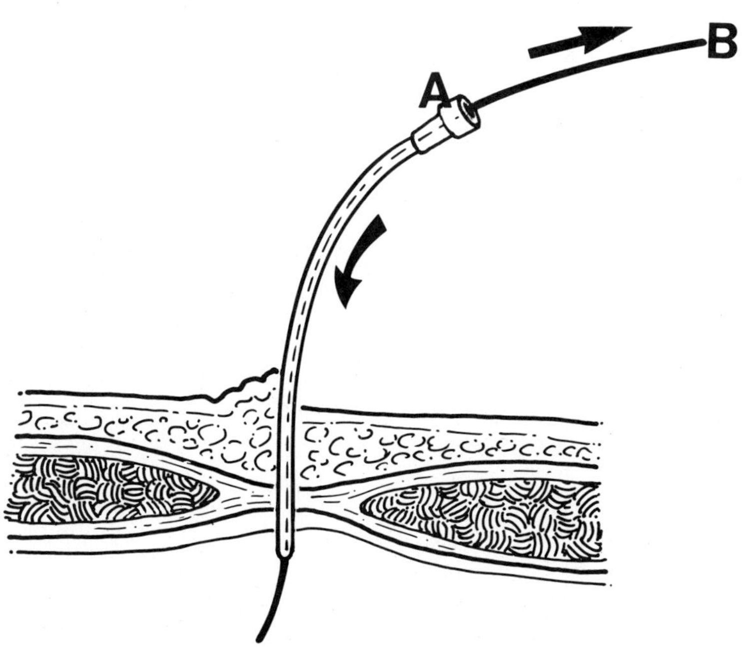

FIGURE 9–11. *A,* Catheter; *B,* guidewire.

5. Many patients with ascites are also coagulopathic. The risk versus benefit of paracentesis in these patients has to be weighed individually. Lidocaine with epinephrine will discourage bleeding from the skin but will not influence bleeding within the peritoneal cavity.
6. If a catheter through the needle system is used, do not remove the catheter from the patient without first removing the needle. This will prevent shearing the tip of the catheter off inside the patient.

Reference

Extensive experience

Rigid Sigmoidoscopy

E. JAMES RADIN, MD

Indications

Sigmoidoscopy is performed to assess the distal 15 to 20 cm of the rectosigmoid colon for the following:

Obstructing mass	Source of hemorrhage	Ischemia
Perforation	Infection	Abnormal mucosa

Contraindications

Known tear
Immunosuppression (relative)
Clotting disorders (relative)

Equipment

Sigmoidoscope and obturator (Figure 9–12)
Light source (Figure 9–13)

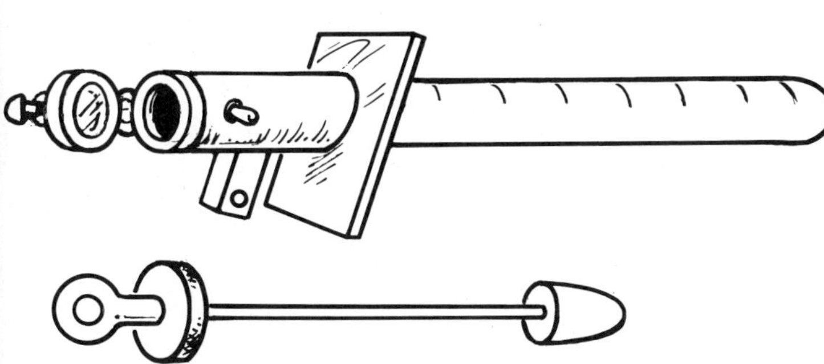

FIGURE 9–12. Sigmoidoscope and obturator.

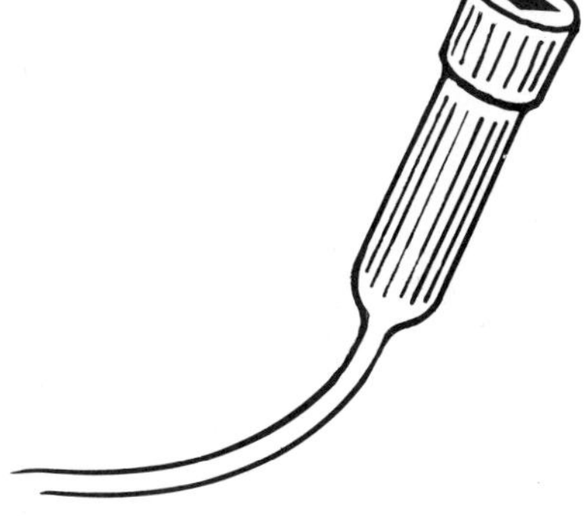

FIGURE 9–13. Light source.

Suction and suction probe (Figure 9–14)
Insufflation bag (Figure 9–15)
Appropriate chair and examination table
Cleaning equipment and disinfectant
Guaiac cards
Long cotton pledges (sterile)
Biopsy forceps and specimen containers (formalin and culture) (Figure 9–16)
Protective eye shield, mask, gloves, and gown with plastic apron
Tap water enema

Universal Precautions

1. Wear mask, gown, gloves, and plastic apron.
2. Use an eye shield.

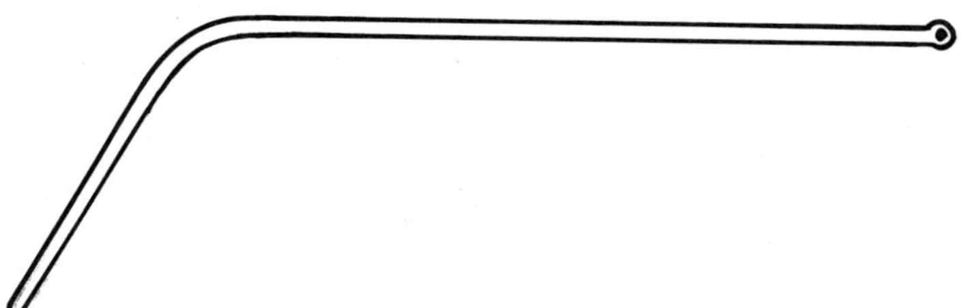

FIGURE 9–14. Suction probe.

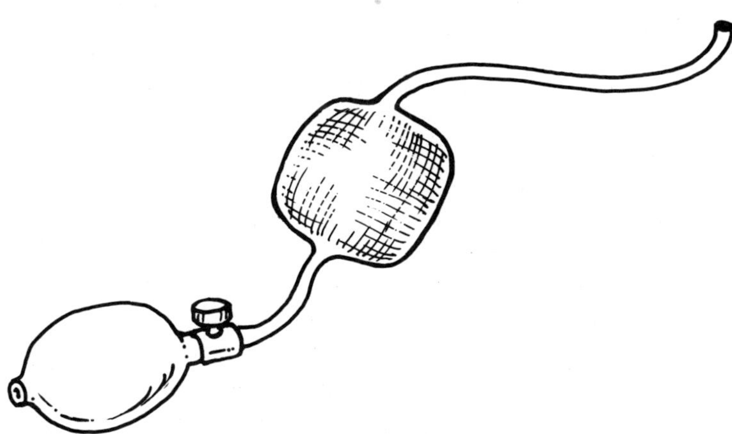

FIGURE 9–15. Insufflation bag.

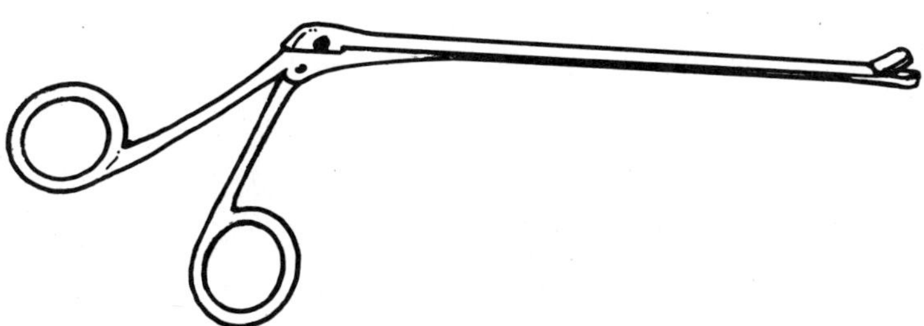

FIGURE 9–16. Biopsy forceps.

Technique

1. Explain the procedure to the patient and obtain consent.
2. Place patient on cardiac monitor and start an intravenous drip with 5% dextrose and water if patient has a history of cardiac problems.
3. Check scope, light source, inflation bag, and suction.
4. Place the patient in a kneeling position on the sigmoid chair/table.
5. Perform perineal and digital rectal examinations, palpating as much of the rectal vault and internal sphincter as possible.
6. Obtain a guaiac stool sample.
7. Change gloves.
8. Lubricate scope with surgical lubricant.
9. With obturator in place, pass scope through sphincter; then remove obturator and close glass.
10. Insufflate air (as small amount as possible).
11. Advance scope fully under direct visualization.
12. Once the scope is maximally advanced, using a circular motion, slowly withdraw the scope, compressing and looking behind *all* folds (Figure 9–17). Obtain specimens and cultures as indicated by observations.
13. Suction all debris that obscures your view.
14. If suction fails to remove blood, stool, and so on, then a tap water enema may be done, remembering that this may obscure any site of bleeding.
15. Repeat procedure after enema.

Complications

Sepsis
Perforation
Bleeding
Vagal stimulation with bradycardia and hypotension
Death

Pearls and Pitfalls

1. Always perform a thorough digital examination first.
2. Check your light source.
3. Flexible procedures are more comfortable and perhaps more accurate, but not in a blood-, clot-, or stool-filled rectum.
4. Do not forget to send sample for culture.
5. Biopsy only the posterior wall or polypoid masses. Do not biopsy other walls with rigid sigmoid biopsy forceps because of the risk of perforation.

Reference

Extensive experience

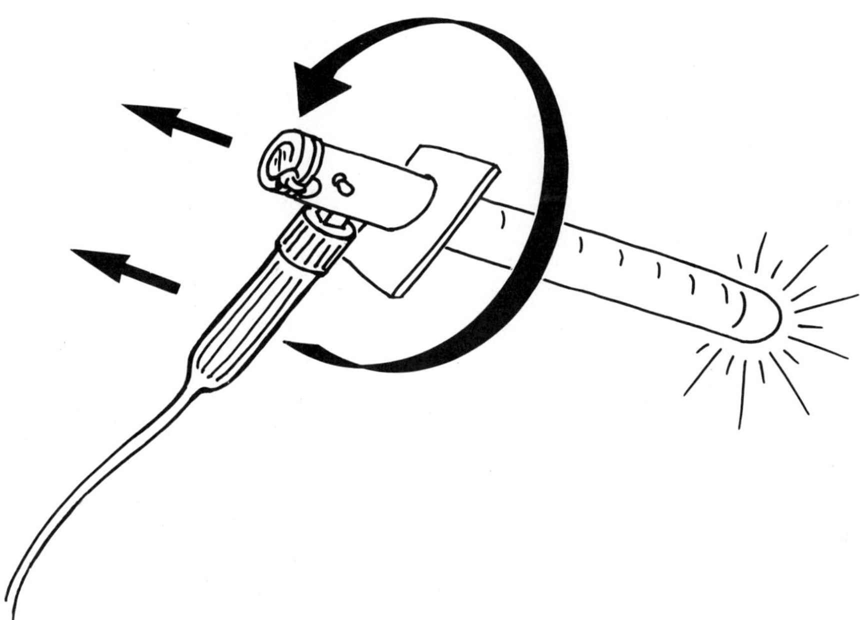

FIGURE 9–17. Sigmoidoscopy.

10

Incision and Drainage

Incision and Drainage of a Felon

W. JOHN ZEHNER, MD

Indication

Drainage of a collection of pus in the pulp space on the volar surface of the distal phalanx

If a felon is not drained or is drained improperly, osteomyelitis, an unstable finger pad, or anesthesia of the fingertip may result.

Contraindications

None

Equipment

5-ml and 20-ml syringes
25-gauge, 1-inch and 20-gauge, 1½-inch needles
Sterile gloves (two pair)
Eye shield
No. 11 blade
Hemostat
Petrolatum gauze
Sterile dressing
Tape
Betadine solution
Finger splint
Local anesthetic solution (without epinephrine)

Universal Precautions

1. Wear sterile gloves and an eye shield.
2. Dispose of needle, syringe, and scalpel properly.

Technique

1. Explain the purpose of the incision and drainage to the patient and obtain consent.
2. Position the patient supine on a stretcher with the affected extremity abducted on an arm board with the palm up.
3. Attempt to localize the "point" of abscess closest to the skin by palpation of the area of most tenderness and fluctuance.
4. Perform a digital block of the involved finger (see Chapter 2).
5. After adequate anesthesia is obtained, clean the distal phalanx with Betadine solution and then wipe any excess solution from the digit.
6. Put on a fresh pair of sterile gloves.
7. If the felon points toward the volar aspect, the anterior (volar) midline approach should be used. Using a No. 11 blade, make a midline volar incision from the fingertip to distal to the distal interphalangeal crease (Figure 10–1).
8. If the felon points to the lateral or medial side of the phalanx, a "hockey stick" incision should be used. The incision is made along the plane just volar to the bony phalanx beginning on the side of the finger just distal to the distal interphalangeal joint and extending to the middle of the fingertip (Figure 10–2).
9. As in any abscess, care must be taken to break up all loculations using a hemostat spread in the plane of the incision, followed by pressure irrigation with 100 to 200 ml of saline using the 20-ml syringe and 20-gauge needle.
10. Place a sterile petrolatum gauze wick in the incision for 24 hours to allow the wound to drain.
11. Splint the finger.
12. Cover with a dry dressing.
13. Start the patient on antistaphylococcal antibiotics for 5 days and give him a prescription for an oral analgesic.

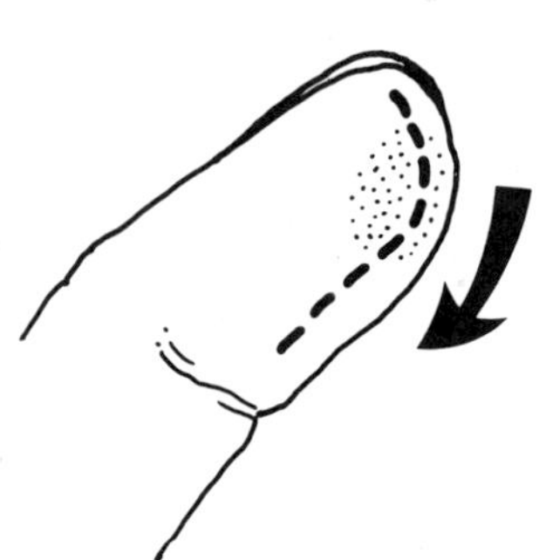

FIGURE 10–1. Drainage of a felon: volar approach.

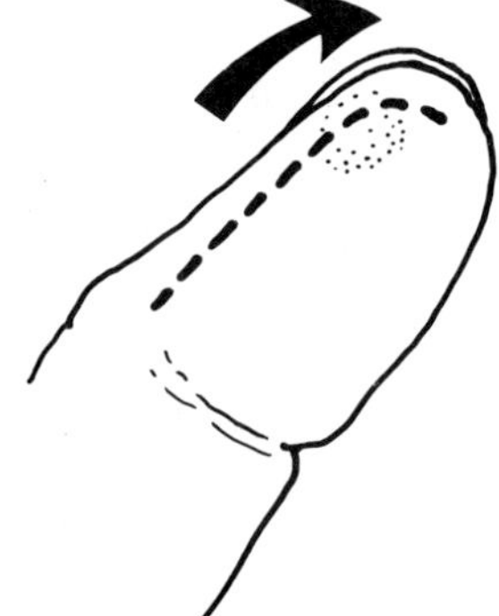

FIGURE 10–2. Drainage of a felon: lateral approach.

Complications

Digital nerve damage resulting in fingertip anesthesia
Damage to the vascular supply of the fingertip
Fingertip pad instability after the fibrous septa are disrupted
Continued infection leading to osteomyelitis

Pearls and Pitfalls

1. There is much controversy as to which technique leads to better results and fewer complications. "Fishmouth" incisions have been associated with a higher incidence of finger pad instability, and lateral connecting incisions have been associated with anesthesia of the fingertip. An approach directing the incision at the area the felon is pointing to is the one recommended here.
2. Application of a tourniquet fashioned from a Penrose drain to the proximal phalanx will give a bloodless field to work in.

References

Mann RJ: Infections of the Hand, pp 21–28. Philadelphia, Lea & Febiger, 1988.
Orban DJ: Hand. In Rosen P (ed): Emergency Medicine—Concepts and Clinical Practice, pp 775–776. St. Louis, CV Mosby, 1988.

Incision and Drainage of External Hemorrhoids

W. JOHN ZEHNER, MD

Indication

Most external hemorrhoids can be treated conservatively with sitz baths, stool softeners, and analgesics. When the hemorrhoids become thrombosed and the patient experiences severe, refractory pain, excision provides immediate, welcomed relief.

Contraindications

Nonthrombosed hemorrhoids
Patient with known coronary artery disease (relative)
Overly anxious and uncooperative patient (may require general anesthesia)

Equipment

Sterile gloves
Scalpel with No. 15 blade
Adson forceps
2-inch tape
10-ml syringe
25-gauge, 1-inch needle
2% lidocaine or bupivacaine with epinephrine
Hemostat
Surgical foam (Gelfoam)
4×4-inch sterile dressing
Betadine

Universal Precautions

1. Wear mask and sterile gloves.
2. Use an eye shield.
3. Dispose of needle, syringe, and scalpel properly.

Technique

1. Explain the procedure and its purpose to the patient and obtain consent.
2. Place the patient prone on a stretcher and stand on the patient's right side.
3. Tape the buttocks to the sides of the stretcher to expose the anus (Figure 10–3).

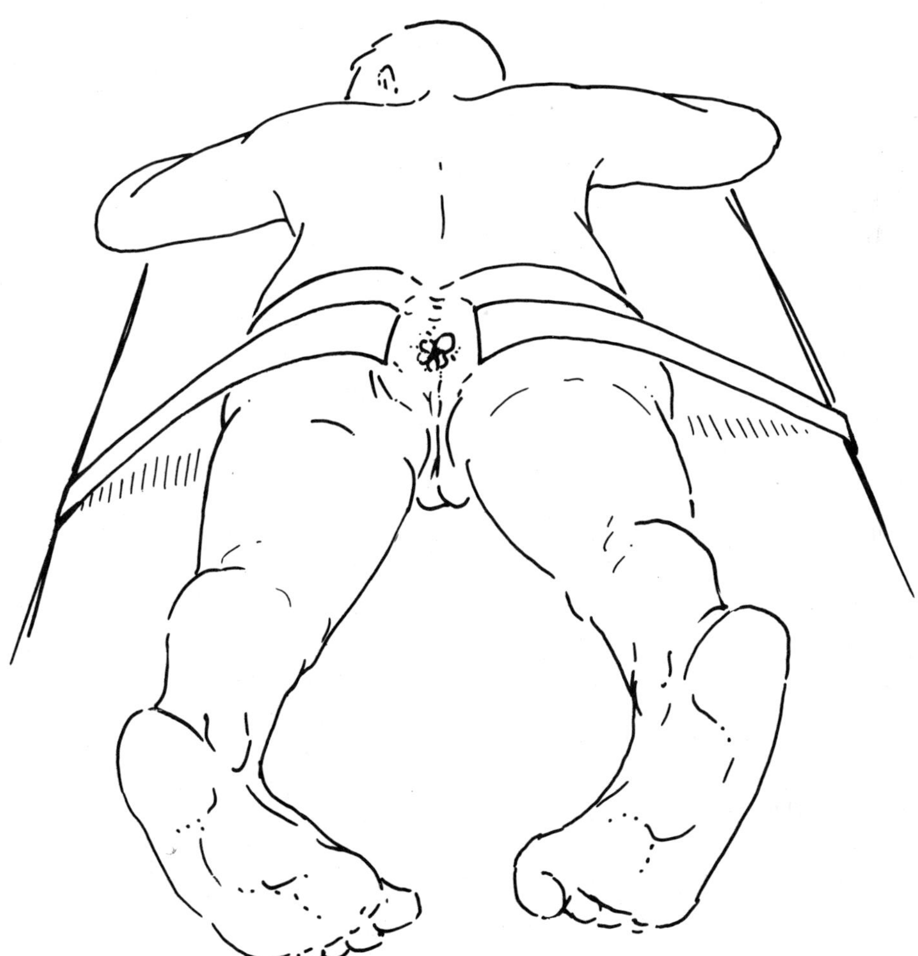

FIGURE 10–3. Hemorrhoid drainage.

4. Cleanse the area with Betadine.
5. Put on mask, eye shield, and sterile gloves.
6. Using a 10-ml syringe and 25-gauge, 1-inch needle with lidocaine or bupivacaine, begin infiltrating the lateral aspect of the hemorrhoid. The medial (anal) aspect may also need to be infiltrated.
7. An unroofing procedure is performed with the scalpel as follows:
   a. Elevate the skin with the Adson forceps, and make an elliptical incision to remove the skin over the hemorrhoid (Figure 10–4). Care should be taken not to extend the incision below the cutaneous layer.
   b. Pick out the thrombosed clot with the hemostat.
   c. Using the hemostat, gently dissect the area looking for more clots.
8. Place a small piece of surgical foam in the wound to promote hemostasis. Leave the wound open and cover with sterile gauze dressing.
9. Advise patient to
   a. Take warm sitz baths three to four times a day for 2 days.
   b. Return for wound check in 2 to 3 days.
   c. Avoid straining and prolonged sitting for several days.
10. Prescribe a stool softener and an oral analgesic.

Complications

Excessive bleeding
Infection

Pearls and Pitfalls

1. Because of the pain and anxiety the patient may be experiencing, administration of systemic analgesia should be considered.
2. Avoid narcotic analgesics if possible because they cause constipation.
3. Antibiotics are not indicated for simple, noninfected, thrombosed external hemorrhoids.

References

Davis SM, Odom MH: Disorders of the anorectum. In Rosen P (ed): Emergency Medicine—Concepts and Clinical Practice, pp 1527–1528. St. Louis, CV Mosby, 1988.

Glauser JM: Thrombosed external hemorrhoids. In Roberts J, Hedges J (eds): Procedures in Emergency Medicine, pp 792–795. Philadelphia, WB Saunders, 1985.

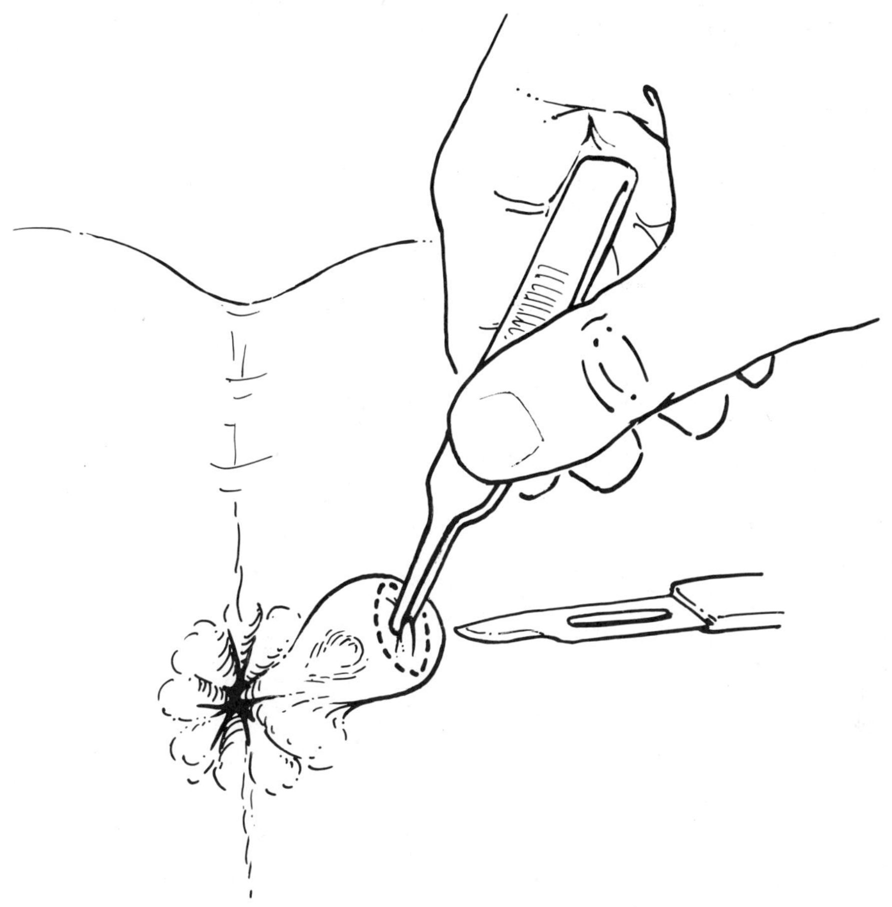

FIGURE 10–4. Hemorrhoid drainage.

Paronychial Drainage

DAVID M. KRUGER, MD

Indication

Infection involving the soft tissue around the fingernail with frank abscess formation

Equipment

Antiseptic solution
Local anesthetic without epinephrine
Sterile gloves
Mask
Eye shield
Hand bowl for soaking
Betadine solution
1 L warm sterile water
Two 18-gauge, 1½-inch needles
25-gauge, 1-inch needle
Scalpel with No. 11 blade
Scalpel with No. 15 blade
Freer elevator or other flat probe
Small dissecting scissors
Sterile drapes
Hand board or Mayo stand
Small sterile gauze wick
2 × 2-inch gauze pads
Kling finger dressing
Antibiotic ointment

Universal Precautions

1. Wear mask and sterile gloves.
2. Use an eye shield.

Technique

1. Explain the procedure to the patient and obtain consent.
2. Confirm the absence of antibiotic and anesthetic allergies.
3. In the hand bowl, mix Betadine solution in 1 L warm sterile water and have the patient soak his or her hand in this solution for 10 minutes before beginning the procedure.
4. Position the patient supine with the affected hand dorsum up on a Mayo stand or hand board covered with a sterile drape.
5. Prepare equipment:
   a. Ensure that all equipment is present and open.
   b. Open the dressing to be used at the completion of the procedure.

6. Put on mask, eye shield, and sterile gloves.
7. At the point of maximum swelling, advance an 18-gauge needle or a No. 11 blade under the eponychium, parallel to the nail, and sweep under the affected paronychium, from proximally toward the finger tip (Figure 10–5).
8. Pus should rapidly escape with relief of pain.
9. Pack a gauze wick beneath the skin fold to keep the cavity open.
10. If the infection is extensive, if there is subungual involvement, or if the above technique fails to release the abscess, proceed with steps 11 through 17.

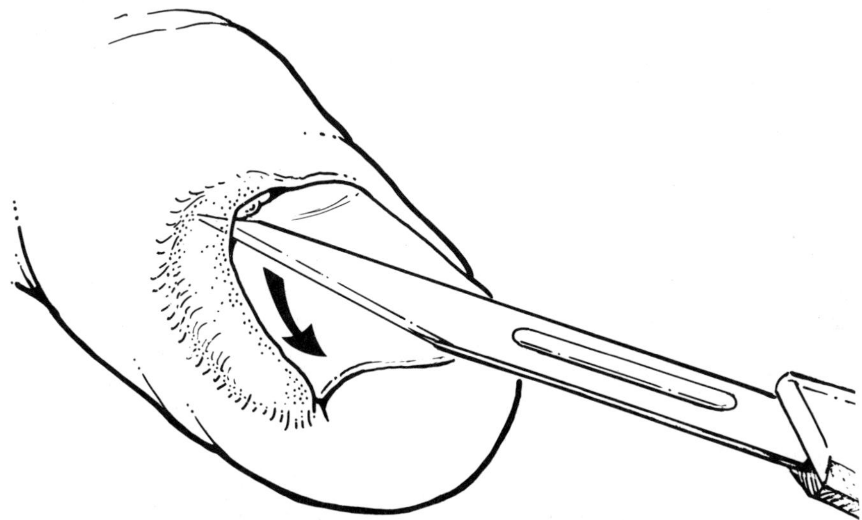

FIGURE 10–5. Paronychial drainage.

11. Perform a digital block of the finger with local anesthetic without epinephrine as described in Chapter 2.
12. Use a No. 15 blade to incise the paronychial fold in line with the lateral edge of the nail proximally toward the base of the nail for approximately 0.5 cm. Introduce the Freer elevator into this incision, and elevate the eponychium and the paronychium.
13. If the pus is incompletely drained or remains subungual, carefully continue with the Freer elevator to elevate the ipsilateral one fourth of the nail from the nail bed without injuring the nail bed itself.
14. Excise the lateral one fourth of the nail with a scissors, carefully avoiding the nail bed.
15. Probe the wound to be certain all the abscess pockets are decompressed.
16. Insert a gauze wick under the nail fold.
17. If the majority of the infection is proximally based, the proximal one third of the nail should be elevated and removed instead of the lateral one fourth. This may be facilitated by making a second incision (as described in step 12) on the other side of the nail.
18. Dress the wound with the 2×2-inch gauze pad and a loosely applied Kling wrap.
19. Instruct the patient to keep his hand elevated.
20. Instruct the patient to begin dressing changes four times a day with warm tap water soaks, followed by reapplication of antibiotic ointment and a gauze dressing 24 hours after the procedure. The wick should be removed with the first soak.
21. Arrange for the first wound check in 2 to 3 days.
22. A broad-spectrum antistaphylococcal antibiotic and an analgesic should be prescribed for 3 to 5 days.

Complications

Incomplete drainage

Damage to nail bed with subsequent nail scarring and deformity

Pearls and Pitfalls

1. When discovered in the early cellulitic stage, paronychia may be successfully treated with warm soaks, elevation of the extremity, and antibiotics, avoiding surgery.
2. Always direct incisions away from the nail fold and parallel to the matrix to minimize the possibility of nail deformity.
3. Warm soaks prior to wick removal minimize patient discomfort.
4. Use of antibiotic ointment prevents painful adherence of the dressing to the nail bed.

References

Lampe EW: Surgical Anatomy of the Hand. Summit, NJ, CIBA Pharmaceutical, 1969.

Neviaser RJ: Infections. In Green DP (ed): Operative Hand Surgery, vol 1, pp 772–773. New York, Churchill-Livingstone, 1982.

Warren TM: Dermatology. In Roberts JR, Hedges JR (eds): Clinical Procedures in Emergency Medicine, pp 993–994. Philadelphia, WB Saunders, 1985.

Incision and Drainage of a Subcutaneous Abscess

SAMMY F. SURIANI, RPA-C, EMT-P

Indication

Abscesses are walled-off areas of infection and collections of purulent material that may appear anywhere on the body. Regardless of location, the primary treatment is incision and drainage to aid in healing and relieve pain caused by the abscess. When an abscess is ready for drainage, it is termed *fluctuant* and will normally develop a soft area near its center.

Contraindications

None

Equipment

Betadine solution
Lidocaine 1% for local anesthesia
Sterile drapes
Hemostat
Scalpel and No. 11 blade
Saline irrigation solution
Culture swabs
Iodoform packing gauze
4 × 4-inch gauze pads
Mask
Eye shield
Sterile gloves
3-ml syringe
25-gauge, 1-inch needle
20-ml syringe
19-gauge, 1½-inch needle

Universal Precautions

1. Wear a mask and sterile gloves.
2. Use an eye shield.

Technique

1. Explain the procedure to the patient and obtain consent.
2. Determine the fluctuance of the abscess.
3. The procedure should be performed aseptically. Prepare the affected area with a topical agent such as Betadine, and drape the area.
4. Using an appropriate-sized injection needle (25- or 27-gauge), introduce the anesthetic in a regional field block technique. The injection should be approximately 1 cm away from the perimeter of the erythematous border of the abscess, taking care to inject subcutaneously. Then inject a small amount into the roof of the abscess in a linear fashion along the projected incision line. Intravenous sedation and analgesia should be considered in children and uncooperative adults and when the abscess is large (Figure 10–6).
5. Once anesthesia has been achieved, use the scalpel to make an incision long and deep enough along the skin tension line to allow for drainage to occur (Figure 10–7).
6. Once purulent material drains, obtain a culture for Gram stain and antibiotic sensitivity.

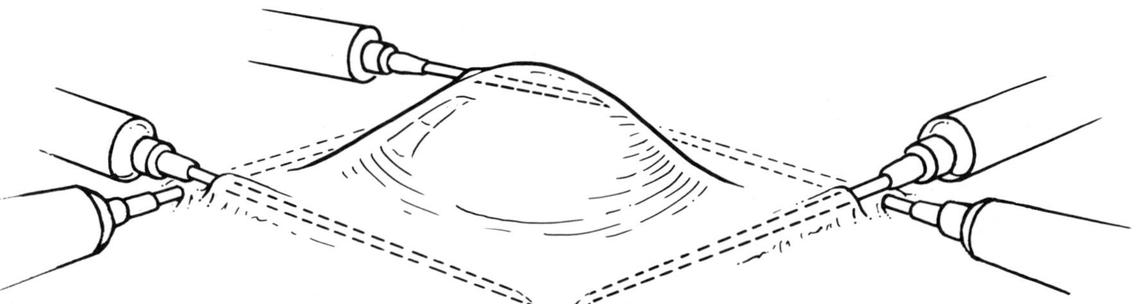

FIGURE 10–6. Anesthesia to drain a subcutaneous abscess.

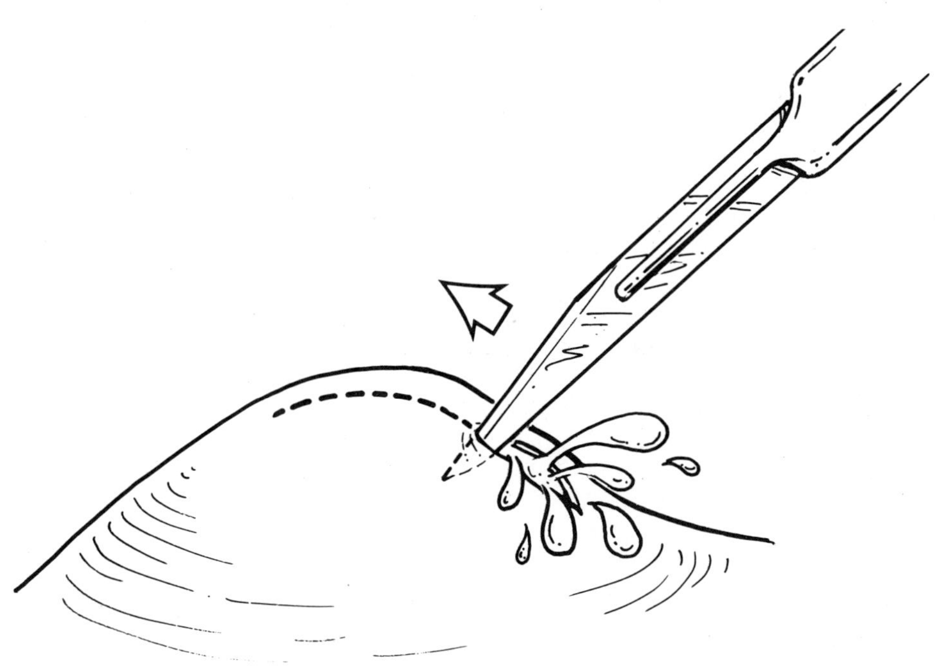

FIGURE 10–7. Drainage of a subcutaneous abscess.

7. Insert a sterile hemostat into the cavity and spread it to break up loculations and release any further pockets of purulent material (Figure 10–8).
8. Irrigate the cavity with a sufficient amount of normal saline solution using the 20-ml syringe and 19-gauge needle.
9. Insert iodoform gauze into the site to fill all areas of the cavity. Allow 1 to 2 cm of gauze to exit the site to allow for adequate drainage and to prevent the incision from sealing over (Figure 10–9).
10. Apply 4 × 4-inch sterile gauze pads over the site.

Complications

Introduction of new bacteria into the wound

Incision size not large enough to allow for adequate drainage

Site not explored completely with some loculated areas left, resulting in continued infection

Systemic sepsis

Bleeding

Pearls and Pitfalls

1. Some infections such as those in the hand, fingers, or perineum can be urgent medical problems and may require the assistance of a specialist.
2. Have the patient return in 1 to 2 days for removal of the packing and for wound check.
3. After packing removal, have the patient apply warm, wet soaks several times daily.
4. Instruct the patient to be aware of the signs of systemic infection.
5. The incision should heal in 7 to 10 days.
6. Incision and drainage alone is adequate therapy for a simple subcutaneous abscess. Antibiotics are not needed.
7. Antibiotic therapy is indicated if there is coexisting cellulitis, if the patient is immunocompromised, or if the patient has an intravascular foreign body (e.g., vascular graft, Hickman catheter, artificial cardiac valve). In these circumstances (especially intravascular foreign bodies), appropriate broad-spectrum antibiotic therapy, based on likely pathogens for the site of infection, should precede the incision and drainage.

References

Grossman JA: Minor Injuries and Disorders: Surgical and Medical Care, pp 207–209. Philadelphia, JB Lippincott, 1984.

Simon RB, Brenner BE: Emergency Procedures and Techniques, 2nd ed, pp 337–339. Baltimore, Williams & Wilkins, 1987.

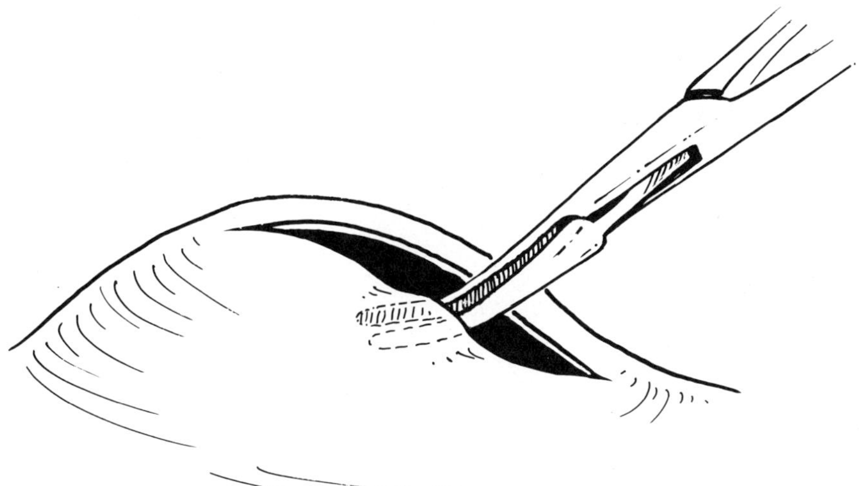

FIGURE 10–8. Drainage of a subcutaneous abscess.

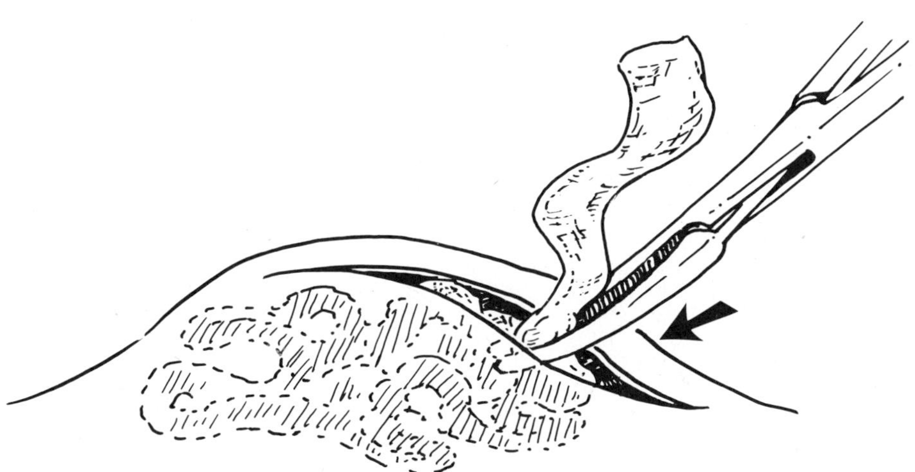

FIGURE 10–9. Packing a subcutaneous abscess.

11

Invasive Vascular Pressure Monitoring

RAE NADINE SMITH, RN, MS

Indications

To assist in diagnosis, define therapy, and evaluate a patient's response to selected therapies

To obtain continuous or intermittent direct pressure measurements

To derive advanced hemodynamic parameters

To develop hemodynamic profiles

To access the cardiovascular system for rapid infusion of fluids or drug therapy

To obtain access for blood sampling, blood gas analysis, and blood flow measurements

To measure pressures not detectable with noninvasive techniques

Vascular Measurements

Systemic arterial blood pressure
Central venous pressure
Right atrial pressure
Right ventricular pressure
Pulmonary artery pressure
Pulmonary capillary wedge pressure
Left atrial pressure
Cardiac output
Right ventricular ejection fraction
Blood gases
Derived parameters

Contraindications

Coagulopathies/septicemia
Hyperinflated lungs
Radiation to insertion site
Cancer (neck, lung)
Anatomic anomalies
Thrombosis of the superior vena cava

Equipment

Note: A variety of satisfactory components are available preassembled in sterile kits.

- Sterile gloves
- Gown
- Mask
- Eye shield
- Transducer, disposable or reusable
- Intravenous normal saline solution with heparin
- Minidrop (microdrop intravenous administration set [60 drops/ml] with air filter)
- Pressure tubing, male-female
- Continuous flush device
- Three three-way stopcocks
- Female cap or deadhead
- Transducer pole or patient mount
- Pressure administration cuff
- Intravenous setup pole

Universal Precautions

1. Wear gown, mask, eye shield, and sterile gloves.

Technique (Figure 11–1)

1. Turn pressure monitor on and attach transducer.
2. Prepare intravenous flush solution (0.25 to 1.0 unit heparin per milliliter of normal saline: optional).
3. Extract all air from the solution, insert a minidrop infusion set, and place the solution into a pressure infusor bag or pump.
4. Gravity-fill system until it is completely air free.
5. Inflate the pressure infusor bag to 300 mm Hg.
6. Place the transducer/flush system into the mount, positioning the balancing (venting) port level with the patient's right atrium (~midaxillary).
7. Vent the balancing port to air, balance the transducer to zero, and calibrate as required (actual procedure depends on the brand of monitor).
8. Close the system, placing a sterile cap on the venting port. Check to be certain the system is completely air free.
9. Activate the fast-flush valve and connect the system to the patient's cannula or catheter.
10. Flush by activating the fast-flush system, checking the waveform for optimal dynamic response (Figure 11–2*A*). Confirm the flush rate is 3 to 6 minidrops per minute and the pressure infusor is at 300 mm Hg.

Complications

- Infection
- Thrombosis
- Emboli
- Hemorrhage
- Vessel and chamber perforation
- Ventricular dysrhythmias
- Fluid overload
- Pneumothorax
- Cardiac valve damage
- Pulmonary infarction
- Electrical microshock
- Erroneous data due to system malfunction and user error

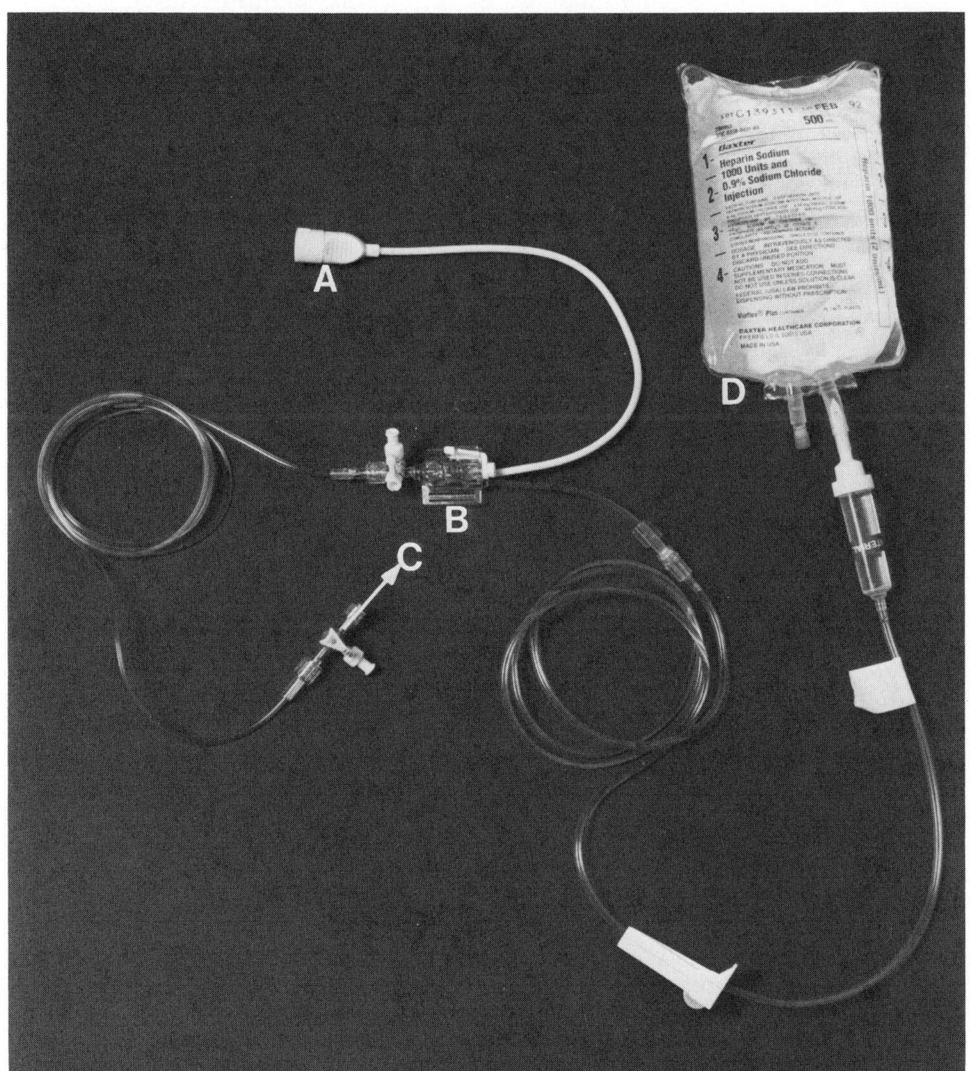

FIGURE 11–1. *A,* Transducer/connection to monitor; *B,* continuous flush device; *C,* arrow indicates direction toward patient; *D,* flush solution.

Pearls and Pitfalls

1. Risks associated with vascular lines can be kept to a minimum by a skilled critical care team with adequate instrumentation.
2. The use of premixed heparin flush solution and a preassembled sterile kit reduces the risk of setup contamination.
3. For accuracy, correct transducer position, balancing, and optimal dynamic response should be confirmed routinely (per shift and as needed).
4. Dynamic response, the ability of a monitoring system to accurately reproduce a pressure signal on a monitor, is affected by the compliance, fluid mass, and resistance of the fluid-filled catheter system between the pressure transducer and the patient. The dynamic response characteristics of a monitoring system may be tested at the bedside by doing a "square-wave" test. Once the transducer is balanced and calibrated at the level of the right atrium, the accuracy of the system may be confirmed by activating the fast-flush valve of a low-compliance continuous flush system and observing the "square wave" that occurs when the transducer senses the pressure of the flush system. The square-wave test provides a means of assessing the natural frequency and damping coefficient to determine the presence and degree of pressure measurement distortion. Figure 11–2*A* illustrates an accurate (optimally damped) waveform. The test is performed by activating and quickly releasing the fast-flush valve. As the fast-flush valve is opened a rapid increase in pressure indicates the transducer sensing the pressure of the flush solution. On closure of the fast-flush valve there is a rapid return to baseline. An optimal response consists of the waveform extending sharply below the baseline with just one or two oscillations (minimal ringing) and a quick return to the pressure waveform.

   Figure 11–2*B* illustrates an overdamped waveform. The "square-wave" waveform does not extend below the baseline, has no ringing (oscillations), and returns slowly to the pressure waveform. Clinically significant characteristics of an overdamped pressure waveform include a diminished or absent dicrotic notch and a false low-systolic and a false high-diastolic pressure measurement. Overdamping is caused by compliance in the system (air bubbles, leaks in the monitoring line, compliant components), and/or occlusion of the catheter/cannula (clots, kinks, positioning of catheter, stopcocks).

   Figure 11–3 illustrates an underdamped waveform. Underdamping is characterized by numerous amplified oscillations above and below the baseline with a delayed return to the pressure waveform. Clinically, underdamped waveforms are characterized by overshoot (ringing artifact) and a false high-systolic pressure reading. This may be caused by small air bubbles (usually in the transducer dome), an inappropriate combination of monitoring components, or, most commonly, pathophysiologic alterations. It may be corrected with variable damping devices or the reduction of pathophysiologic alterations, such as hypothermia, vasoconstriction, and low cardiac output. It cannot be corrected by the use of electronic amplifier filters.
5. The optimal hemodynamic monitoring system should be as simple as possible, have minimal connecting tubing and stopcocks, contain the least compliant components available, and be air free. For accuracy, it must be periodically balanced and calibrated, with dynamic response ("square-wave") testing used to ensure optimal dynamic response. As with all clinical variables, pressure measurements should be integrated into the overall clinical picture before being used as the basis for major therapeutic interventions.

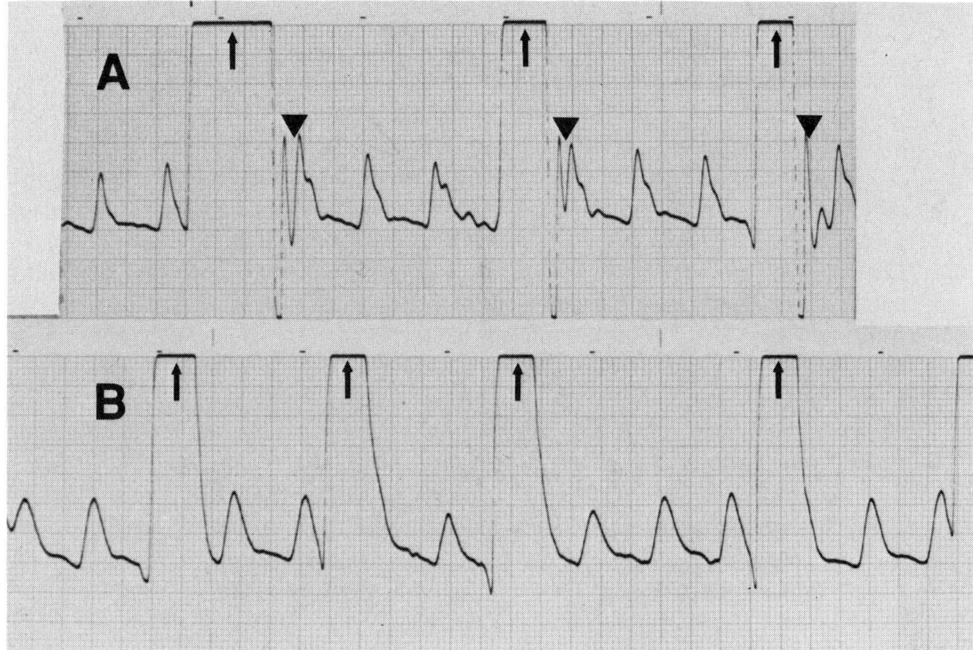

FIGURE 11–2. *A,* Normal pressure response to a fast flush. *B,* Overdamped response to a fast flush. Arrows point to square waves. Arrowheads point to oscillations.

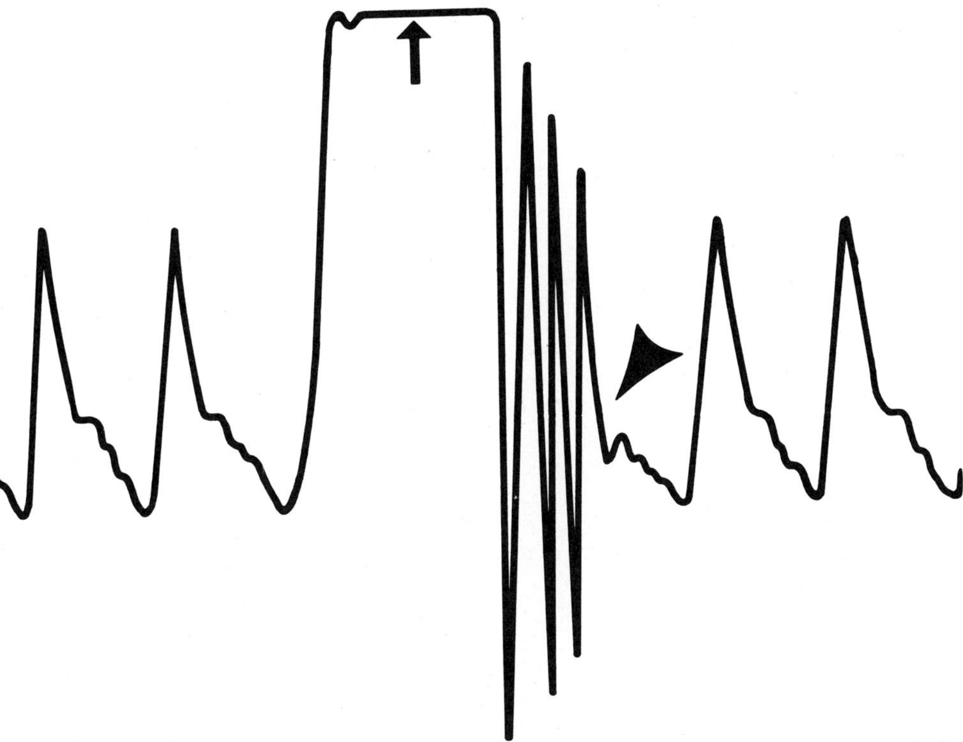

FIGURE 11–3. Underdamped response to a fast flush. Arrow points to a square wave. Arrowhead points to oscillations.

Troubleshooting

1. False low reading
   Cause: Transducer positioned above right atrium, incorrect balancing and calibration, overdamping
   Intervention: Position transducer approximately midaxillary, vent to air; balance and calibrate; eliminate overdamping.
2. Overdamping (usually false low-systolic and false high-diastolic readings)
   Cause: Air bubbles, loose connections, back bleeding, clotting, compliant components, partially occluded system
   Intervention: Check plumbing for kinks, cracks, air, or loose connections; flush solution; confirm pressure cuff at 300 mm Hg; correct flush technique.
3. False high reading
   Cause: Transducer positioned below right atrium, incorrect balancing and calibration, continual flush greater than 8 ml/hr, underdamping
   Intervention: Position transducer approximately midaxillary; vent to air; balance and calibrate; eliminate underdamping.
4. Underdamping
   Cause: System dynamics
   Intervention: Use variable damping device.
5. Erratic traces
   Cause: Patient movement, damaged or incorrectly mounted transducer
   Intervention: Limit movement; use pole mount; use solid-state transducer.

References

Bolgiano CS, et al: The effect of two concentrations of heparin on arterial catheter patency. Crit Care Nurse 19:47–56, 1990.

Henneman EA, Henneman PL: Intricacies of blood pressure measurement: Reexamining the rituals. Heart Lung 18:263–273, 1989.

Smith RN, de Asla R: Instrumentation. In Kinney M, Packa D, Dunbar S (eds): AACN's Clinical Reference for Critical-Care Nursing, pp 33–82. New York, McGraw-Hill Book Company, 1988.

12

Laceration Repair

MICHAEL S. JASTREMSKI, MD

Indications

Control of hemorrhage
Irrigation and debridement to reduce the incidence of infection
Restoration of the functional integrity of the skin and minimization of subsequent scarring

Contraindications

There are no absolute contraindications, however delayed closure may be prudent in highly contaminated wounds or when there has been a long interval (approximately 24 hours for the face and 12 hours for the rest of the body) since the time of injury.

Equipment

Sterile saline for irrigation
Betadine solution
Local anesthetic
25-gauge, 1-inch and 19-gauge, 1½-inch needles
3-ml and 50-ml syringes
Sterile drapes
Assorted suture material (Table 12–1)
Hemostats
Adson forceps
Needle holder
Suture scissors
Iris scissors
Scalpel with No. 11 blade
4 × 4-inch gauze pads
Sterile basin
Topical antibiotic ointment
Nonadherent dressing material
Gauze
Tape

Universal Precautions

1. Wear mask and gloves.
2. Use an eye shield.

Technique

1. Explain the procedure to the patient and obtain consent.
2. Have you done the following?
   a. Checked for drug allergies
   b. Asked about tetanus immunization
   c. Obtained an x-ray film and looked at it if there is any possibility of fracture or foreign body
   d. Checked motor and sensory function before anesthesia
3. Position the patient lying comfortably on a stretcher with the injured area easily accessible.
4. Stand or sit next to the injured area.
5. Make sure the injured area is well lighted. A high-intensity focusable operating room–type light works best.
6. Prep the area with Betadine and place sterile drapes.
7. Anesthetize the wound using a regional block or local infiltration into the wound. If using local infiltration, the following measures will minimize pain:
   a. Use a small 25- or 27-gauge needle on a 3- or 5-ml syringe.
   b. Inject deep to the dermis through the wound, rather than through intact skin.
   c. Inject slowly.
   d. Wait several minutes before proceeding to ensure that anesthesia has occurred.
8. Debride devitalized tissue using the iris scissors or scalpel.
9. Pressure irrigate the wound using 250 to 500 ml of normal saline directed into all areas of the wound using a 19-gauge needle on a 50-ml syringe. Have your assistant pour the saline for irrigation into the sterile basin so you can easily draw it up. Alternatively, you may use one of the commercially available wound irrigation kits, but they are relatively expensive.

Debridement and irrigation are the key to preventing wound infection.

---

10. Carefully visualize the entire wound looking for foreign bodies or damage to deeper structures such as tendons or joints. These injuries may be missed unless you have the patient move the potentially injured tendon or joint through its full range of motion as you observe it in the wound. Repair of deep structures is beyond the scope of this book. For deeper injuries or complex areas such as the lip or eyelid margin seek consultation unless you are sure you know how to care for them.
11. Close the subcutaneous fascial layers, if lacerated, with interrupted absorbable sutures. Be careful to reestablish anatomic approximation since good approximation of the deeper layers helps ensure good approximation of the skin (Figure 12–1).
12. Close the skin.
   a. Choose the appropriate size of suture and needle (see Table 12–1).
   b. Grasp the needle with the needle holder as shown in Figure 12–2 and hold the needle holder with the thumb and fourth finger of your dominant hand. This relationship of hand, needle holder, and needle will result in the proper passage of the needle through the skin edges.
   c. Hold the Adson forceps in your nondominant hand. This forceps will

TABLE 12–1. Guide to Suturing

	Skin	Skin Suture Removal*	Subcutaneous Tissue and Muscle	Stitch Used
Face	6-0 nylon or polypropylene	3–5 days	4-0, 5-0 Dexon or Vicryl	Simple, simple running, or subcuticular
Scalp	4-0 nylon or polypropylene	5–8 days	3-0, 4-0 Dexon or Vicryl	Simple, simple running
Trunk	4-0 nylon or polypropylene	7–10 days	3-0, 4-0 Dexon or Vicryl	Simple, vertical mattress, running simple or vertical mattress
Extremities	4-0 nylon or polypropylene	7–10 days	4-0 Dexon or Vicryl	Simple, vertical mattress, running simple or vertical mattress
Hands/Feet	4-0, 5-0 nylon or polypropylene	10–14 days	4-0, 5-0 Dexon or Vicryl	Simple, vertical mattress
Mucous Membranes			4-0, 5-0 Dexon or Vicryl	Inverted simple
Tendon			4-0 nylon or wire	Figure eight

*Use the longer interval if the laceration is under tension or across an area of motion.

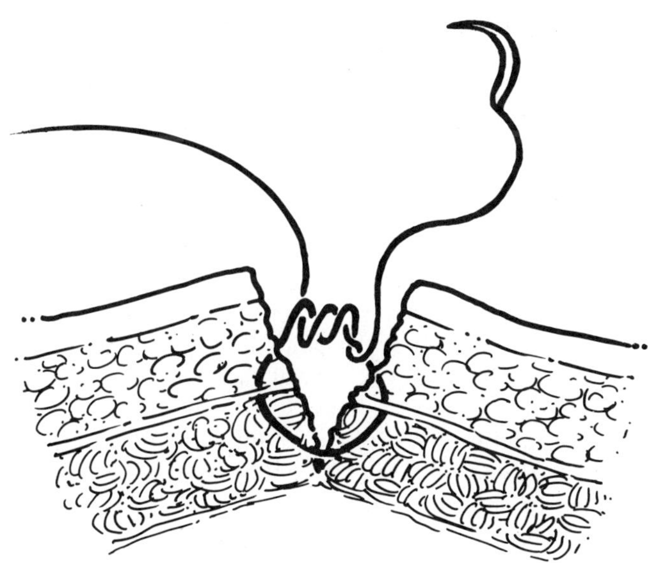

FIGURE 12–1. Closure of deep layers.

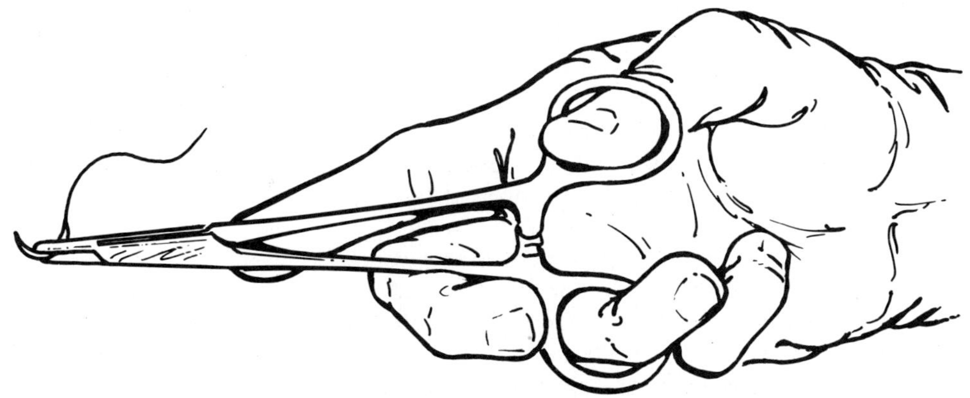

FIGURE 12–2. Hand position on the needle holder.

be used to grasp the skin edges for traction and to pull the needle through. Your fingers should never be near the wound while you are suturing!

d. Short wounds are closed by starting at one end and working to the other. Long wounds are best closed by starting in the middle and successively dividing the wound in half. Use skin landmarks (e.g., wrinkles, vermillion border of the lip) to help ensure that the wound closes evenly.

e. Simple sutures are placed as follows (Figure 12–3):
   1) Hold the skin edge with the Adson forceps.
   2) Position the tip of the needle perpendicular to the skin at an appropriate distance from the end of the wound and the skin edge. The best cosmetic results are obtained by placing the sutures close to the wound edge and close together using small-sized needles and suture material. Thus facial wounds are closed with small-sized sutures using more sutures per inch than trunk or extremity wounds.
   3) Twist your wrist to advance the needle through the skin on one side of the wound and out the skin on the other side. The distances from the end of the wound, the skin edge, and the depth in the wound should be the same on both sides. As the needle passes through the wound, reposition the Adson forceps to steady the second skin edge. When the wound is wide in relation to the needle size it will not be possible to advance the needle through both sides with one pass. In this case, pass the needle through one side; visualize the tip in the wound, grasp it with the Adson forceps, release the needle holder, and pull the needle out of the wound; reclamp it with the needle holder; and then pass the needle through the second skin edge starting in the wound at the same depth as the first side so the needle exits perpendicular to the skin at the same distance from the wound end and skin edge as on the first side.
   4) Tie the suture using a surgeon's knot with adequate tension to slightly invert the skin edges. Words cannot teach you how to tie knots; get someone to show you the one-hand, two-hand, and instrument tie, and then practice until you are adept at tying them.

f. The mattress suture may be necessary when the wound is long and/or wide such that there is considerable tension on the skin edges in the center of the wound. Mattress sutures may be used to divide the wound into halves, quarters, or eights, and then the spaces between the mattress sutures closed with simple sutures. In areas such as the shin where the skin is tight with little subcutaneous tissue, it may also be necessary to undermine the skin so it will be looser and pull together more easily. Figure 12–4 illustrates the route followed by the needle when placing a mattress suture.

13. Use a 4×4-inch gauze pad moistened with some of the irrigating solution to cleanse the area around the wound, and blot the wound dry with a dry 4×4-inch gauze pad.
14. Apply topical antibiotic ointment to the wound.
15. Dress the wound using a nonadherent pad and gauze wrap. I try to avoid using tape since it hurts when removed. It is best to leave facial and scalp wounds uncovered.
16. Before you discharge the patient:
    a. Tell the patient how to care for the wound

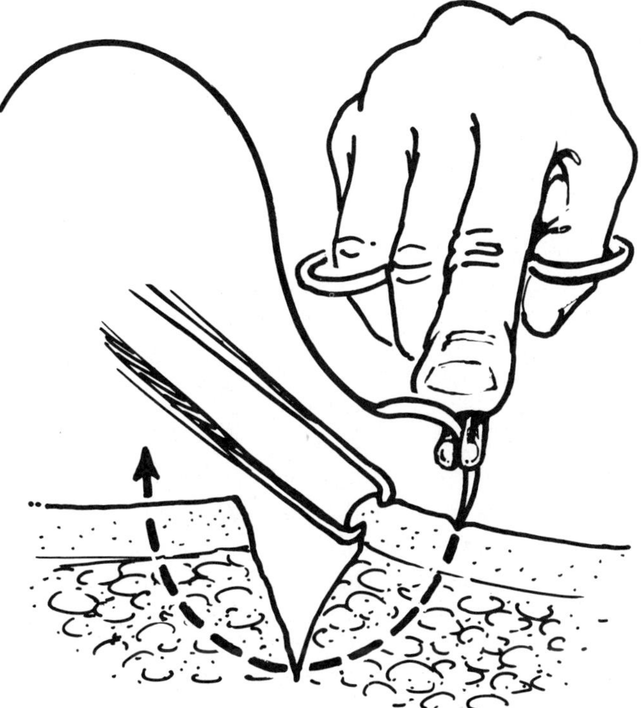

FIGURE 12–3. Skin closure.

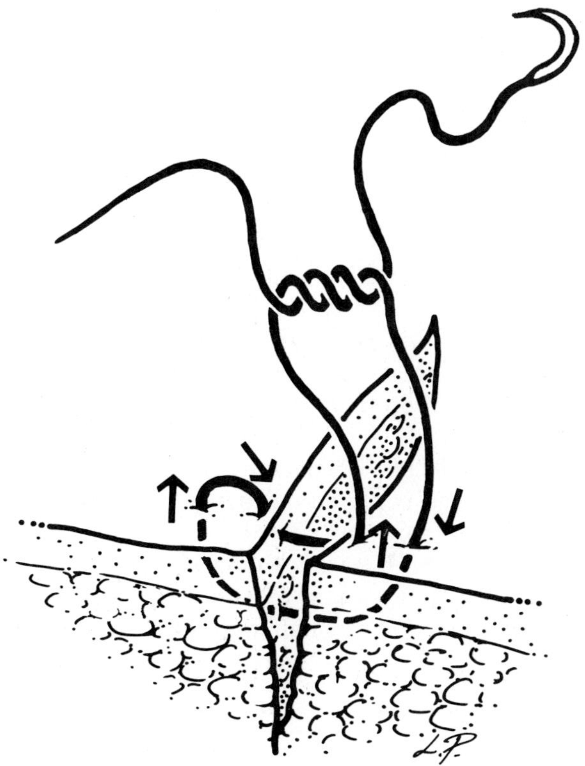

FIGURE 12–4. Mattress suture.

b. Explain the signs of infection
c. Arrange for suture removal
d. Consider the need for tetanus immunization and a prescription analgesic

Complications

Infection
Hematoma
Wound dehiscence
Retained foreign body
Missed injury to deeper structures

Pearls and Pitfalls

1. "Prophylactic" systemic antibiotics do not reduce the incidence of wound infection and are not indicated for routine laceration care. A short course of antibiotics may be beneficial when the laceration is very contaminated or associated with a fracture or joint penetration. Debridement, pressure irrigation, and a topical antibiotic prevent wound infections.
2. Many short, simple lacerations (especially on the face) are readily closed without tension by surgical tapes (e.g., butterfly bandages or Steri-strips). These closures are less traumatic, especially for children, probably less prone to infection, and may give a better cosmetic result. This closure should not be used in moist areas or for lacerations under tension or across joint lines.
3. The number of suture knots needed to prevent slippage varies with the type of suture material:
   a. Wire (2)
   b. Silk, braided (3)
   c. Multifilaments, nylon, Vicryl, Dexon, catgut (4)
4. Hemostasis is best achieved by local pressure. It is almost never necessary to clamp and tie bleeders in simple skin lacerations. The skin sutures will control them.
5. Laceration closure by staples gives good results and is faster than sewing, so you might want to consider this technique for long lacerations on the trunk or extremities.
6. Your laceration repairs will go faster if you learn how to hold and use the needle holder and suture scissors at the same time so you do not have to put one down, pick up the other, use it, put it down, pick up the other, etc (Figure 12–5).
7. A nice dressing for digits can be made by cutting a square dressing as shown in Figure 12–6. The digit is placed on the wide part of the dressing with the tip at the base of the narrow part. The narrow part is then folded back over the digit and finally the wide part is wrapped around the digit.
8. Curved or jagged lacerations may be difficult to align. Start the closure where you can rejoin clear-cut landmarks on each side of the wound.

Reference

Extensive experience

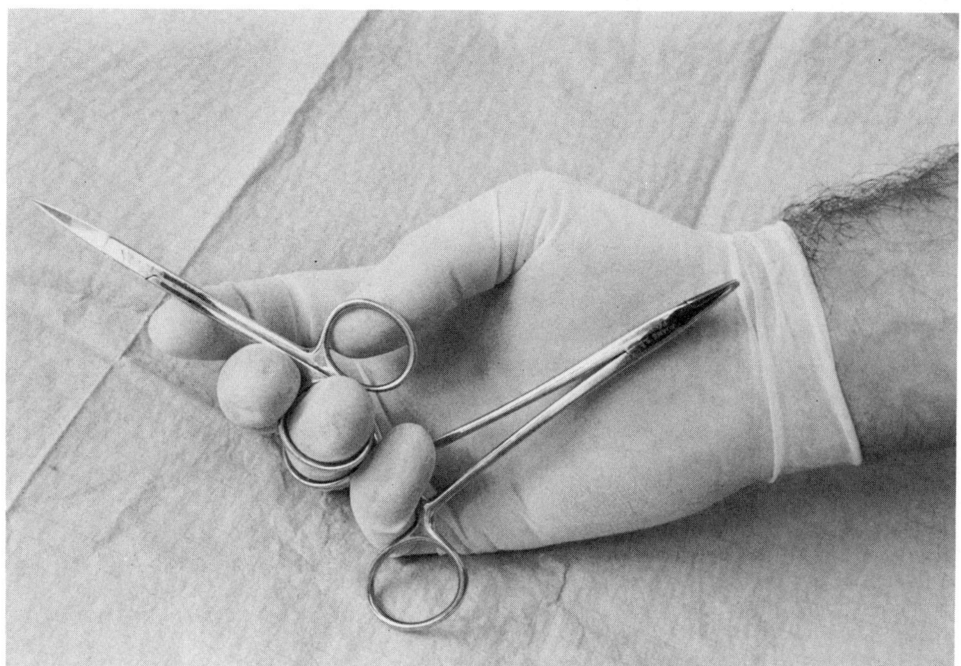

FIGURE 12–5. Holding the instruments.

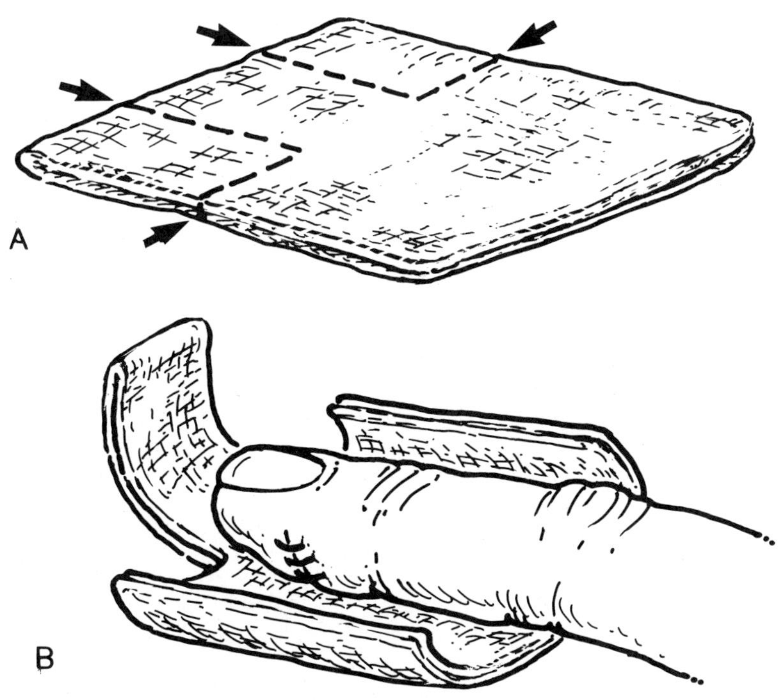

FIGURE 12–6. Finger dressing.

13 Nasal Packing

MICHAEL S. JASTREMSKI, MD

Indication

Control of nasal hemorrhage

Contraindications

Ability to control hemorrhage by simple means

Granulocytopenia (relative—severity of hemorrhage needs to be weighed against risk of life-threatening infection)

Equipment

Examining chair

Headlight (or ENT mirror and light source)

Nasal speculum

Kidney basin

Suction

Cotton-tipped applicators

4 × 4-inch gauze pads

Drape to protect the patient's clothing

Bayonet forceps

Hemostats

Silver nitrate sticks

Surgical foam (Gelfoam)

Prepackaged ½-inch × 6-foot petrolatum gauze strips with antibiotic ointment

Scissors

Local anesthetic

Mask

Gown

Eye shield

Gloves

For posterior packing, above equipment plus the following:

Specifically designed balloon device for nasal tamponade

or

Foley catheter (No. 16 with 5-ml balloon)

or

Gauze

Surgical tubing

Umbilical clamp (or hemostat)

1-0 silk suture

Rubber suction catheter

Forceps

Universal Precautions

1. Wear mask, gown, and gloves.
2. Use an eye shield.

Technique

1. Obtain a careful history and examination to discover treatable causes (e.g., hypertension, coagulopathy) or other injuries. Check the patient's blood pressure and lower it if it is elevated (as a rough guide, systolic > 180 or diastolic > 90). Obtain blood for type and cross-match and coagulation studies if clinically indicated. Obtain nasal x-ray film if patient has a history of acute trauma.
2. Start an intravenous drip of Ringer's lactate if massive hemorrhage, unstable vital signs, or a need to acutely lower the blood pressure is present.
3. While doing steps 1 and 2, have the patient (or do it yourself if the patient cannot) maintain constant pressure by pinching the nose between the thumb and first finger as close to the facial bones as possible.
4. Explain the procedure to the patient and obtain consent.
5. Position the patient sitting in the examination chair and stand facing the patient.
6. Cover the patient's clothes with a drape or gown and hand him or her the kidney basin to spit in.
7. Make sure that the suction and headlight are working.
8. Put on mask, eye shield, gown, headlight, and gloves.
9. Determine the site of bleeding.
   a. Localize the bleeding to one naris (although both sides may be simultaneously bleeding, especially with trauma).
   b. Determine if the bleeding site is anterior, superior, or posterior. Anterior bleeding from Kiesselbach's area on the nasal septum accounts for 90% of epistaxis, is usually due to nasal irritation, and is usually easily controlled. Superior and posterior epistaxis is more likely to be associated with another medical problem, is more common in older patients, and may be difficult to control.
   c. Careful examination, aided by removal of blood with cotton-tipped applicators or suction, should reveal the bleeding site. Anterior hemorrhages are easily visualized. With superior hemorrhages, the bleeding site will not be visualized but blood will be seen dripping from above the superior turbinate. Posterior hemorrhages are usually brisk with lots of blood flowing out both anteriorly and into the nasopharynx.
10. Control of anterior bleeding
    a. If the bleeding persists after the initial effort at pressure control (step 3), repeat this yourself.
    b. If the bleeding stops with pressure, advise the patient to relax and not cough, sneeze, blow, or pick the nose. Tell them you will be back in 30 minutes to make sure the bleeding has not restarted. Go see other patients, have dinner, read a journal, or otherwise amuse yourself for 30 to 60 minutes. Then return and recheck the patient. If the bleeding has not restarted, discharge the patient with instructions to pinch the nose for 10 minutes by the clock if the bleeding resumes before returning to the emergency department; not to cough, blow, sneeze, or pick the

nose; and to use a humidifier or saline spray if the cause was nasal drying and cracking.

c. If the bleeding persists after you have personally applied pressure for at least 5 minutes, then the active bleeding site should be cauterized. This is best done chemically with a silver nitrate stick.
   1) Dry the bleeding site with a cotton-tipped applicator or suction.
   2) Then touch the silver nitrate–coated portion of the stick to the bleeding site for several seconds, being careful not to touch any normal mucosa.
   3) After cautery, place a small patch of Gelfoam in the bleeding site to absorb any pinpoint bleeders.
   4) Do as instructed in step 10b above.
d. If the nose is still bleeding after pressure and cautery, then an anterior nasal pack should be placed.
   1) Explain the procedure to the patient.
   2) Open the prepackaged container of ½-inch × 6-foot petrolatum gauze for nasal packing with the scissors.
   3) Hold the nasal speculum in your nondominant hand and use your dominant hand to manipulate the bayonet forceps.
   4) Grasp the gauze strip with the bayonet forceps, forming a loop that leaves the end of the packing outside the nose (Figure 13–1).

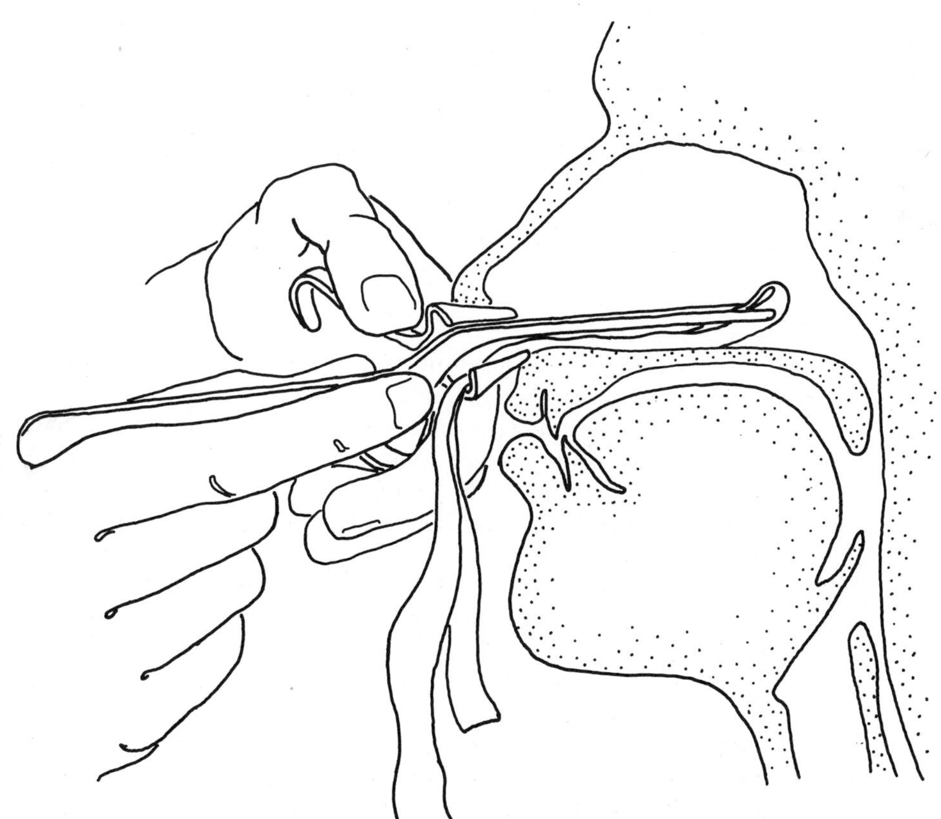

FIGURE 13–1. Anterior nasal pack, 1.

5) The anterior nasal cavity is then packed from *top* to *bottom* by inserting successive loops of packing into the nose. Each loop should be placed under the previous loops and as far posterior as possible (Figure 13–2).
6) Fill the nostril, but not too tightly since excessive pressure may cause ischemic necrosis.
7) When the nostril is fully packed, trim any remaining gauze with the scissors, leaving an inch of packing at each end outside the nose to facilitate removal.
8) Arrange for the patient to be seen in 12 to 24 hours for removal of the pack and provide the patient with a prescription for an analgesic such as acetaminophen (Tylenol) with codeine since these packs are uncomfortable. (Do not prescribe aspirin or other nonsteroidal anti-inflammatory agents because of their effect on platelet function.)

11. Control of superior bleeding. Superior epistaxis that does not respond to pressure will need to be controlled with an anterior nasal pack placed as described above. Cautery should not be attempted since the bleeding site cannot be directly visualized.
12. Control of posterior bleeding
    a. Posterior bleeding requires a posterior and anterior pack to control.
    b. Anesthetize the nose by inserting long cotton strips soaked with topical anesthesia (e.g., 2% cocaine) deep within the affected nostril. Leave these strips in place for 5 minutes and repeat the application if the anesthesia is not sufficient. Remember to leave an end outside the nose so the cotton strips can be easily removed when anesthesia is achieved. This is a very uncomfortable procedure so systemic sedation is often necessary to supplement the local anesthesia.
    c. If using a specifically designed nasal tamponade balloon catheter:
        1) Lubricate the device.
        2) Pass the tip into the bleeding naris well into the posterior pharynx.
        3) Inflate the posterior balloon with the recommended volume of air (check the package insert for this information).
        4) Gently pull the catheter out of the nostril until the posterior balloon is impacted in the posterior choana.
        5) Inflate the anterior balloon.
    d. If using a Foley catheter:
        1) Cut a 1-inch piece of surgical tubing and slide it over the balloon end of the catheter up to the valve at the other end.
        2) Lubricate the Foley catheter and pass it into the bleeding naris until the tip is visible in the nasopharynx.
        3) Inflate the balloon with 10 to 15 ml of air.
        4) Gently pull the catheter out of the nostril until the balloon is impacted in the posterior choana.
        5) While keeping the Foley catheter in the middle of the naris and under constant traction, place an anterior pack around the catheter.
        6) Slide the surgical tubing down snugly against the anterior pack and place an umbilical clamp (or hemostat) distal to the surgical tubing to hold the catheter in place.
    e. If using a conventional gauze pack:
        1) Fold a gauze 4×4-inch pad into a cone-shaped pack, secure it with umbilical tape or 1-0 silk suture (do not cut the ends), and lubricate it with a broad-spectrum antibiotic ointment.

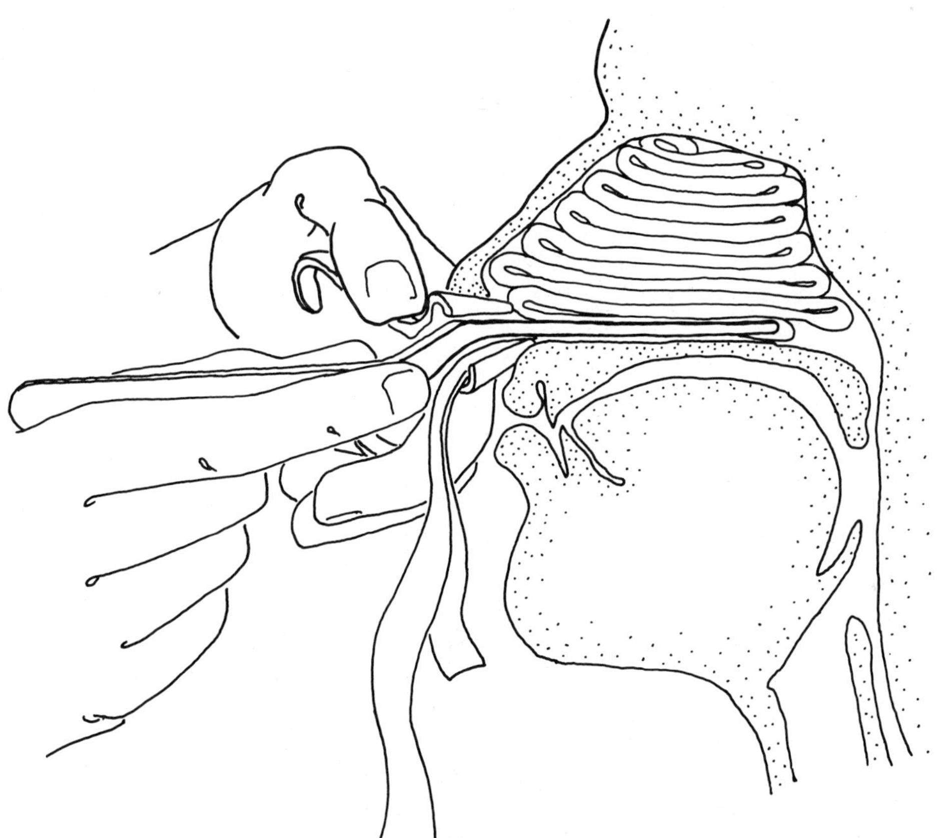

FIGURE 13–2. Anterior nasal pack, 2.

2) Pass a small lubricated suction catheter through the affected naris into the posterior pharynx where it can be grasped with a forceps and pulled out the mouth (Figure 13–3).
3) Tie the gauze pack to the suction catheter with an end of the umbilical tape or suture. Leave the other end of the tape or suture long enough to come out of the mouth. This will be used to retrieve the pack when it is removed (Figure 13–3).
4) Pull the suction catheter out the nose, grasp the tape or suture, and gently pull on it to impact the gauze pack in the posterior choana (Figure 13–4). It may be helpful to use a finger through the mouth to push the pack up into the nasopharynx.
5) Place an anterior pack.
6) Tie the end of tape or suture coming from the nose around a rolled-up gauze pad held firmly against the anterior pack (Figure 13–5).
7) Tape the end of the suture or umbilical tape coming from the mouth to the patient's cheek.

13. Place the patient on systemic prophylactic antibiotics.
14. All patients with a posterior nasal pack require admission to the hospital.

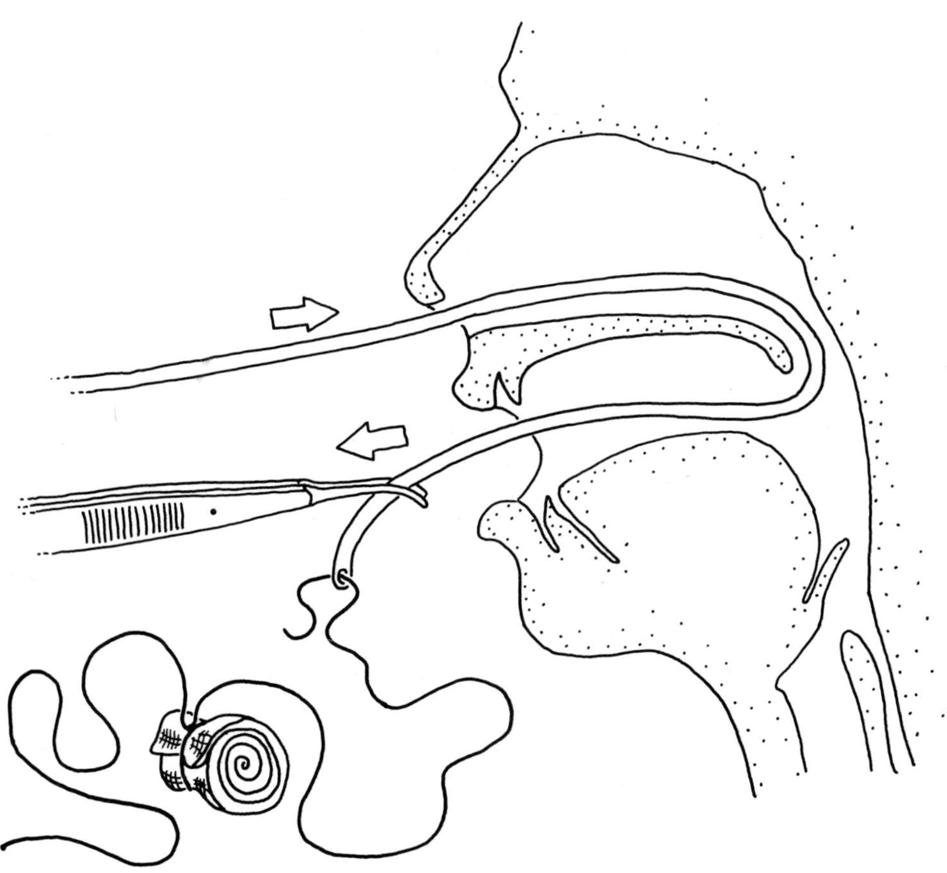

FIGURE 13–3. Posterior nasal pack, 1.

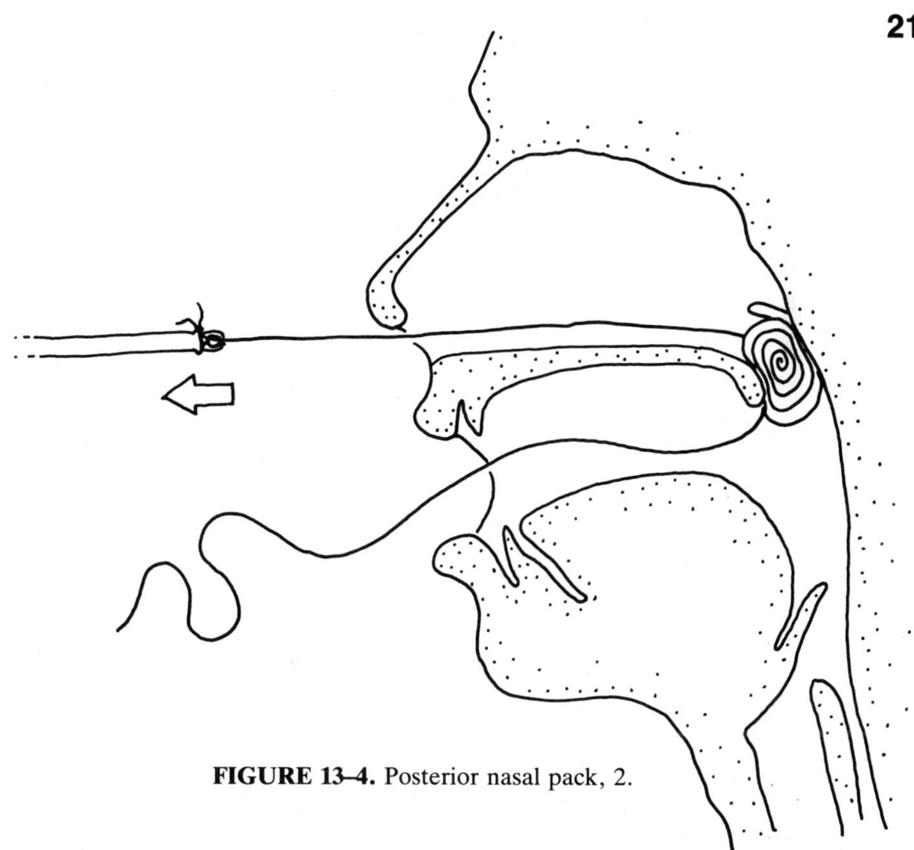

FIGURE 13–4. Posterior nasal pack, 2.

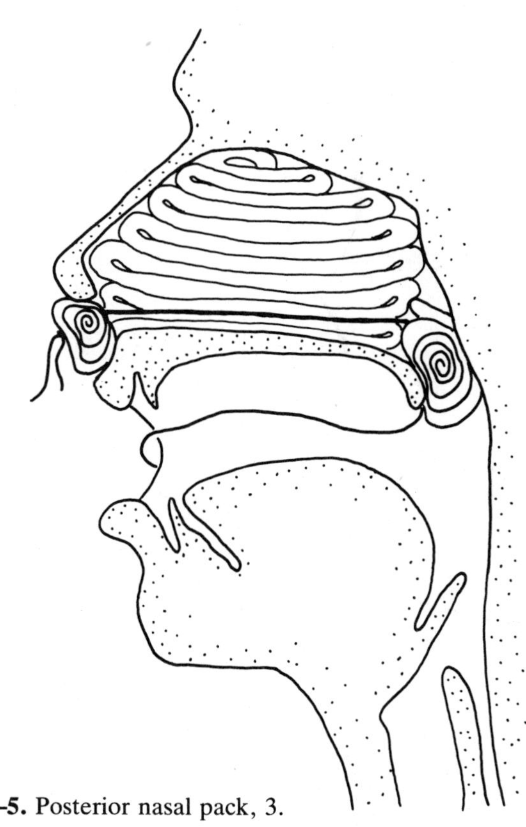

FIGURE 13–5. Posterior nasal pack, 3.

All persons caring for a patient with a posterior nasal pack should know how to remove it should it become dislodged and obstruct the airway.

Complications

Infection
Continued bleeding
Airway obstruction
Ischemic necrosis of nasal and palatal structures
Pain
Hypoventilation and hypoxia
Dysphagia
Death

Pearls and Pitfalls

1. Properly applied pressure will stop almost all anterior hemorrhages.
2. The specially designed balloon catheters for posterior packing are simple to use and should be tried first if available. However, they have a lower success rate than a conventional gauze pack, which should be the next step if bleeding persists after placement of a balloon catheter.
3. Some epistaxis will not stop even with perfectly applied packing. These patients need surgical intervention.
4. Cocaine provides excellent anesthesia and vasoconstriction. However, it has a narrow therapeutic to toxic ratio and there currently is a severe shortage of medicinal cocaine. Lidocaine 4% and epinephrine in combination may be used as an alternative to cocaine.
5. Do not use a vasoconstrictor until you have identified the bleeding site.

Reference

Abelson TI, Witt WJ: Otolaryngologic procedures. In Roberts JR, Hedges JR (eds): Clinical Procedures in Emergency Medicine, pp 927–936. Philadelphia, WB Saunders, 1985.

14

Neurologic

Emergency Temporal Burr Hole in Patients with Clinical Signs of Progressive Tentorial Herniation

JEFFREY WINFIELD, MD, PhD

Although contemporary management of severe head injuries always includes early emergency department stabilization and urgent computed tomography, delays in patient transfer to a hospital with computed tomography, or to the admitting hospital's computed tomography suite may interpose a detrimental time delay until the needed surgical decompression of the brain stem in patients with progressive signs of tentorial herniation. Up to 70% of patients with clinical signs of "progressive" brain stem herniation have a surgical intracranial mass, most of which will be extra-axial (either an epidural or subdural hematoma). More important than its diagnostic value is *early therapeutic decompression,* preventing further irreversible brain stem injury.

Indications

The initial emergency department management of increased intracranial pressure, following airway protection with cervical spine stabilization and blood pressure stabilization, includes

1. Hyperventilation to a P_{CO_2} of 28 to 30 mm Hg
2. Intravenous furosemide (0.1 mg/kg) and mannitol (1.0 g/kg)

The majority of patients will have stabilization of their neurologic status following these medical measures; however, there is a group of patients who will show continued deterioration. In this clearly definable group of patients, consideration for the placement of a temporal fossa burr hole should be given.

Clinical Signs

A patient has the following presenting sign or progresses to this neurologic status following medical measures to control intracranial pressure: *unilateral dilated and fixed pupil without response to light.*

These pupillary findings invariably occur in association with either a contralateral or, less commonly, an ipsilateral hemiparesis or hemiplegia. The patient can alternatively exhibit motor responses of either decorticate or decerebrate posture.

In the patient older than age 30 who presents following a low velocity head injury, such as from a fall or from being struck by a car, with a single fixed and dilated pupil there is an extremely high probability of an extra-axial mass lesion on the side of the dilated pupil.

The burr hole should always be made on the side of the dilated pupil and/or the side of the obvious direct trauma.

Contraindications

Flaccid motor exam with bilateral fixed and dilated pupils. In one review of 100 patients treated with emergency burr holes prior to computed tomography, there were only three survivors who presented to the emergency department with this neurologic status. Furthermore, the results suggest that in patients younger than 30 and with "a high velocity head injury" such as occurs from a motor vehicle accident, the burr hole exploration was also less likely to be positive.

Immediate availability of a neurosurgeon

Equipment

- Razor
- Cap, mask, and eye shield
- Sterile gown
- Sterile gloves
- Suture material (3-0 chromic, 4-0 nylon)
- Sterile drapes
- Betadine skin preps
- Adequate light source
- Sterile marking pen
- Monopolar disposable coagulator
- Sterile saline for irrigation
- 20-ml syringe
- 20-gauge angiocatheter
- Burr hole set, which includes
  - Hemostats and dissectors
  - Knife with No. 15 and No. 10 blades
  - Trephine device
  - Sterile suction
  - Bone wax
  - Small self-retaining retractor
- Sterile scissors

Universal Precautions

1. Wear cap, mask, eye shield, and sterile gown and gloves.

Technique

1. Informed consent may not be possible. This is an acute life-threatening emergency.
2. Position the patient supine on a stretcher with the head turned 90 degrees so that the side of the head with the dilated pupil is parallel to the floor and is the up side. Place a rolled towel under the ipsilateral shoulder to facilitate positioning. Stand at the side of the stretcher facing the patient's head (Figure 14–1).

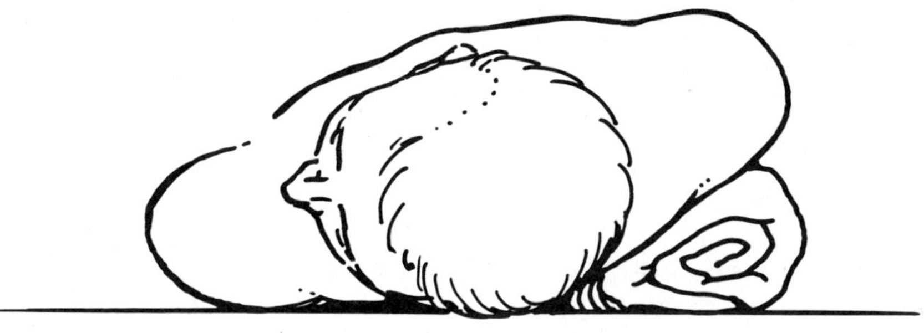

FIGURE 14–1. Patient position for emergency temporal burr hole.

3. Shave the area overlying the temporalis muscle in front of the ear down to the zygomatic arch (removing all sideburns).
4. Put on cap, mask, sterile gown, eye shield, and sterile gloves.
5. Thoroughly scrub the area for 5 minutes with a Betadine prep. The surgical field is then draped.
6. Palpate the superficial temporalis artery so that you know its course in the skin. *The skull will be drilled at a point 2 fingerbreadths in front of the ear and 2 fingerbreadths above the zygomatic arch* (Figure 14–2). Mark the skin

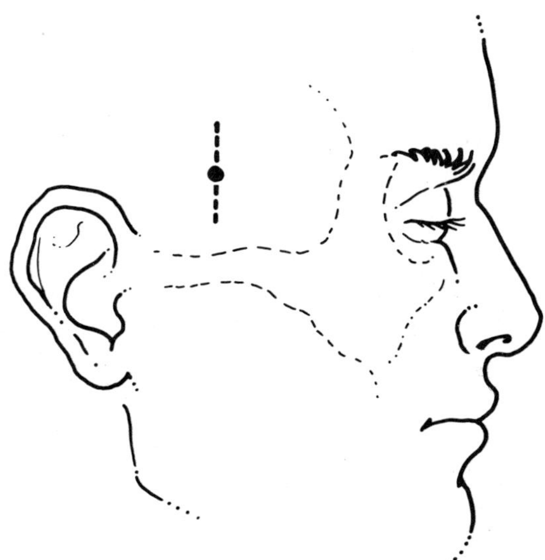

FIGURE 14–2. Location of incision for emergency temporal burr hole.

at this point. Then make a vertical skin incision approximately three-fourths of an inch above and below the drill point. The incision can be carried down through the underlying soft tissue and muscle layers to the bone. Place the self-retaining retractor in the incision, deep enough to retract all soft tissue layers. Spreading it wide open will usually result in complete hemostasis. Hemostats or cautery can be used to stop point source bleeding in the scalp edges and underlying muscle.

7. Using a dissector, scrap the periosteum off the bone.
8. Then, using the drill/trephine, make a hole in the skull. The skull is only 3 to 8 mm thick at this point. Since the skull has three layers (outer cortical layer, diploë, and inner table), the drilling usually will have three phases —hard, easy, and then hard again. The drill will often bind up as it passes through the inner table, at which point the drill is withdrawn (Figure 14–3).
9. Irrigate the wound using a 20-ml syringe and 20-gauge angiocatheter and gently begin suction in the burr hole. If an epidural hematoma is present, there will be an immediate excrescence of dark clotted blood. Tease out further clot using suction and additional irrigation. If the exposed dura begins to pulsate, then the procedure is complete. The incision is closed in several layers using a standard scalp laceration suturing technique.
10. If the dura is visualized and no clot extrudes, then carefully nick the dura using the tip of the monopolar cautery after it has turned "red hot." If you are rewarded with a clot, the dural incision can be enlarged with the cautery to the edges of the burr hole. Carefully suction and irrigate out the clot. Because of increased intracranial pressure, both epidural and subdural clots will usually self-extrude with little assistance required. The dural incision can be left open and the scalp incision closed as above (Figure 14–4).
11. If no clot is found, repeat the procedure on the other side.
12. Manage other injuries as needed. Obtain a computed tomographic scan of the head.

Complications

Bleeding
Infection

Note: The risk of infection or further brain injury from this procedure is low considering the extremely high mortality in this patient population.

References

Andrews B, Pitts L, Lovely M, Bartkowski H: Is computer tomography scanning necessary in patients with tentorial herniation? Neurosurgery 19:408–414, 1986.

Andrews B, Ross A, Pitts L: Surgical exploration before computer tomography scanning in children with traumatic tentorial herniation. Surg Neurol 32:434–438, 1989.

Mahoney B, Rockswold G, Ruiz E, Clinton J: Emergency twist drill trephination. Neurosurgery 8:551–554, 1981.

McKissock W, Richardson A, Bloom W: Subdural haematoma: A review of 389 cases. Lancet 1:1365–1369, 1960.

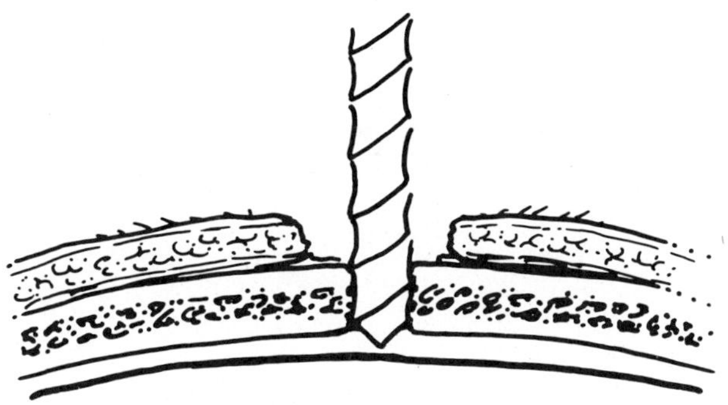

FIGURE 14–3. Drilling the skull.

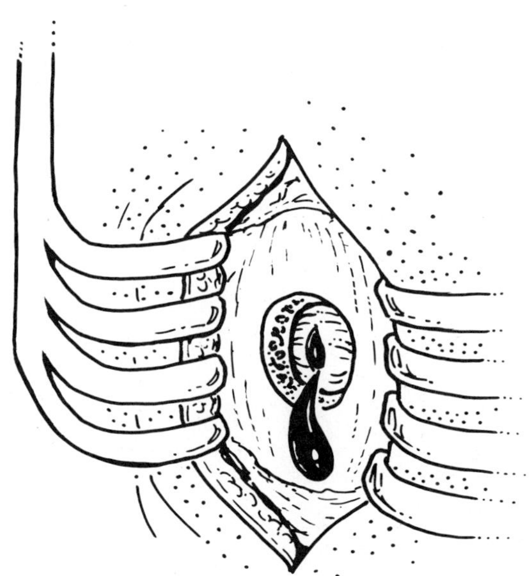

FIGURE 14–4. Dural incision.

Intracranial Pressure Monitoring

CONNIE WALLECK, RN

Indications

Traumatic brain injury
Space-occupying lesions
Suspected intracranial hypertension
Identification of intracranial pressure waves
Measurement of brain compliance
Calculation of cerebral perfusion pressure
Assessment of interventions for increased intracranial pressure

Contraindications

Known ventriculitis (do not use intraventricular monitoring)
Severe coagulopathy

Equipment

Razor
Local anesthetic
Ventriculostomy tray, which includes:
- Twist drill (sterile)
- Knife with No. 11 blade
- Needle holder
- Hemostats
- Sterile suction
- Self-retaining retractor
- Bone wax
- Sterile scissors
- Monopolar coagulator
- Suture material (3–0 chromic and 4–0 nylon)

Monitoring device—intraventricular catheter, subarachnoid bolt, epidural transducer, or fiberoptic catheter

Transducer setup (except with epidural transducer or fiberoptic catheter)

Stopcocks

Sterile saline solution without preservatives (to flush transducer and prime tubing)

Dressing materials

Drainage bag (if intraventricular catheter is being used)

Betadine scrub

Betadine solution

Sterile drapes

Mask, gown, and eye shield

Sterile gloves

Topical antibiotic ointment

Universal Precautions

1. Wear mask, cap, and sterile gown and gloves.
2. Use an eye shield.

Technique (Intraventricular Catheter)

1. Explain procedure to the patient or surrogate and obtain consent.
2. Ideal positioning is with patient supine with head of bed elevated to 45 to 90 degrees (Figure 14–5).

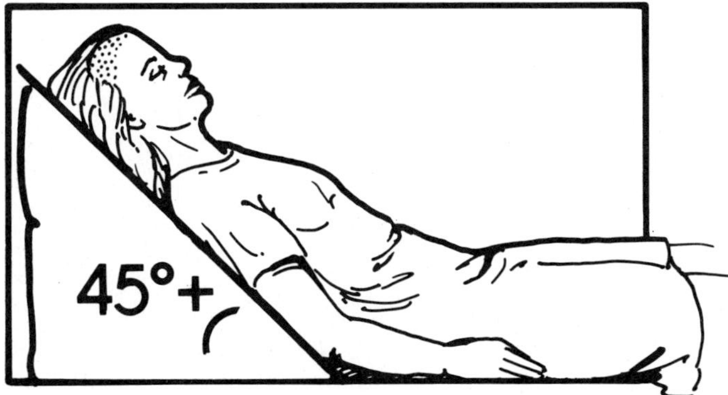

FIGURE 14–5. Patient position for insertion of an intracranial pressure monitor.

3. Stand at top of bed facing patient's head.
4. Shave scalp over right frontal hemicranium.
5. Assemble transducer and drainage bag.
6. Open sterile ventriculostomy tray.
7. Put on mask, cap, eye shield, and sterile gown and gloves.
8. Prep scalp with Betadine.
9. Infiltrate scalp down to the periosteum with local anesthetic at the incision site.
10. Make an incision and then a twist drill hole through the skull 2.5 cm to the right of the midline and 1.5 cm in front of the coronal suture (Figure 14–6).
11. Open dura, arachnoid, and pia with a nick from the No. 11 blade.
12. Introduce catheter (or No. 5 or No. 8 pediatric feeding tube) through the twist drill hole with a stylette into the right frontal horn of the lateral ventricle (a distance of approximately 5 cm) (Figure 14–7).
13. Remove the stylette.
14. Tunnel the catheter under the scalp and bring it out through a separate puncture wound behind the twist drill incision.
15. Connect catheter to stopcock and T port attached to the transducer.
16. Balance and calibrate the transducer.
17. Connect T port to drainage system.
18. Suture catheter to scalp and close the incision.
19. Apply antibiotic ointment and a sterile dressing covering incision and exit point up to the stopcock.
20. Obtain a lateral skull x-ray film to check catheter position.

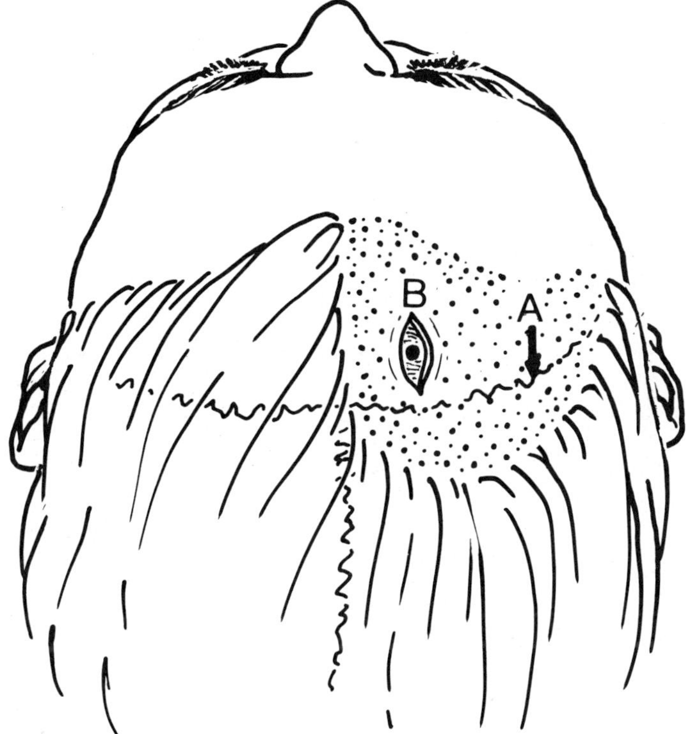

FIGURE 14–6. *A,* Coronal suture; *B,* incision.

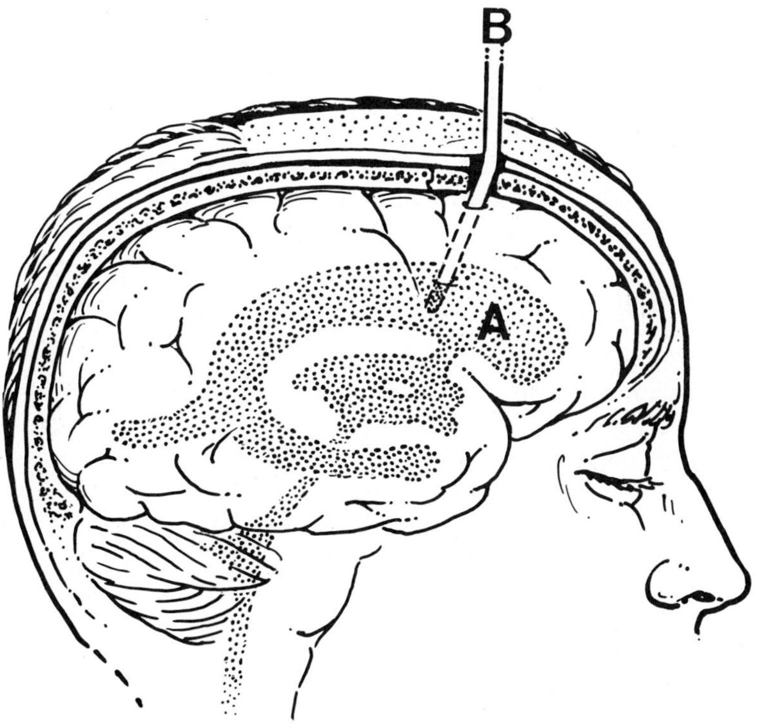

FIGURE 14–7. *A,* Lateral ventricle; *B,* catheter.

CHANGING THE INTRAVENTRICULAR CATHETER DRAINAGE BAG

Indications

Routine change at least every 24 hours
Full drainage bag
Poor drainage due to clots in the tubing
Contamination of the drainage bag

Equipment

New drainage bag
Sterile 4 × 4-inch gauze pads
Safety pin
Tape
Sterile gloves
Mask

Universal Precautions

1. Wear mask and sterile gloves.

Technique

1. Close clamp on T port to prevent inadvertent drainage of cerebrospinal fluid.
2. Open T port/drainage bag connection (avoid tugging on intraventricular catheter).
3. Disconnect old drainage bag.
4. Insert top of new drainage bag into T port.
5. Connect T port to bag tightly. Secure with tape.
6. Pin the drainage bag to bed linen with the level of the highest point of the system being 7 to 20 cm (usually 15 cm) above the level of the ventricles.

Complications

Inadvertent removal of intraventricular catheter
Fall of nonsecured bag to the floor, causing rapid draining of the ventricles leading to their collapse
Subdural or subarachnoid hemorrhage
Infection
Inaccurate drainage measurements

REMOVAL OF INTRAVENTRICULAR CATHETER

Indications

Suspected infection
No need for continued monitoring

Equipment

Sterile specimen cup
Sterile 4 × 4-inch gauze pads
Sterile scissors
Suture removal set
Tape
Sterile gloves
Mask

Universal Precautions

1. Wear mask and sterile gloves.

Technique

1. Remove sutures around the intraventricular catheter.
2. Remove the catheter.
3. Cut off tip of the catheter with sterile scissors and drop the tip into the sterile cup.
4. Dress the incision and exit wound with 4 × 4-inch gauze pads.
5. Send the catheter tip to the laboratory for culture.

INSERTION OF SUBARACHNOID/SUBDURAL BOLT

Indications

Traumatic brain injury
Space-occupying lesions
Suspected intracranial hypertension
Identification of intracranial pressure waves
Measurement of brain compliance
Calculation of cerebral perfusion pressure
Assessment of interventions for increased intracranial pressure

Contraindication

Intracranial pressure greater than 60 mm Hg, since this will obliterate the subdural space

Equipment

- Subarachnoid/subdural bolt with screwdriver
- Ventriculostomy tray, which includes:
  - Twist drill (sterile)
  - Knife with No. 11 blade
  - Needle holder
  - Hemostats
  - Sterile suction
  - Self-retaining retractor
  - Sterile scissors
  - Monopolar coagulator
  - Bone wax
  - Suture material (3-0 chronic, 4-0 nylon)
- Razor
- Local anesthetic
- Transducer
- Stopcock
- Sterile saline solution to prime bolt and transducer
- Betadine solution
- Betadine scrub
- Sterile drapes
- Dressing materials
- Mask, cap, eye shield
- Sterile gown and gloves
- Topical antibiotic ointment

Universal Precautions

1. Wear mask, cap, and sterile gown and gloves.
2. Use an eye shield.

Technique

1. Explain the procedure to the patient or surrogate and obtain consent.
2. Ideal positioning is with patient supine with head of bed elevated to 45 to 90 degrees (see Figure 14–5).
3. Stand at top of bed facing the patient's head.
4. Shave scalp over right frontal hemicranium.

5. Assemble transducer.
6. Open sterile ventriculostomy tray.
7. Put on mask, cap, eye shield, and sterile gown and gloves.
8. Prep scalp with Betadine.
9. Infiltrate scalp down to the periosteum with local anesthetic.
10. Make a 2-cm skin incision and then a twist drill hole through the skull 2.5 cm to the right of the midline and 1.5 cm in front of the coronal suture (see Figure 14–6).
11. Once twist drill hole is made, cut through dura with an X incision using the No. 11 blade.
12. Insert bolt to level of dural incision or slightly lower to penetrate the arachnoid space.
13. Ensure bolt is tightly in place with no fluid leak around bolt (Figure 14–8).
14. Instill 1 ml of normal saline through bolt.
15. Attach transducer to stopcock at the top of the bolt.
16. Apply antibiotic ointment and a sterile dressing around bolt.

Complications

Scalp infection

Debris blocking tip of bolt, causing dampened waveform

Meningitis

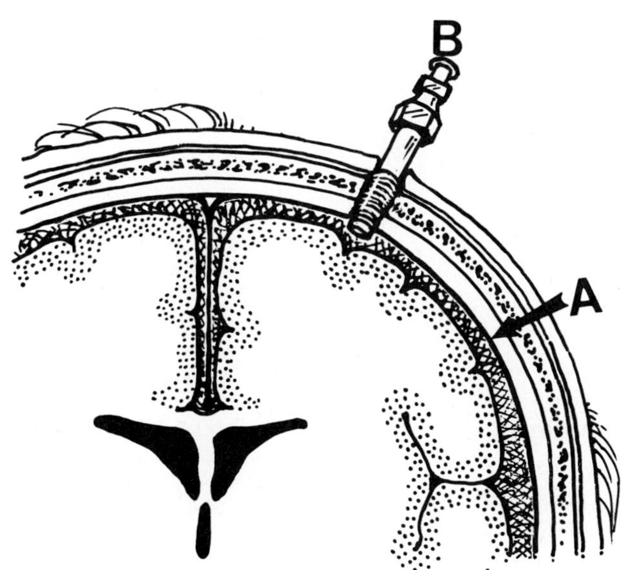

FIGURE 14–8. *A,* Dura; *B,* monitoring bolt.

INSERTION OF EPIDURAL TRANSDUCER

Indications

Traumatic brain injury
Space-occupying lesions
Suspected intracranial hypertension
Identification of intracranial pressure waves
Measurement of brain compliance
Calculation of cerebral perfusion pressure
Assessment of interventions for increased intracranial pressure

Contraindication

Intracranial pressure greater than 60 mm Hg (readings may be inaccurate)

Equipment

- Razor
- Local anesthetic
- Ventriculostomy tray, which includes:
  - Twist drill (sterile)
  - Knife with No. 11 blade
  - Needle holder
  - Hemostats
  - Sterile suction
  - Self-retaining retractor
  - Sterile scissors
  - Monopolar coagulator
  - Bone wax
  - Suture material (3-0 chromic, 4-0 nylon)
- Monitoring device—epidural transducer or fiberoptic catheter
- Stopcocks
- Dressing materials and topical antibiotic ointment
- Betadine scrub
- Betadine solution
- Sterile drapes
- Mask, cap, eye shield
- Sterile gown and gloves

Universal Precautions

1. Wear sterile gown and gloves, mask, and cap.
2. Use an eye shield.

Technique

1. Explain the procedure to the patient or surrogate and obtain consent.
2. Ideal positioning is with the patient supine with head of bed elevated to 45 to 90 degrees (see Figure 14–5).
3. Stand at top of bed facing patient's head.
4. Shave scalp over right frontal hemicranium.

5. Assemble transducer.
6. Open sterile ventriculostomy tray.
7. Put on mask, cap, eye shield, and sterile gown and gloves.
8. Prep scalp with Betadine.
9. Infiltrate scalp down to the periosteum with local anesthetic.
10. Make a 2-cm skin incision and then a twist drill hole through the skull 2.5 cm to the right of the midline and 1.5 cm in front of the coronal suture (see Figure 14–6).
11. Slide self-contained transducer above dura. Transducer must be zero balanced prior to insertion (Figure 14–9).
12. Suture scalp incision around transducer wire.
13. Dress scalp wound using topical antibiotic ointment and a sterile occlusive dressing.

Complications

Inaccurate readings due to inability to rebalance transducer
Scalp infection

Pearls and Pitfalls

1. Do not connect an irrigation system to ventricular or bolt system.
2. Realign and rebalance transducer if bed level changes (or at least every 8 hours).
3. Check the monitoring system for leaking.
4. Sedate agitated patients adequately to prevent disconnection of system or dislodgement of monitoring device.

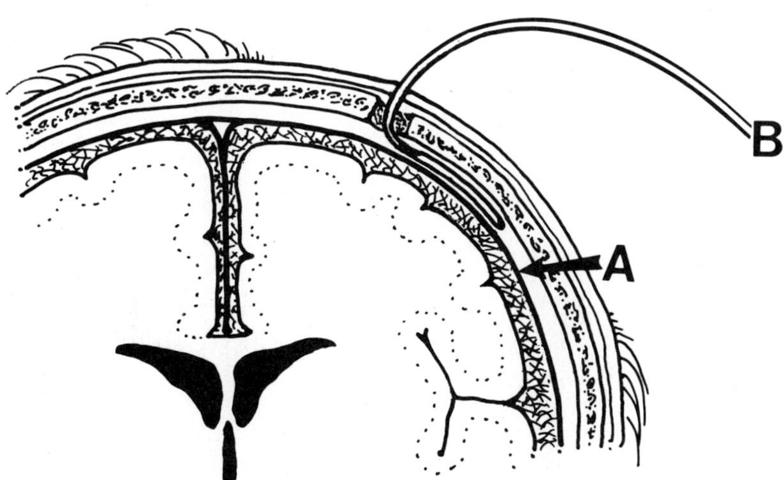

FIGURE 14–9. *A,* Dura; *B,* epidural transducer.

5. Measure brain compliance, if intraventricular catheter or bolt is being used, at least once a day.
   a. Introduce a small amount of sterile saline without preservative (1–2 ml) over 1 second and measure pressure. A 1-ml injection over 1 second causing less than 2 mm Hg increase in intracranial pressure is considered normal.
6. Daily testing of cerebrospinal fluid for cells and culture to identify infection with a ventricular catheter should be done.
7. Irrigation of an intraventricular catheter or bolt may be necessary if waveform is dampened.
   a. Irrigation should be done judiciously by a physician. The smallest amount of fluid to clear the blockage should be used. A spinal needle can be inserted through a bolt for irrigation purposes using 1-ml boluses of saline until no resistance is met.
8. Recognition of "A" or plateau waves is critical in management of these patients. "B" waves may be precursors of "A" waves and should be documented as well.

References

Hickman KM, Muwaswes M: Intracranial pressure monitoring: Review of risk factors associated with infection. Heart Lung 19:84–90, 1990.

Maryland Institute for Emergency Medical Services Systems, Baltimore, Maryland, Nursing Procedure Manual, 1984.

Robinet K: Increased intracranial pressure management with an intraventricular catheter. Neurosurg Nurs 17(6):95–104, 1985.

Lumbar Puncture

MARCY LAYTON, MD

Indications

Removal of cerebrospinal fluid for microscopic and chemical analysis.

In emergency setting the primary indication is to rule out infectious meningitis. Remember the meningitis pentad of fever, altered mental status, nuchal rigidity, headache, and photophobia.

Contraindications

Coagulopathy (relative)
Localized infection in lumbar region

Equipment

Note: The following usually come in a prepackaged kit.

20- or 22-gauge spinal needle with stylette
Betadine
1% lidocaine
Sterile field
Manometer with three-way stop-cock for pressure management
Four sterile tubes
Gauze sponges
5-ml syringe
25-gauge, 1-inch needle
20-gauge, 1½-inch needle
Sterile gloves
Mask and eye shield

Universal Precautions

1. Wear mask and sterile gloves.
2. Use an eye shield.

Technique

1. Explain the procedure to the patient and obtain consent.
2. Rule out increased intracranial pressure by fundoscopic examination or computed tomographic scan (if there is a very high index of suspicion).
3. Proper positioning of the patient is the key to success. The usual position is on one side, in the fetal position, with maximum neck and lower extremity flexion and the spinal column parallel to the table (Figure 14–10*A*).
4. Select and mark the L4–L5 or L3–L4 interspace.
5. Put on mask, eye shield, and sterile gloves.
6. Prep field with Betadine. Drape sterile field.
7. Anesthetize area with 1% lidocaine, first intradermally with the 25-gauge needle, followed by subcutaneous injection between the spinous processes with the longer 20-gauge needle.
8. Enter interspace with spinal needle/stylette, 20-gauge recommended. (Use 22-gauge or 25-gauge if concerned about increased intracranial pressure or a coagulopathy.) Entry site should be in the vertical middle of the interspace toward distal vertebra with needle parallel to the axis of the spine aimed toward the umbilicus (Figure 14–10*B*).
9. Once needle "pops" into the subarachnoid space, remove the stylette and attach the stopcock and manometer to the needle to measure the opening pressure. The patient's legs and neck should be straightened before measuring the pressure. If a free flow of cerebrospinal fluid is not obtained, try gently rotating the needle 180 degrees.
10. Obtain samples of fluid (1 ml per tube appropriately, except if cytology is needed try for 5 ml in one tube).
11. Measure closing pressure.
12. Remove catheter and place bandage over site.
13. Patient should remain prone for at least 4 hours to avoid post–lumbar puncture headache.
14. Fluid should be sent for appropriate analysis:
    a. Tube 1—Gram stain and bacterial culture (fungal, viral, acid-fast bacillus if indicated)
    b. Tube 2—Chemistry (protein, glucose, lactate dehydrogenase)
    c. Tube 3—Serology, cytology, or immunoelectrophoresis if indicated
    d. Tube 4—Cell count and differential

Complications

Headache
Infection
Nerve damage
Herniation if unsuspected mass lesion
Spinal epidural hematoma

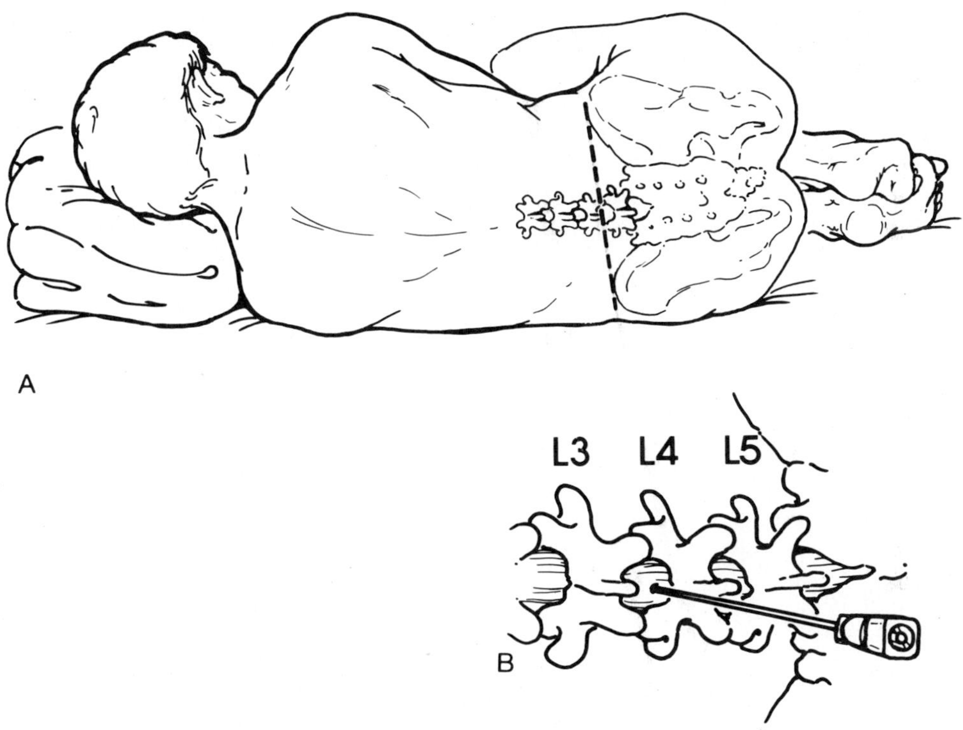

FIGURE 14–10. Lumbar puncture.

Pearls and Pitfalls

1. Appropriate positioning is the key to success. If the patient is delerious, extra personnel to help hold the patient are essential.
2. The procedure may also be performed with the patient seated and leaning forward on a pillow placed on a bedside stand. In fact, it is often easier to find the landmarks and accomplish a difficult lumbar puncture using this position.
3. If unsuccessful on the first attempt, withdraw the needle from the skin and reattempt at a slightly different angle. Striking bone indicates that the needle is being directed away from the midline.
4. Sometimes twisting the needle 90 to 180 degrees will initiate flow.
5. If the ligaments are extremely calcified in an elderly patient, it may feel like you are hitting bone.
6. If the patient has had previous spinal surgery or an infectious process in the lumbar region, a neurosurgery consultation may be needed to obtain fluid from the cervical spinal canal.
7. If there is a strong suspicion of bacterial meningitis, antibiotics should be given before the lumbar puncture. (In our emergency department one of our quality assurance monitors is institution of antibiotic therapy within 30 minutes of the time of presentation when meningitis is suspected.) This will not affect the subsequent results of cerebrospinal fluid culture if the lumbar puncture is accomplished within 3 to 4 hours.

Reference

Extensive experience

Ventriculoperitoneal/Atrial Shunt Tap

JEFFREY WINFIELD, MD, PhD

Indications

Shunt obstruction with acute brain stem herniation

Except in the single clinical presentation of progressive loss of brain stem reflexes, there are no emergent situations that would warrant the tapping of a ventriculoperitoneal/atrial shunt. The suspicion of a shunt infection is not an indication for a shunt tap, and the patient can be expediently referred to a hospital with a neurosurgeon. In more than 70% of proven shunt obstructions, the ventricular end is the obstructed portion of the shunt, necessitating the need for a direct ventricular puncture when the patient presents *in extremis*.

Clinical Presentation

A patient with a ventriculoperitoneal shunt obstruction presents to the emergency department with a *rapidly* progressive decline in mental status reported by the caretaker. The patient is unresponsive to verbal commands; vital signs may show hypertension and bradycardia (Cushing reflex = increased intracranial pressure) and a respiratory pattern indicative of central hyperventilation or Cheyne-Stokes breathing.

Examination of brain stem reflexes shows the following:

1. Enlarged and often oval pupils that are sluggishly reactive to light.
2. Corneal and gag reflexes may also be depressed.
3. Response to central or extremity painful stimulus may be either decorticate or decerebrate posturing.

This picture is synonymous with impending brain stem herniation, which, if it occurs, will be heralded by sudden respiratory arrest and the patient becoming flaccid with fixed and dilated pupils. Patients with obstructed ventriculoperitoneal shunts who progress to central herniation have an extremely poor prognosis, and, therefore, even direct ventricular puncture can be justified in this specific clinical setting.

Contraindication

None if the above clinical picture exists.

Equipment

Razor
Cap, mask, and gown
Sterile gloves
Betadine skin preps
23-gauze butterfly needles
Eye shield
2×2-inch gauze pads
5- and 10-ml syringes
20-gauge spinal tap needle
Preservative-free normal saline
Sterile drape with a center hole cut

Universal Precautions

1. Wear mask, cap, and sterile gloves and gown.
2. Use an eye shield.

Technique

1. Obtain a lateral skull x-ray film. Irrespective of the manufacturer of the shunt, the shunt will have either a "Rickam reservoir" or a right-angle connector at the exit point of the ventricular catheter from the skull. A piece of tubing will then run posterior to a shunt valve, which will have a pliable reservoir in it. The Rickam reservoir should be tapped if present; otherwise the valve can be tapped. Figure 14–11*A* and *B* shows a lateral skull x-ray film of a patient with and without a Rickam reservoir, respectively.
2. Shave a 50 cent piece–sized area over the tap sight.
3. Put on cap, mask, eye shield, and sterile gloves and gown.
4. Proceed to sterilize the skin with several applications of Betadine prep solution. Then place the sterile drape to cover the unshaven hair.
5. Using the 23-gauge butterfly needle, pass the needle through the skin and into the reservoir. Uncap the distal end of the butterfly needle after holding the tubing straight up vertically to create a manometer column with the tubing. If cerebrospinal fluid squirts out under pressure, then the distal end of the shunt is obstructed and a syringe can be attached to the tubing and 20 to 40 ml of cerebrospinal fluid safely removed (Figure 14–12).
6. If there is no sudden flow of cerebrospinal fluid into the butterfly tubing, then the proximal end (ventricular catheter) is obstructed. Do not panic!
7. Attach a 5-ml syringe that is one-half full of preservative-free normal saline to the butterfly needle. Vigorously withdraw and instill the fluid into the shunt. Be sure to hold the butterfly needle in position when this is done, since a sudden installation of fluid into the butterfly needle can cause it to be propulsed out of the reservoir. If cerebrospinal fluid begins to flow, then withdraw 20 to 40 ml.

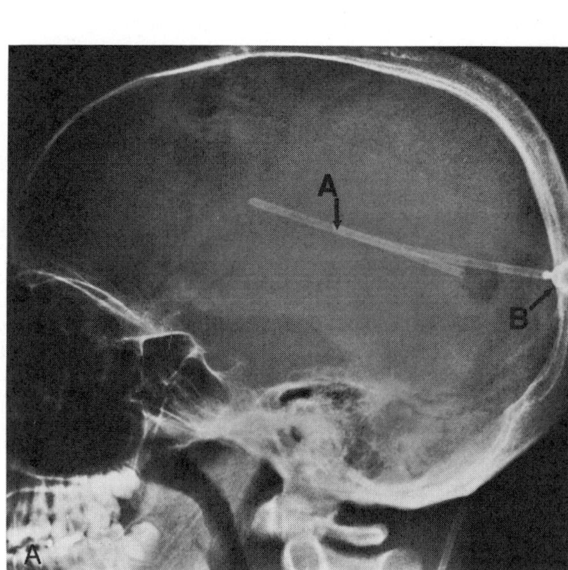

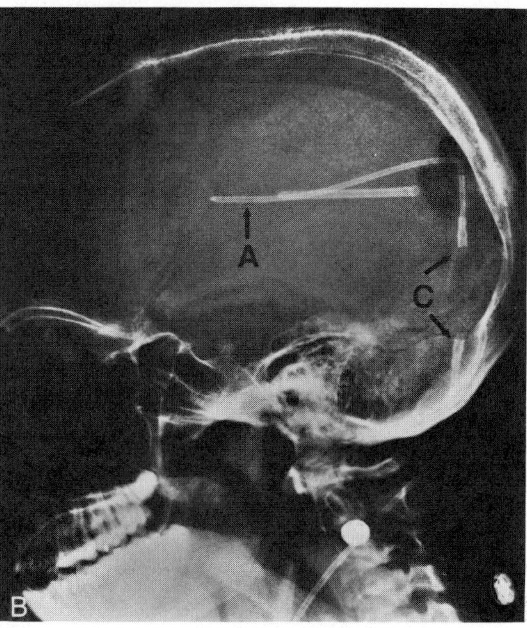

FIGURE 14–11. A, Shunt with Rickam reservoir. *A,* previous, now unconnected, ventricular catheter; *B,* Rickam reservoir. **B,** Shunt without Rickam reservoir. *A,* previous, now unconnected, ventricular catheter; *C,* shunt valve and reservoir; *D,* right angle connector.

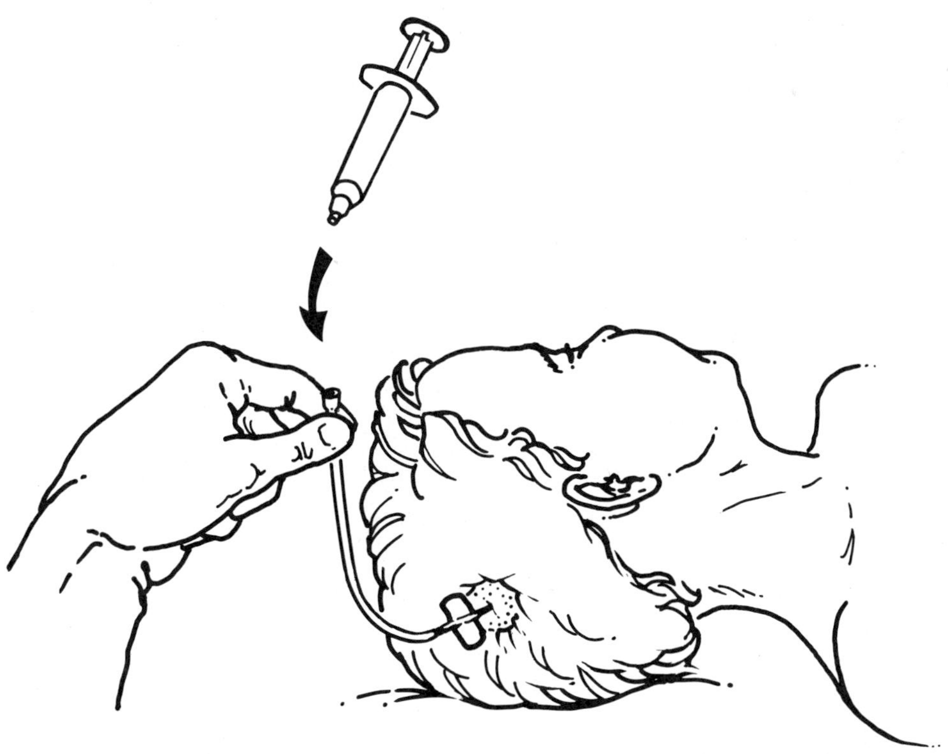

FIGURE 14–12. Tapping a Rickam reservoir.

If no cerebrospinal flow is established, then a critical decision must be made. The patient needs to be intubated, hyperventilated, and given furosemide (0.1 mg/kg) and mannitol (0.5 g/kg). Intubation should be performed by skilled hands, with temporary paralysis with a short-acting paralytic. The patient should be given a dose of diazepam (0.1 mg/kg) and morphine (0.1 mg/kg). These measures should significantly reduce the intracranial pressure and allow time for rapid transport to a hospital with a neurosurgeon.

If several hours will be required before transfer to a neurosurgeon can be completed, then the ventricle may need to be directly tapped. In this unusual situation, proceed as follows:

1. After the patient has been intubated and given the above medical treatment, the area overlying the skull exit of the ventricular catheter (location of the Rickam reservoir or right-angle connector) should be reprepped and draped as above.
2. The preexisting burr hole for shunt placement will be used to pass the spinal needle through the skull and into the ventricular system. The spinal needle can be passed directly through the center of the Rickam reservoir or adjacent to the right-angle connector.
3. Take the spinal needle with the obturator in place and gently with a slow, continuous motion pass the needle through the skin and into the brain.
   a. If the "tap sight" is located posterior, aim the needle at the contralateral inner canthus of the eye (Figure 14–13).
   b. If the "tap sight" is a frontal burr hole, then aim the needle tangental to the skull and medially at the inner canthus of the contralateral eye and slightly anterior to the external auditory meatus of the ipsilateral ear (Figure 14–14).
   c. When the needle has been advanced to 5.5 cm, remove the obturator. If cerebrospinal fluid returns, drain 20 to 40 ml and remove the needle. If no cerebrospinal fluid returns, replace the obturator and advance the needle another 1 cm and again remove the obturator to see if the ventricle has been entered.

At either ventricular tap sight, the ventricle should be reached by a depth of no greater than 6.5 cm. If cerebrospinal fluid is not obtained at this point slowly withdraw the needle and redirect it. Do not pass the needle deeper than 7.0 cm.

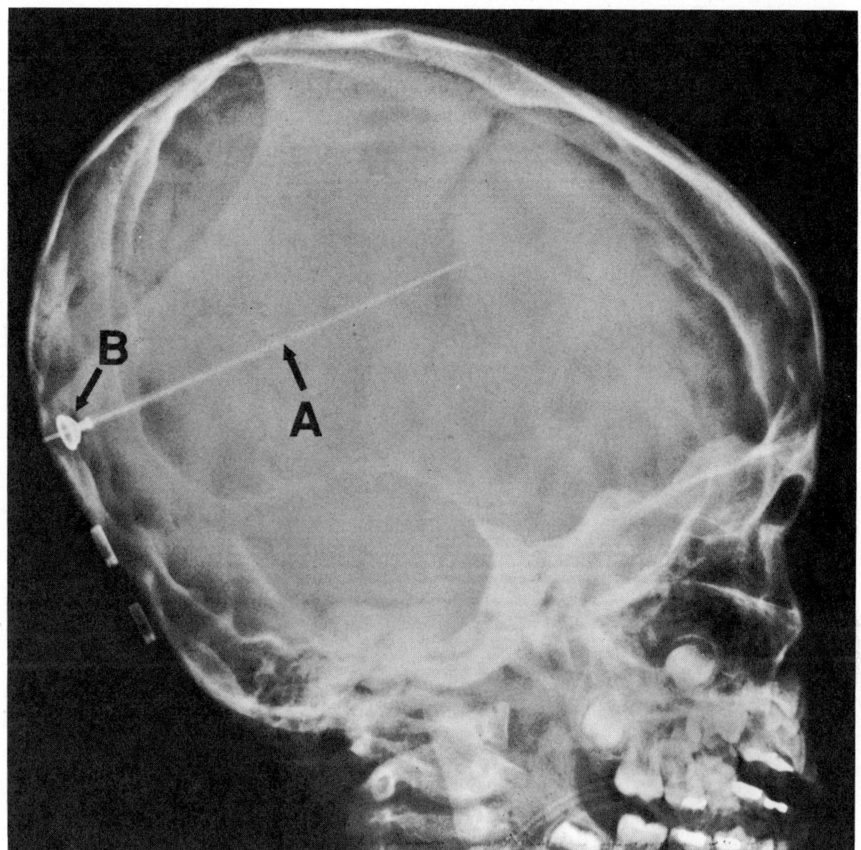

FIGURE 14–13. Ventriculostomy through a Rickam reservoir: Posterior approach. *A*, Needle; *B*, Rickam reservoir; *C*, valve.

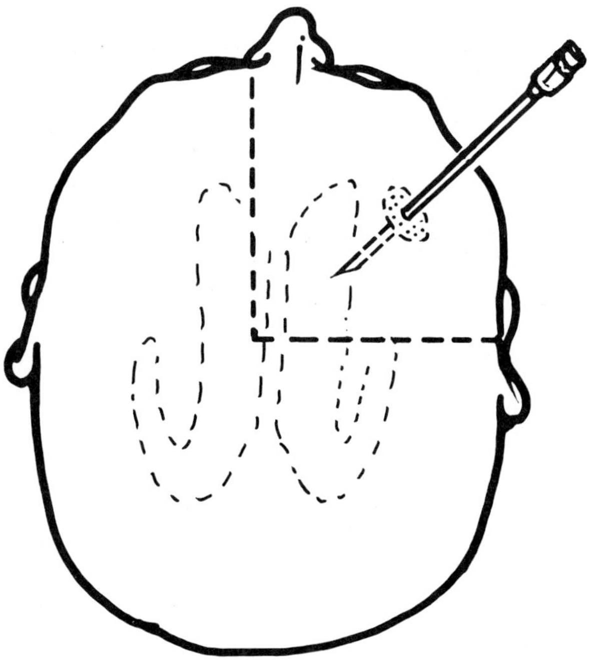

FIGURE 14–14. Ventriculostomy through a Rickam reservoir: Anterior approach.

Complications

Tapping the shunt has very low risks, including a 1% to 2% chance of infection with good sterile technique and damage to the shunt, which is irrelevant since the shunt will need to be revised!

Direct ventricular puncture has the obvious risk of brain hemorrhage and the same low risk of infection. In my experience, children eventually transferred to a university hospital following herniation from an obstructed shunt have at least a 25% mortality and greater than a 50% chance of remaining in a chronic vegetative state. Although, rapid clinical deterioration, necessitating the above measures is unusual, tapping of the shunt by an emergency physician is warranted, given the high morbidity and mortality, should the patient present to the emergency department with the signs of progressive herniation.

Reference

Madsen MA: Emergency department management of ventriculoperitoneal cerebrospinal fluid shunts. Ann Emerg Med 15:1330, 1986.

15

Ocular Tonometry

MICHAEL S. JASTREMSKI, MD

Indication

Measurement of intraocular pressure to diagnose glaucoma

Contraindications

Penetrating injury of the globe
Corneal abrasion or burn
Infection
Corneal distortion (edema, scarring)
Nystagmus
Uncontrolled coughing

Equipment

Topical anesthesia
Schiotz tonometer

Universal Precautions

None

Technique

1. Explain the procedure to the patient and obtain informed consent.
2. Position the patient supine or sitting with head back. Clothing around the neck should be loose.
3. Anesthetize the eyes with a topical anesthetic solution.
4. Make sure the instrument is clean. Check the calibration of the instrument by placing the plunger on the test block supplied with the tonometer. The pointer should be at zero; if not, adjust it by loosening the set screw and turning the frame. (Refer to the instructions specific for the tonometer you are using.)

5. Stand at the patient's side facing the patient.
6. Attach the 5.5-g weight to the tonometer.
7. Have the patient fix his gaze on a distal spot (ceiling or wall) and instruct him not to hold his breath.
8. Retract the patient's lids, without pressing on the globe, with your hand that is lateral to the eye (i.e., right hand for left eye and left hand for right eye).
9. Holding the tonometer vertically with your other hand that is resting on the patient's forehead for stability, slowly place the plunger of the tonometer on the center of the cornea (Figure 15–1).
10. Lower the handle of the tonometer until it is free, line up the pointer with its mirror image, and take a reading.
11. Add weights until the scale reading is between 4 and 10. (Note the 5.5-g weight is the zero reference, so adding, for example, a 7.5-g weight is considered a total load of 7.5 g when using the table to convert scale reading to pressure.)
12. Use the table supplied with the tonometer to convert scale reading to intraocular pressure. The normal range is 10 to 20 mm Hg.
13. Clean the instrument after each use according to the manufacturer's instructions.

Complications

Infection

False readings due to

- Diurnal variation (pressures highest at 4 to 7 AM)
- Myopia
- Cyclitis
- Detachment of choroidal or ciliary body
- Dehydration
- Hyperglycemia
- Stenosis of ipsilateral carotid artery
- Myotonic dystrophy

Pearls and Pitfalls

Acute glaucoma is a life-threatening emergency that requires immediate ophthalmologic consultation. The usual presentation is acute loss of vision with a unilateral red, painful eye whose pupil is fixed and dilated. However, acute glaucoma may cause severe nausea and vomiting such that the gastrointestinal symptoms may overshadow the ocular problem and fool the unwary physician.

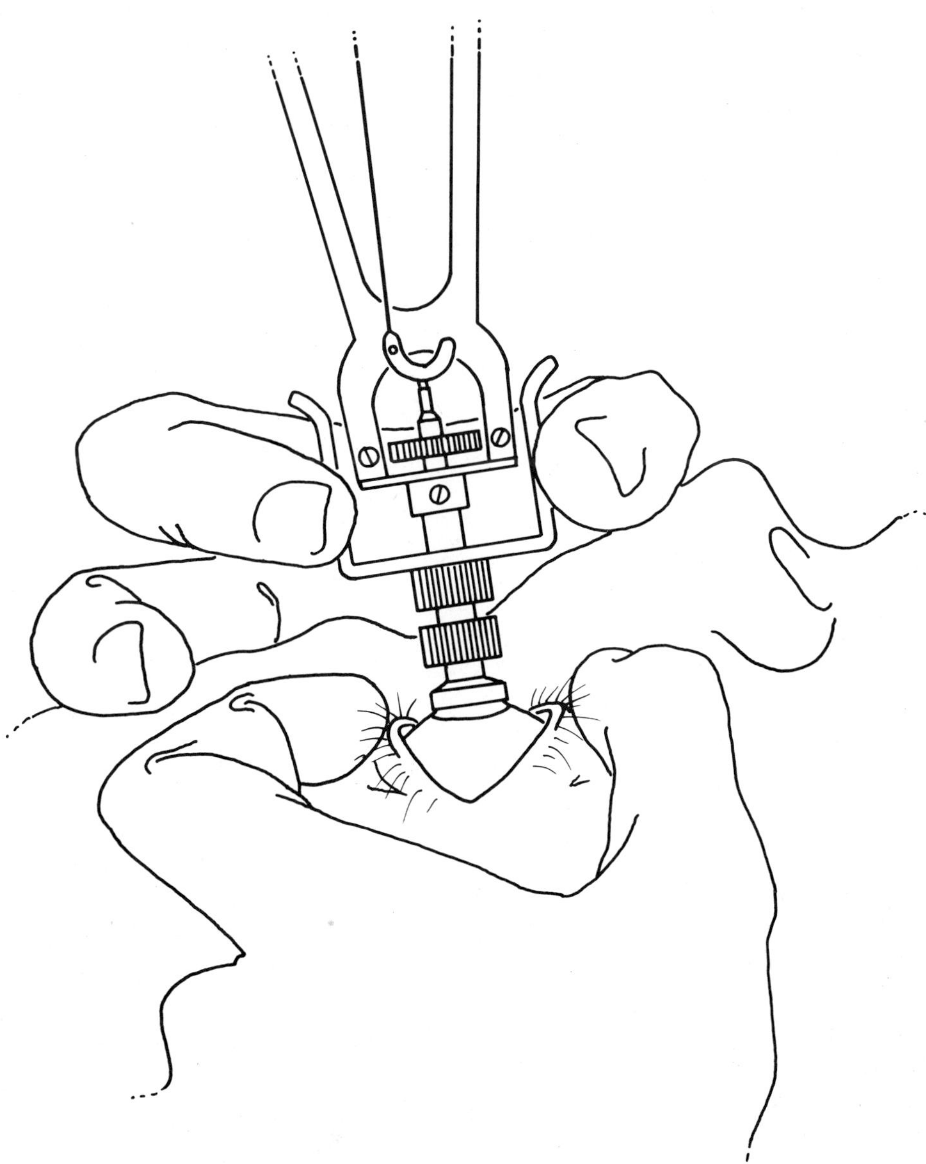

FIGURE 15–1. Ocular tonometry.

16

Orthopedic

Amputations

MICHAEL S. JASTREMSKI, MD

Indication

Preservation of severed body parts for possible replantation, including digits, arms, legs, penis, ears, and nose

Contraindications

None. Not all severed body parts can be reattached, especially if severely crushed or mutilated; but this decision is best left to an experienced replantation surgeon.

Equipment

- Sterile dressings—4 × 4-inch gauze pads and wrap
- Ringer's lactate solution (or normal saline)
- 50-ml syringe
- 19-gauge needle
- Ice
- Ice chest
- Dry, sterile container
- Sterile gloves
- Mask
- Eye shield

Universal Precautions

1. Wear mask and sterile gloves
2. Use an eye shield.

Technique

1. General care of the patient
   a. Perform a primary and then a secondary survey per Advanced Trauma Life Support guidelines, and provide resuscitation as indicated.
   b. Explain the problem to the patient and obtain consent. Be careful not to make any absolute promises or raise false hopes about the possibility of replantation or ultimate functional outcome. Let an experienced replantation surgeon explain the odds to the patient.
   c. Start an intravenous line and begin fluid therapy with Ringer's lactate.
   d. Determine need for tetanus prophylaxis, and administer Hyper-tet and dT as needed.
   e. Administer a dose of a broad-spectrum antibiotic.
   f. Consider giving systemic analgesia, depending on overall patient status.
2. Care of the stump
   a. Put on mask, eye shield, and sterile gloves.
   b. Pressure irrigate the stump with lactated Ringer's to remove dirt and debris using a 50-ml syringe and 19-gauge needle. Control bleeding with pressure and elevation. Do not clamp any bleeding vessels unless absolutely necessary.
   c. Apply a sterile gauze dressing and elevate the stump.
3. Care of the amputated part
   a. Put on mask, eye shield, and sterile gloves.
   b. Pressure irrigate the amputated part with cold Ringer's lactate to remove dirt and debris using a 50-ml syringe and 19-gauge needle.
   c. Wrap the amputated part in dry, sterile gauze and place it in a dry, sterile container (Figure 16–1).

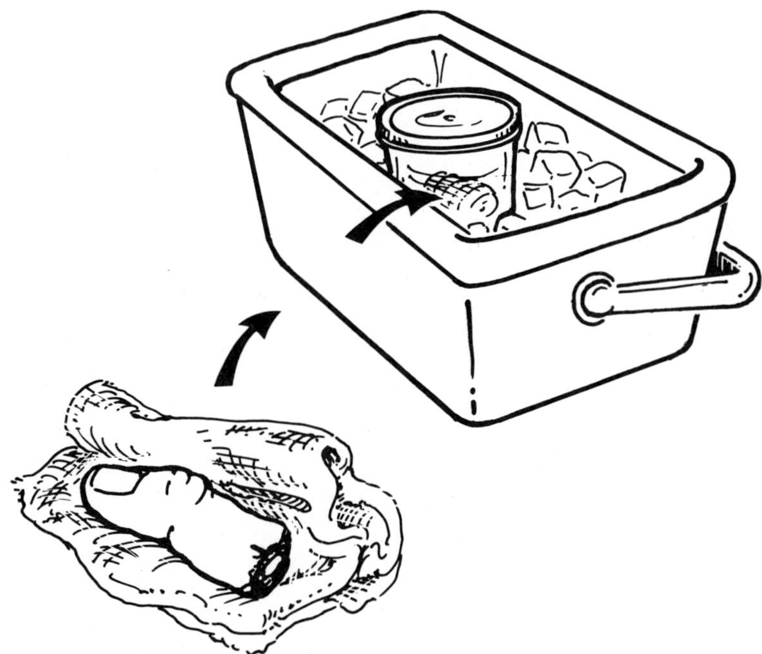

FIGURE 16–1. Preservation of amputated part.

d. Place the container holding the amputated part in a second container holding ice. Do not let the amputated part come in direct contact with the ice since this may cause an additional frostbite injury.

4. Care of a partially amputated extremity (Figure 16–2)
   a. Put on mask, eye shield, and sterile gloves.
   b. Pressure irrigate with 500 to 1000 ml chilled sterile Ringer's lactate to remove dirt and debris using a 50-ml syringe and 19-gauge needle.
   c. Cover the wound with dry, sterile gauze.
   d. Splint the site of injury.
   e. Wrap the injured extremity with dry, sterile gauze to form a bulky dressing.
   f. Cool the distal extremity and wound area by placing ice in plastic bags around the wrapped extremity. *Do not* allow the injured extremity to come in direct contact with the ice.
5. Arrange for transfer to the care of a replantation specialist.

Pearls and Pitfalls

1. Do not let the obvious amputation distract you from more serious life-threatening injuries.
2. Only an experienced replantation surgeon can determine if a part can be salvaged. Do not make the mistake of either discarding a salvageable part or giving false hope about the possibility of replantation. The emergency physician should simply tell the patient that he or she and the severed part are being sent to an expert who will determine if it can be saved.
3. Time is crucial. The longer the severed or nearly severed part is ischemic, the less the chance of salvage. Management and transfer must be carried out expeditiously. If possible, someone should be making contact with the replantation surgeon while the patient and amputated part are being resuscitated and prepared for transport.
4. Do not apply ice or any other cold material directly to the amputated part, since this may increase the extent of tissue injury.

Reference

Morgan RF, Reisman NR, Curtis RM: Preservation of upper extremity devascularization and amputations for replantation. Am Surgeon 48:481, 1982.

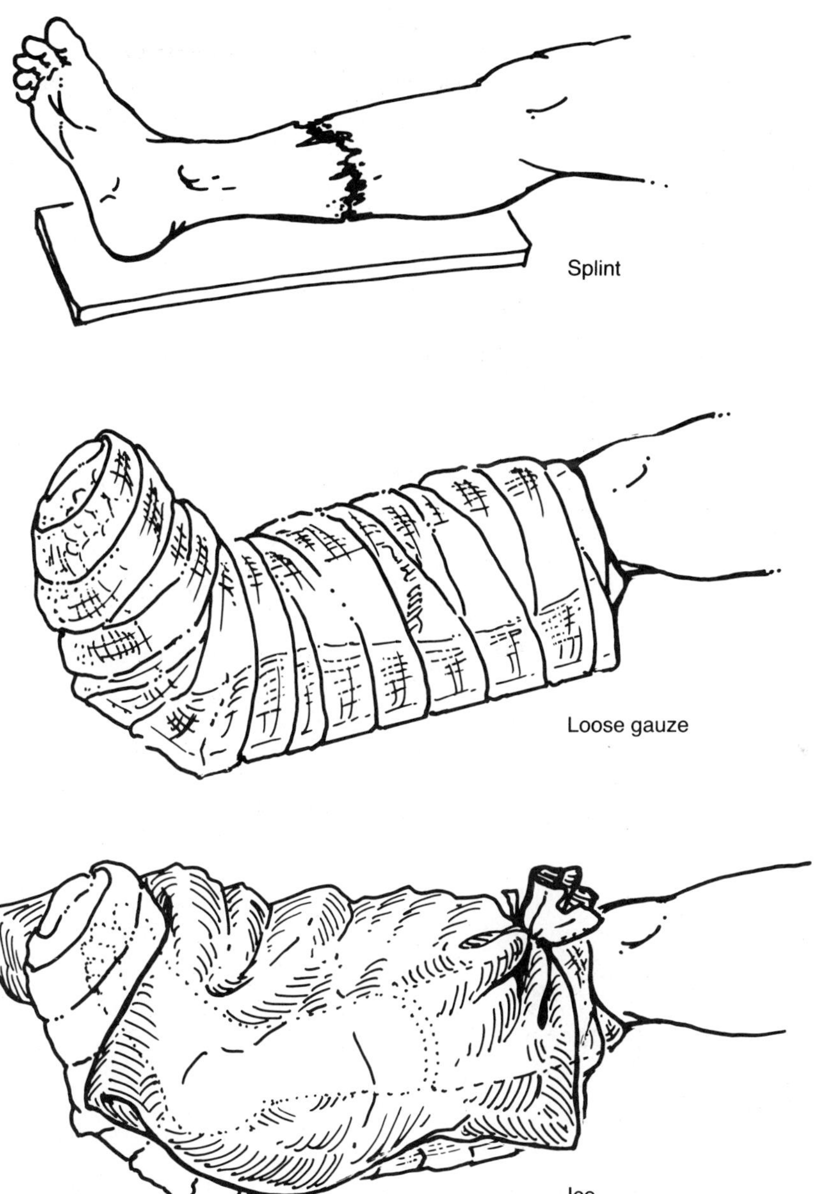

FIGURE 16–2. Care of a partially amputated extremity.

Arthrocentesis

E. JAMES RADIN, MD

Indication

Diagnostic assessment of any acutely inflamed joint or bursa, primarily to diagnose sepsis

Contraindications

Coagulopathy (relative)

Equipment

Two 10-ml syringes
5-ml syringe
Two 3-ml syringes
4 × 4-inch gauze pads
2% lidocaine
Heparin flush solution (100 U/ml)
Needle assortment (gauge and length depend on joint)
20-gauge spinal needle
Two microscope slides for Gram stains
Sterile gloves
Sterile drape
Dressing for puncture site

Universal Precautions

1. Wear sterile gloves.

Technique

Knee (Figure 16–3)

1. Explain procedure to patient and obtain consent.
2. Check equipment to ensure that all is present.
3. Position patient sitting with the leg hanging freely.
4. Stand on the side of the arthrocentesis, facing the knee.
5. Put on sterile gloves.
6. Pretreat collection syringes with heparin flush solution.

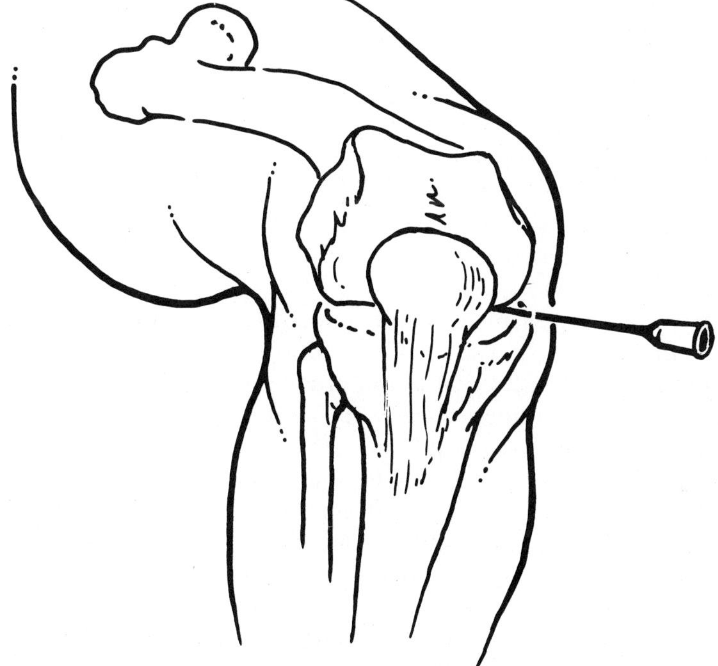

FIGURE 16–3. Knee arthrocentesis.

7. Prep and drape the medial aspect of the joint.
8. Locate the site for aspiration over the joint line 2 to 3 fingerbreadths posterior from the patella.
9. At the aspiration site, infiltrate the skin and subcutaneous tissues including the periosteum with local anesthetic using a 5-ml syringe and a 25-gauge, 1½-inch needle.
10. Use the anesthetic syringe and needle to locate the easiest route to the synovial fluid and the proper angle and depth. Do not be too traumatic!
11. Use a 10-ml syringe coated with a small amount of heparin and an 18-gauze, 1½-inch needle to aspirate a sample of joint fluid.
12. Place samples into red-topped, lavender-topped, and culture tubes. Place a drop of synovial fluid on a microscope slide for Gram stain.
13. Ensure hemostasis and bandage.
14. Review the Gram stain yourself prior to any intra-articular treatments, especially therapy with corticosteroids.

Shoulder (Figure 16–4)

1. Explain procedure to patient and obtain consent.
2. Check equipment to ensure that all is present.
3. Position patient sitting with arms relaxed.
4. Stand facing the patient.
5. Put on sterile gloves.
6. Pretreat collection syringes with heparin flush solution.
7. Prep with Betadine and drape the anterior shoulder.
8. Locate the site of aspiration at the groove palpated along the anterior and medial edge of the humerus below the acromioclavicular joint approximately halfway to the axilla.
9. Using a 25-gauge, 1½-inch needle and 5-ml syringe, locally infiltrate the skin and subcutaneous tissue with anesthetic down to the medial edge of the humeral head. Then walk the needle around the medial edge of the humerus into the shoulder joint.
10. Once the joint space is localized, use an 18-gauge, 1½-inch needle on a 10-ml syringe coated with heparin to aspirate fluid.
11. Ensure hemostasis and bandage.
12. Place samples into red-topped, lavender-topped, and culture tubes. Place a drop of synovial fluid on a microscope slide for Gram stain.
13. Send the specimen to the laboratory for Gram stain and analysis of the fluid.

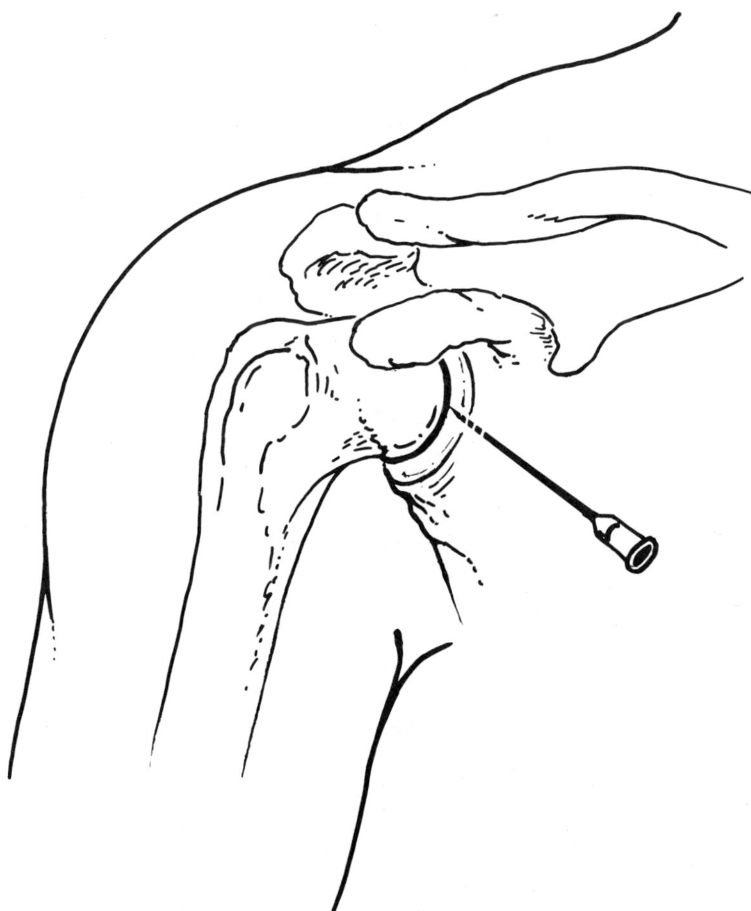

FIGURE 16–4. Shoulder arthrocentesis.

Ankle (Figure 16–5)

1. Explain procedure to patient and obtain consent.
2. Check equipment to ensure that all is present.
3. Position patient supine with the foot neutral.
4. Stand on the side for arthrocentesis facing the ankle.
5. Put on sterile gloves.
6. Pretreat collection syringes with heparin flush solution.
7. Prep with Betadine and drape.
8. The lateral malleolus is palpated and local anesthesia performed with a 5-ml syringe and 25-gauge needle by superficially anesthetizing the skin with 1 to 3 ml of 2% lidocaine 2.5 cm proximal and 1.3 cm medial to the distal tip of the lateral malleolus.
9. Advance an 18- or 20-gauge needle on a 5- to 10-ml syringe coated with heparin through this window into the articular space and aspirate joint fluid.
10. Place samples into red-topped, lavender-topped, and culture tubes. Place a drop of synovial fluid on a microscope slide for Gram stain.
11. Ensure hemostasis and bandage.
12. Look at the Gram stain.

Elbow (Figure 16–6)

1. Explain procedure to patient and obtain consent.
2. Check equipment to ensure that all is present.
3. Position patient supine with the arm abducted 45 to 90 degrees and the shoulder and elbow flexed 90 degrees with the palm flat on a table.
4. Stand at the side of arthrocentesis facing the elbow.
5. Put on sterile gloves.
6. Pretreat collection syringes with heparin flush solution.
7. Prep with Betadine and drape.
8. Locate the space between the lateral epicondyle of the humerus and the radial head and infiltrate this area with 1 to 3 ml of 2% lidocaine delivered with 25-gauge, 1-inch needle and 5-ml syringe.
9. Advance an 18- or 20-gauge needle on a 5- to 10-ml syringe coated with heparin through this window into the articular space and aspirate joint fluid.
10. Place samples into red topped, lavender topped, and culture tubes. Place a drop of synovial fluid on two microscope slides for Gram stain.
11. Ensure hemostasis and bandage.
12. Look at the Gram stain.

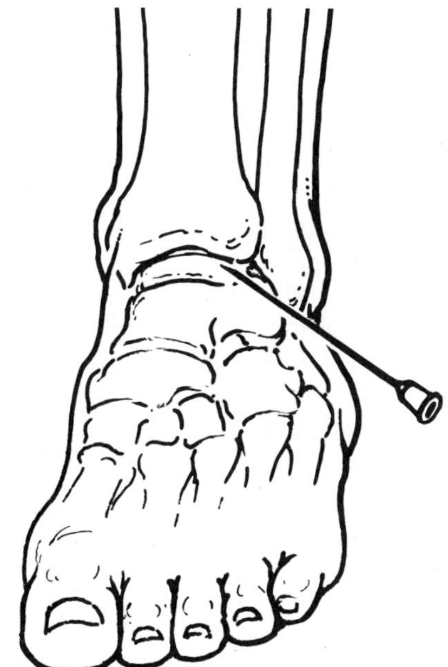

FIGURE 16–5. Ankle arthrocentesis.

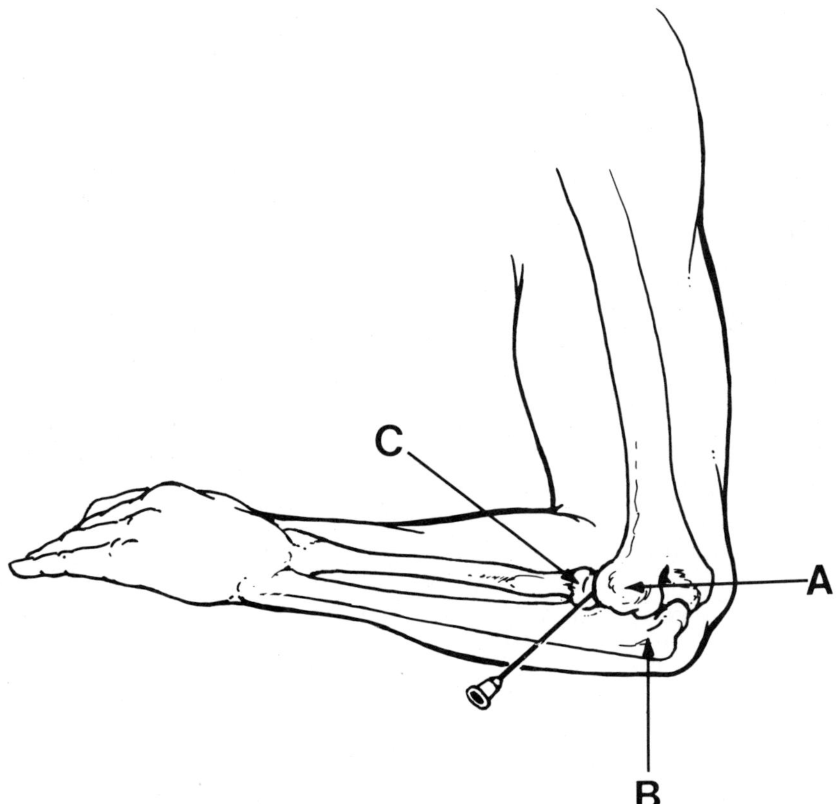

FIGURE 16–6. Elbow arthrocentesis. *A*, Lateral epicondyle; *B*, olecranon; *C*, radial head.

Wrist (Figure 16–7)

1. Explain procedure to patient and obtain consent.
2. Check equipment to ensure that all is present.
3. Position patient with the wrist and arm flat on table, palm down.
4. Stand on the side of arthrocentesis facing the wrist.
5. Put on sterile gloves.
6. Pretreat collection syringes with heparin flush solution.
7. Prep and drape the wrist.
8. Locally anesthetize with 1 to 3 ml of 2% lidocaine, using a 25-gauge, 1-inch needle on a 5-ml syringe, superficially and deep, just ulnar to the extensor pollicis longus tendon at the radial carpal junction into the palpable articular space.
9. Aspirate synovial fluid with a 20-gauge needle on a 5-ml syringe coated with heparin.
10. Place samples into red-topped, lavender-topped, and culture tubes. Place a drop of synovial fluid on two microscope slides for Gram stain.
11. Ensure hemostasis and bandage.
12. Look at the Gram stain.

Digits (Figure 16–8)

1. Explain procedure to patient and obtain consent.
2. Check equipment to ensure that all is present.
3. Position the patient's hand palm down with fingers spread.
4. Stand facing the hand.
5. Put on sterile gloves.
6. Pretreat collection syringes with heparin flush solution.
7. Prep whole digit and hand with Betadine and drape, exposing the involved digit.
8. Use your nondominant hand to flex the joint 20 to 30 degrees while applying distal traction (or have an assistant wearing a sterile glove do this).
9. Superficially infiltrate 1 to 2 ml of 2% lidocaine at the site just medial or lateral to the dorsal tendon at the point where the tendon crosses the joint space using a 25-gauge, 1-inch needle and 3-ml syringe.
10. Perform the aspiration with a 22-gauge, 1-inch needle inserted into the joint space on a 5-ml syringe coated with heparin.
11. Place samples into red-topped, lavender-topped, and culture tubes. Place a drop of synovial fluid on two microscope slides for Gram stain.
12. Ensure hemostasis and bandage.
13. Look at Gram stain.

Alternately, a digital block may be performed to provide anesthesia for digital joint aspiration (see Chapter 2).

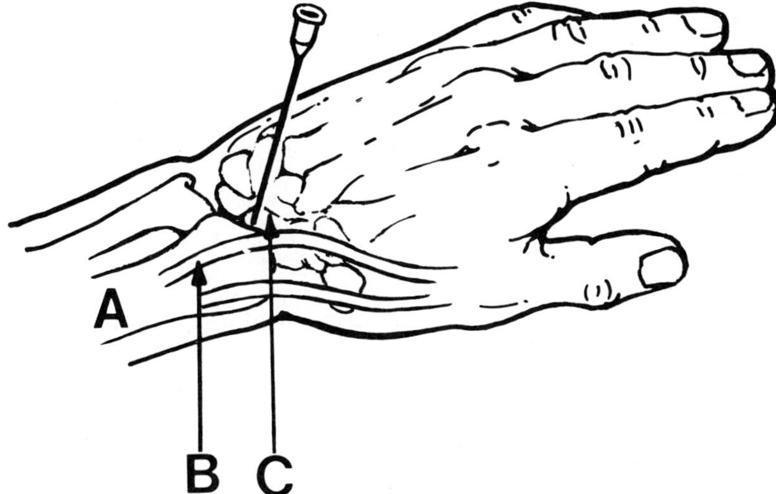

FIGURE 16–7. Wrist arthrocentesis. *A*, radius: *B*, extensor pollicis longus tendon; *C*, scaphoid.

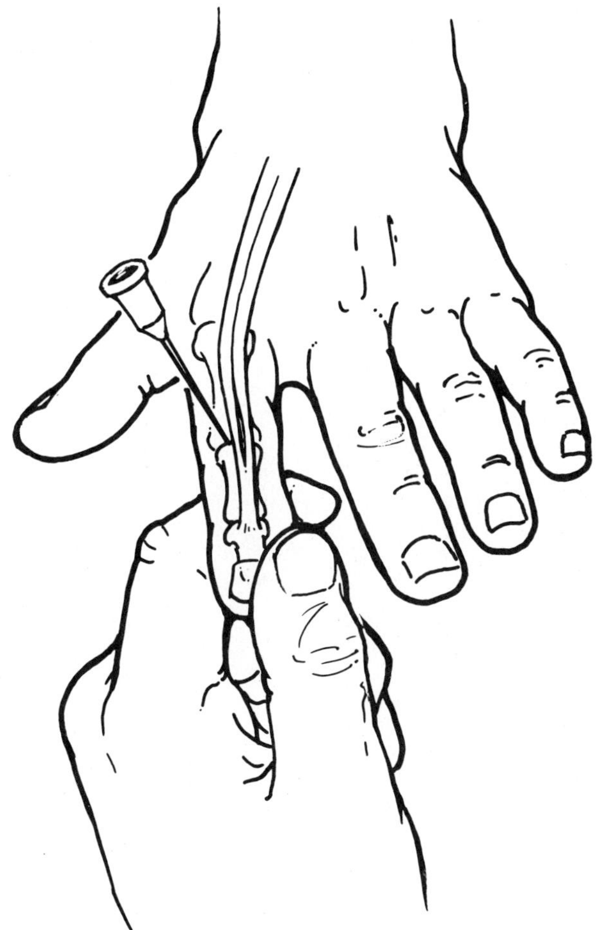

FIGURE 16–8. Digital arthrocentesis.

Complications

Bleeding—intra-articular or extra-articular
Trauma to cartilage and meniscus
Infection—intra-articular or extra-articular

Pearls and Pitfalls

1. Sometimes it is easier to send fluid samples in a lavender-topped tube for cell count and differential; a red-topped tube for viscosity, crystals, and chemistries, and a culturette for culture and sensitivity and Gram stain.
2. *Always* look at the Gram stain *yourself.*
3. Slight flexion and traction will open the joint space and may facilitate the procedure.
4. Arthrocentesis of the hip is difficult, often requires fluoroscopic guidance, and is best left to the specialist.

References

Extensive experience.
Kobernick M: Arthrocentesis. In Roberts JR, Hedges JR (eds): Clinical Procedures in Emergency Medicine, pp 687–697. Philadelphia, WB Saunders, 1985.

Ankle Dislocation Reduction

KEVIN FERGUSON, MD

Ankle dislocations only occasionally occur without associated fracture(s). Many will require urgent surgical repair. All will need orthopedic referral. Associated injuries, if any, will influence the rapidity of definitive repair. Unless there is evidence of vascular compromise, full radiologic evaluation of the injury with anteroposterior, lateral, and oblique views should be completed prior to any attempted reduction.

Ankle dislocations are classified by the direction of displacement of the foot relative to the tibia. Therefore, there are posterior, anterior, lateral, and superior dislocations.

Posterior dislocations are relatively common. They may be associated with fractures of one or both malleoli. The typical mechanism of injury involves posterior to anterior force to the distal tibia, usually from a direct blow. This causes plantar flexion of the foot and the appearance of a shortened foot.

Anterior dislocations are not as common. They are usually associated with a fracture of the anterior tibia. The mechanism of injury is typically either an anteroposterior-directed force to the tibia with a fixed foot causing posterior displacement of the tibia or forced hyperdorsiflexion.

Lateral dislocations are the most frequently seen and are *always* associated with fractures of the malleoli or fibula. The limb is obviously deformed with the foot deviated laterally. These fracture-dislocations can destroy the mortise structure and represent a potential threat to the vascularity of the foot and future function of the joint. Careful assessment of vascular integrity is mandatory.

Superior dislocations (diastases) are uncommon and usually result from vertical compaction. They are often associated with articular surface damage.

Indications

Dislocation with vascular compromise
Dislocation and orthopedic consultation unavailable within an acceptable time

Contraindications

Acute, life-threatening injury that requires more immediate attention
Rapid availability of orthopedic consultation

Equipment

Analgesic and muscle relaxant medications, or a regional block such as a Bier block

Splinting materials to make a molded splint after reduction.

An assistant to provide countertraction on the lower leg is helpful but not necessary.

Universal Precautions

1. Wear gloves if open wounds are present.

Technique

The specific technique of reduction varies with the type of dislocation. The basic technique maneuvers the articular surfaces and fractured bones back to their anatomic positions (Figure 16–9), with the direction of the force for reduction being opposite the direction of the dislocation. This motion is preceded by a maneuver to minimize the bone-on-bone grinding.

Anterior Dislocations (Figure 16–10)

1. Explain the procedure to the patient and obtain consent.
2. Position the patient supine on a stretcher.
3. Evaluate and document neurovascular function of the affected foot.
4. Administer intravenous analgesia and/or sedation. A benzodiazepine and a narcotic are a good combination.
5. Have an assistant stand at the patient's knee facing the foot and grasp the patient's lower leg in the mid-calf region. The assistant then picks the leg up to flex the knee and hip.
6. You stand at the foot of the stretcher facing the patient and hold the injured foot with one hand under the heel and the other on the dorsum over the metatarsals.
7. Dorsiflex the foot to disengage the talus, pull the foot toward you as the assistant applies counteraction, and then push the foot directly downward into its normal position.
8. Reevaluate neurovascular function.
9. Splint the foot and ankle.
10. Obtain a postreduction x-ray film and look at it.
11. Arrange for orthopedic consultation.

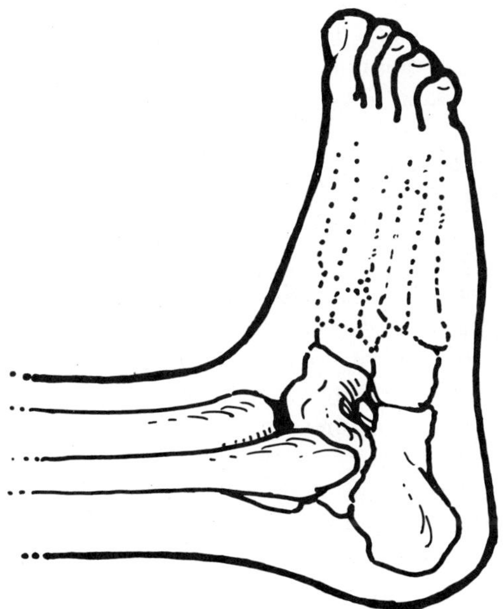

FIGURE 16–9. Normal anatomy of ankle joint.

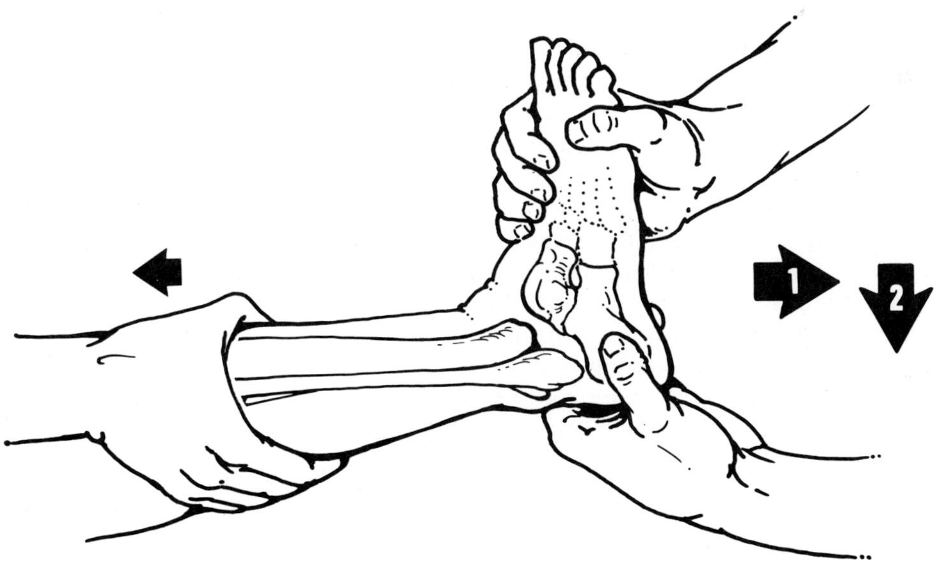

FIGURE 16–10. Reduction of anterior ankle dislocation.

Lateral Dislocation (Figure 16–11)

1. Explain the procedure to the patient and obtain consent.
2. Position the patient supine on a stretcher.
3. Evaluate and document neurovascular function of the affected foot.
4. Administer intravenous analgesia and/or sedation. A benzodiazepine and a narcotic are a good combination.
5. Have an assistant stand at the patient's knee facing the foot and grasp the patient's lower leg in the mid calf region. The assistant then picks the leg up to flex the knee and hip.
6. You stand at the foot of the stretcher facing the patient and hold the injured foot with one hand under the heel and the other on the dorsum over the metatarsals.
7. While the assistant applies countertraction, pull the foot distally to disengage the tibia, then push it immediately back into position. *Note:* Almost all lateral dislocations require open reduction for definitive repair. This is a temporary measure to restore vascular integrity.
8. Reevaluate neurovascular function.
9. Splint the foot and ankle.
10. Obtain a postreduction x-ray film and look at it.
11. Arrange for orthopedic consultation.

Posterior Dislocation (Figure 16–12)

1. Explain the procedure to the patient and obtain consent.
2. Position the patient supine on a stretcher.
3. Evaluate and document neurovascular function of the affected foot.
4. Administer intravenous analgesia and/or sedation. A benzodiazepine and a narcotic are a good combination.
5. Have an assistant stand at the patient's knee facing the foot and grasp the patient's lower leg in the midcalf region. The assistant then picks the leg up to flex the knee and hip.
6. You stand at the foot of the stretcher facing the patient and hold the injured foot with one hand under the heel and the other on the dorsum over the metatarsals.
7. As the assistant applies countertraction, plantar flex the foot and pull the heel toward you; then push the foot upward (dorsiflex) while still pulling the heel toward you.
8. Reevaluate neurovascular function.
9. Splint the foot and ankle.
10. Obtain a postreduction x-ray film and look at it.
11. Arrange for orthopedic consultation.

Superior Dislocation

Superior dislocations are not reduced emergently by closed technique since they will require surgical repair and rarely cause vascular compromise. The diastasis will keep the reduction from being fixated externally. These injuries should be splinted in place and referred to an orthopedist.

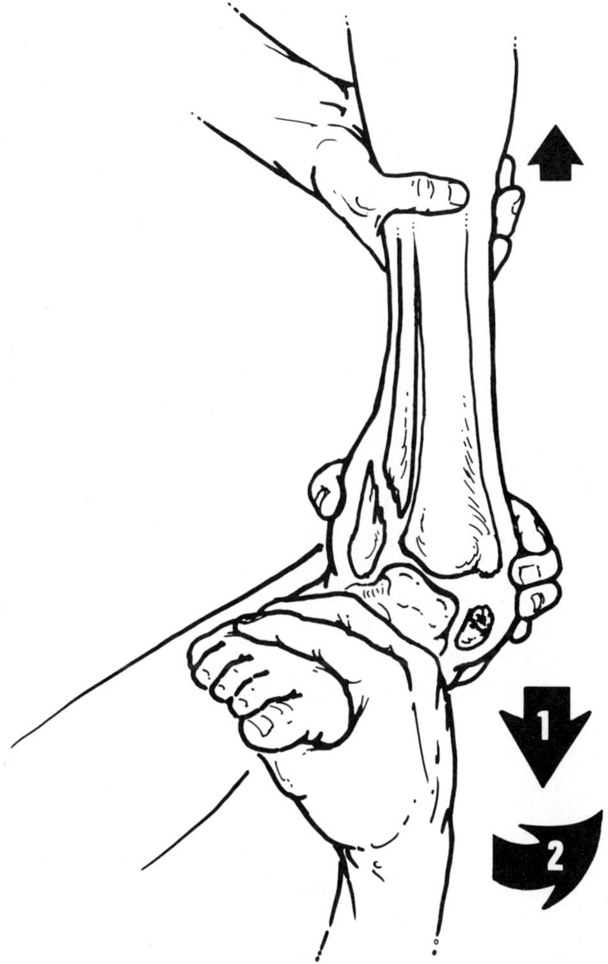

FIGURE 16–11. Reduction of lateral ankle dislocation.

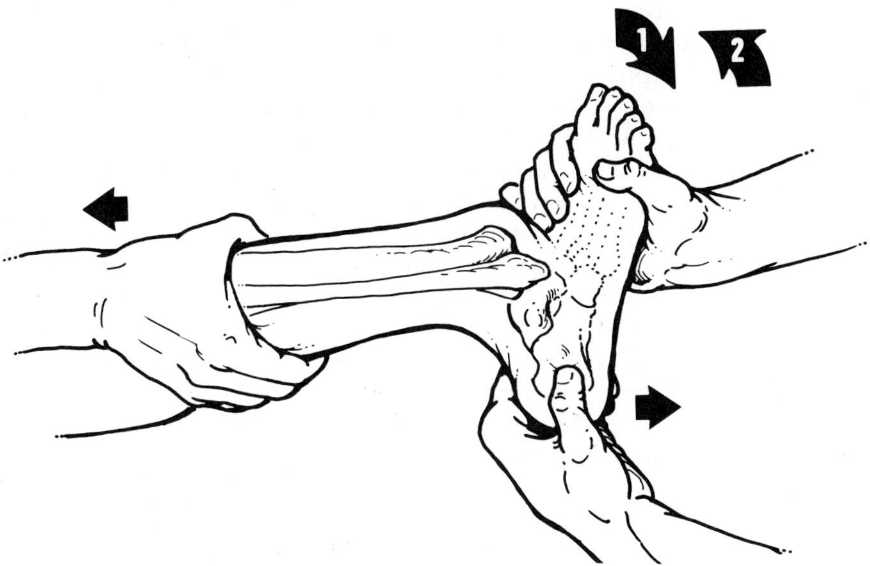

FIGURE 16–12. Reduction of posterior ankle dislocation.

Complications

1. Persistent talar instability is a very common complication of ankle injuries from sprains to fracture-dislocations. Patients sometimes complain of "feeling insecure" standing on the ankle or of it "buckling."
2. Avascular necrosis of the talus has been reported.
3. Patients with elongation of the lateral ligaments are predisposed to chronic ankle sprains.
4. Traumatic arthritis occurs in up to 40% of patients with ankle fractures, especially the elderly.
5. Nonunion occurs in 10% to 15% of ankle fractures treated closed. As with any fracture, malunion can occur with ankle fractures and can be treated surgically if symptomatic.
6. Neurovascular injury is not rare; complications obviously increase and worsen as time to diagnosis increases. Loss of circulation of either anterior or posterior tibial artery flow can lead to tissue loss.
7. Sudek's atrophy is a sympathetic dystrophy caused by ankle fractures which can lead to a rapidly progressive osteoporosis distal to the neural injury. Patients will present with a complaint of burning pain beginning distally. It resolves with return of normal ankle function.
8. Synostosis or ossification of the interosseous membrane is a common complication, and patients may complain of a dull ache or instability in the ankle.

Pearls and Pitfalls

1. Prereduction and postreduction examinations of neurovascular status need to be clearly documented. Serial documentation is advised, and the chart should reflect the time of the reduction attempt(s) relative to vascular assessments.
2. A complete series of ankle x-ray films to document initial injury, an adequate reduction, and the presence or absence of reduction-related injury is mandatory. Especially, be sure to account for any chip fractures since they can frequently be intra-articular and difficult to see.
3. Be suspicious of proximal tibia or fibula fractures. The construction of the lower extremity can transmit forces, particularly torque, from one end of the lower leg to the other. Most experienced othopedists and emergency physicians can relate a case when the majority of physical findings, swelling, ecchymosis, and so on, were in the ankle and only normal ankle x-ray films prompted formal tibia/fibula views and the discovery of the midshaft or proximal fracture. The opposite, major physical findings proximal and fracture distal, is also not uncommon. To avoid missing possible "occult" fractures, the importance of palpation of the entire course of both bones of the lower extremity cannot be overemphasized. Point tenderness of the tibia or fibula alone should create enough concern to warrant more x-ray films.
4. Regardless of x-ray findings, if the physical examination creates concern of significant joint injury the patient should have the joint immobilized and an orthopedic referral.
5. Beware of intra-articular bone fragments since they can potentially complicate the reduction and are another reason to review a full ankle series prior to attempting reduction.

References

Rosen P, Dailey R (eds): Emergency Medicine Concepts and Clinical Practice. St. Louis, CV Mosby, 1983.

Tintinalli J, Krome R (eds): Emergency Medicine: A Comprehensive Review Guide. New York, McGraw-Hill Book Company, 1988.

Radial Head Subluxation (Nursemaid's Elbow)

THOMAS TERNDRUP, MD

Indication

The typical patient is between 1 and 4 years of age and presents with a pronated arm hanging at the side following a distractive force applied to the arm. A child with this finding who refuses to use the affected arm should be suspected to have this injury. There usually are no soft tissue findings, but mild radial head tenderness is found in some patients (Figure 16–13).

Contraindication

Suspected fracture

Equipment

Generally none

Universal Precautions

None

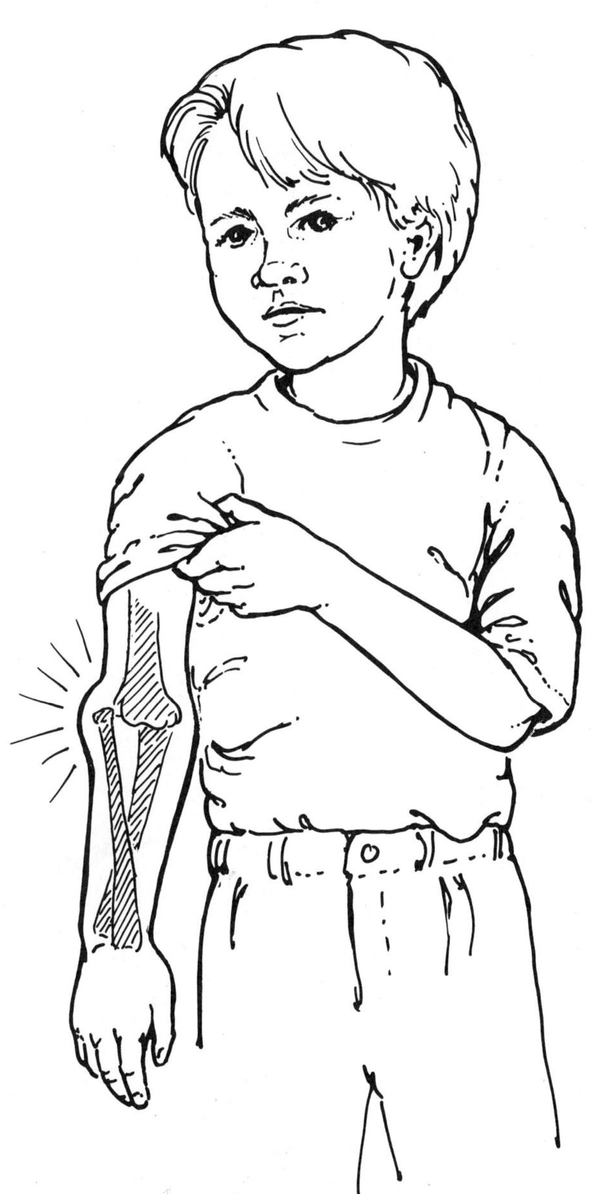

FIGURE 16–13. Nursemaid's elbow.

Technique

1. Explain the procedure to the parent, who should restrain the child in his or her lap; otherwise this can be done by an assistant.
2. Sit facing the child, and cup the affected elbow with the nondominant hand.
3. The affected elbow is fully supinated (Figure 16–14), then flexed with the dominant hand while using the supporting hand as a fulcrum (Figure 16–

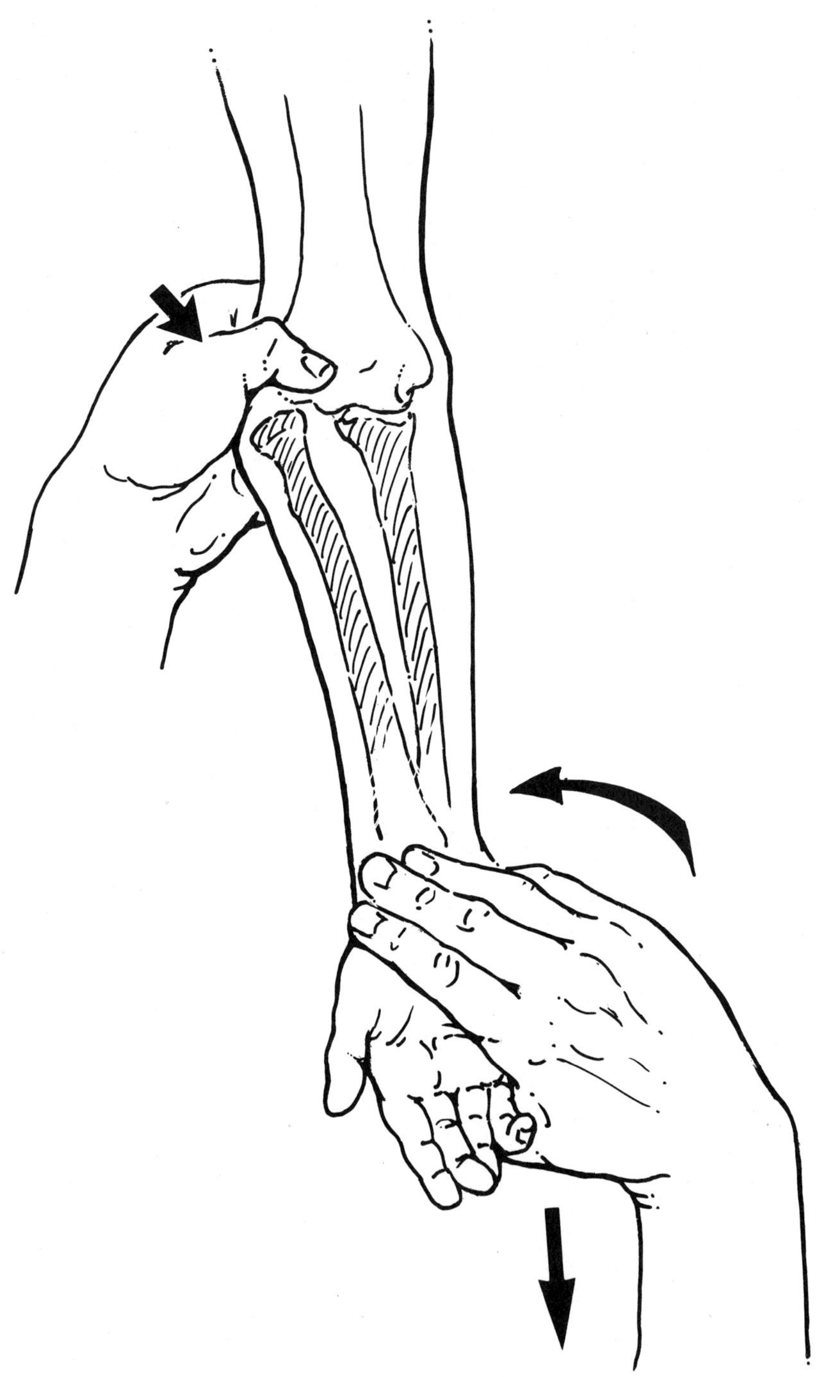

FIGURE 16–14. Reduction of nursemaid's elbow: Step 1.

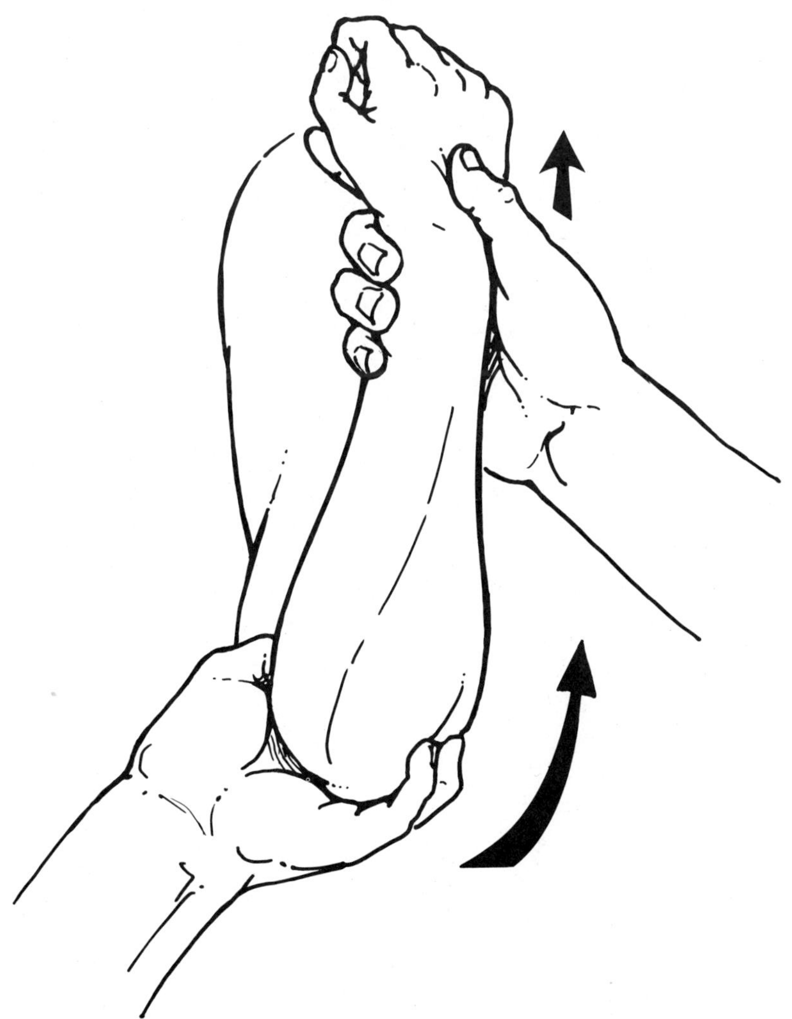

FIGURE 16–15. Reduction of nursemaid's elbow: Step 2.

15). Efficacy can be enhanced by the application of an additional force with the thumb of the nondominant hand directed medially over the radial head during supination (see Figure 16–14). A palpable click is usually appreciated with relocation, typically followed by the child moving the elbow in 10 to 15 minutes.

4. No immobilization is required following reduction.
5. If the child is not moving the arm normally within 10 to 15 minutes, a second attempt at reduction should be performed.
6. X-ray films may be indicated in the child without a typical mechanism of injury who does not improve following attempts at reduction.

Complications

Irreducible dislocations (extremely uncommon)
Neurovascular injury (extremely uncommon)
Avulsion fractures (uncommon)

Pearls and Pitfalls

1. This is a procedure that, when performed correctly, is generally successful and without complications.
2. Careful discussion of the momentary pain associated with the procedure with the accompanying parent will allay anxiety and improve patient relations.
3. Firm pressure over the radial head in the medial direction may improve reduction efficacy.

Reference

Extensive experience

Reduction of Finger Dislocations

THOMAS TERNDRUP, MD

Indications

Finger dislocations are common injuries seen in the emergency department. Most frequently this involves the proximal interphalangeal (PIP) joint, followed by dislocations of the distal interphalangeal (DIP) joint. Dislocations of the metacarpophalangeal joints are uncommon and are generally irreducible, except by open reduction. Most finger dislocations are posterior; some are lateral. All dislocations require an evaluation of the integrity of the collateral ligaments and volar plate. The goals are restoration of normal alignment and optimizing recovery of normal function and stability.

Contraindications

Coexisting fracture—seek orthopedic consultation
Open dislocation

Equipment

Local anesthesia (without epinephrine)
3-ml syringe
27-gauge needle
Gauze pads
Sterile gloves

Universal Precautions

1. Wear sterile gloves.

Technique

1. Explain procedure to the patient and obtain consent.
2. Anesthetize the affected finger with a digital block (see Chapter 2) or local infiltration around the affected joint. Wait 10 to 15 minutes to ensure adequate anesthesia prior to attempts at reduction.
3. Apply distal traction to create distraction at the dislocated joint (Figure 16–16*A*). Then a slight push in the direction opposite of the initial dislocation usually restores normal alignment (Figure 16–16*B*).
4. Following reduction, the joint should be examined for instability in the anteroposterior and mediolateral planes (Figure 16–17). An open or unstable joint mandates orthopedic referral.
5. Immobilization of the relocated PIP or DIP joint at 15 to 20 degrees of flexion in a dorsal foam-padded splint or by simple buddy taping should be continued for 21 days.

Complications

Fracture-dislocation of the affected joint space

Unsuccessful reduction

Failure to refer unstable reductions

Pearls and Pitfalls

1. A majority of PIP or DIP joint dislocations can be managed effectively by the emergency physician.
2. An examination for instability is mandatory following reduction. Any instability, fracture-dislocation, or open dislocation should be considered complex and mandates orthopedic referral.

Reference

Carter P (ed): Common Hand Injuries and Infections. Philadelphia, WB Saunders, 1988.

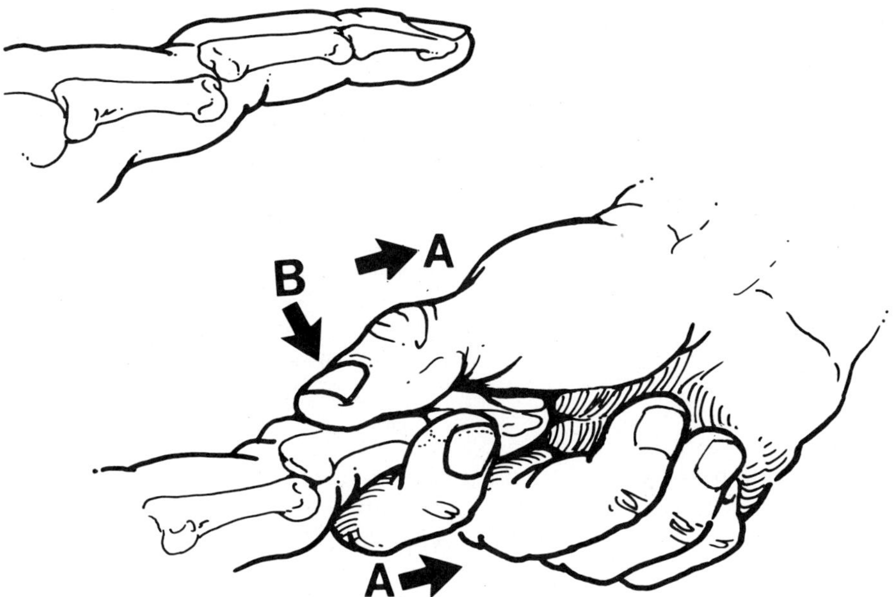

FIGURE 16–16. Reduction of dislocated finger.

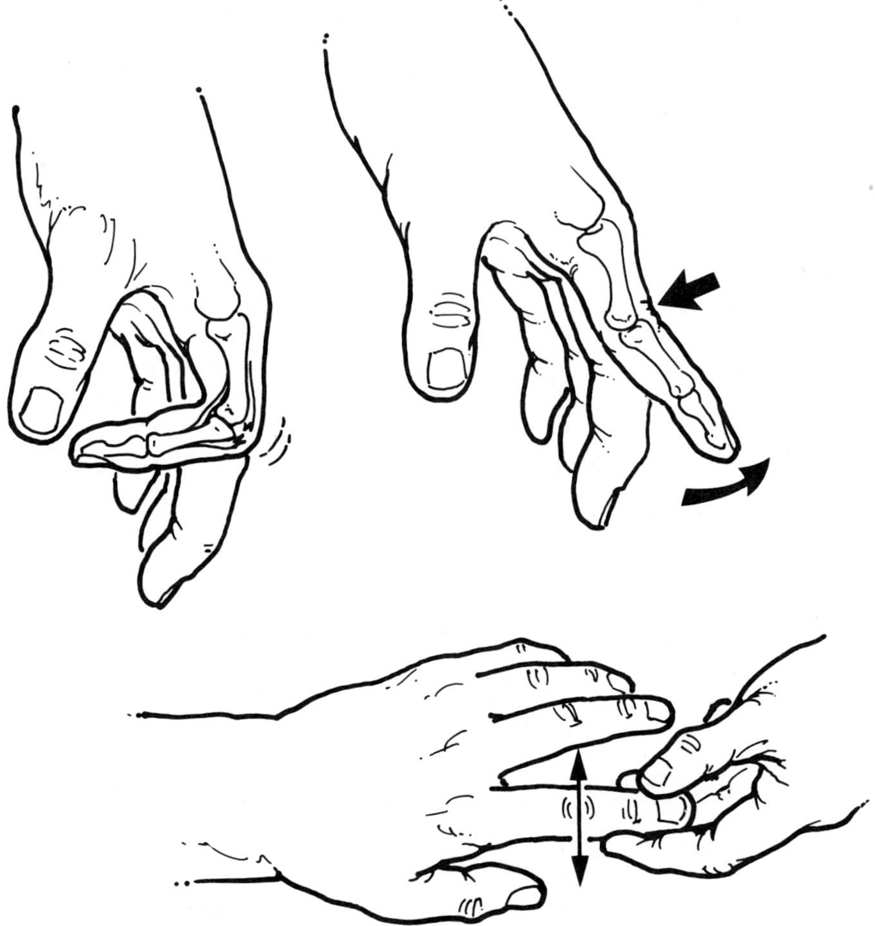

FIGURE 16–17. Examination for joint instability.

Hip Dislocation Reduction

KEVIN FERGUSON, MD

Hip dislocation represents a true orthopedic emergency. The incidence of concurrent injury to the acetabulum and the involved extremity is high, and early reduction reduces the risk of avascular necrosis of the femoral head. Additionally, the forces required to produce dislocation of the hip indicate a very violent mechanism of injury and should initiate the evaluation of the patient as a major trauma victim. Posterior dislocations are the more frequent. Anterior dislocations are not manageable in the emergency department and will likely require general or regional anesthesia. If immediate orthopedic management is not available, posterior dislocations can often be reduced using the technique described below.

Indication

Posterior hip dislocation without immediate orthopedic consultation available

Contraindications

More serious injury to be addressed (i.e., hemodynamic instability or airway compromise)

Immediate availability of an orthopedic specialist

Equipment

Backboard with buckle or Velcro strap restraints

Narcotic analgesic

Intravenous muscle relaxant—midazolam

Leg traction device

Universal Precautions

1. Wear gloves if any bleeding is present.

Technique

1. Explain the procedure to the patient and obtain consent if circumstances allow.
2. The patient should be secured to the backboard and the whole unit lowered to near floor level. This affords a mechanical advantage that will be needed when working against the powerful muscles of the pelvic girdle.
3. The patient should be premedicated with a narcotic and muscle relaxant, assuming there is no hemodynamic compromise or other contraindication, such as a possible surgical abdomen or marginal respiratory status. If significant intra-abdominal or pelvic injury has not been ruled out or at least had an initial surgical evaluation, then this procedure should not be attempted; potentially life-threatening injuries take precedence over reduction. If the patient's hemodynamic stability is in question and/or intravenous analgesics and sedation are contraindicated, then this procedure can be postponed until the patient is stabilized or in the operating room.
4. Procedure (Figure 16–18)
   a. The assistant kneels at the patient's lower abdomen facing the patient's

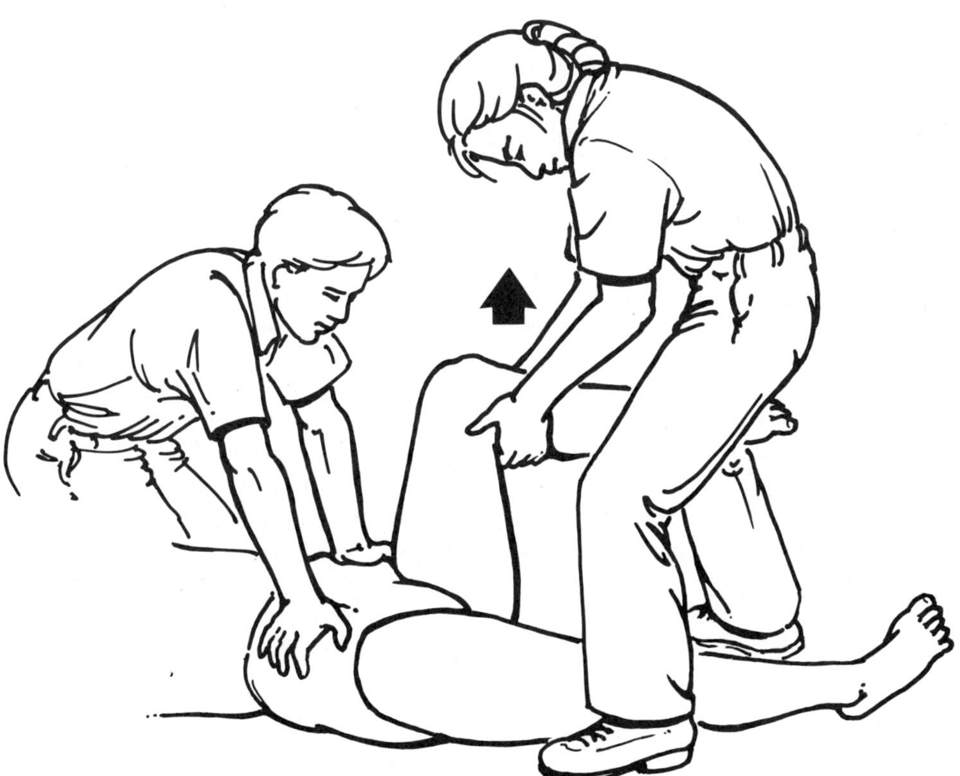

FIGURE 16–18. Reduction of a dislocated hip.

feet, grasps both iliac crests, and applies downward traction on the pelvis, immobilizing it against the backboard.

b. Depending on the side of the dislocation the person effecting the reduction needs to position himself directly over the patient's dislocated hip. Location and positioning are important since the reduction will take time. Often, straddling the patient affords the best angle and position for a long reduction. This may necessitate lowering the stretcher to 20 to 30 cm off the floor and straddling it or getting onto the stretcher with the patient. (The latter choice is not optimal from a personal safety aspect.)
c. Flex the hip and the knee 90 degrees, and then apply traction to the distal femur in line with the deformity. Continued upward traction will effect reduction in most cases. A second person applying traction on the proximal lower leg may also be employed. Keep in mind the muscle groups opposing reduction are powerful, and prolonged traction, muscle relaxation, and fatigue are important allies.
d. After reduction the hip and leg should be placed in anatomic position and traction applied to maintain reduction.
e. Obtain a postreduction x-ray film and look at it.
f. Arrange to have the patient admitted for traction and observation.

Complications

Ligamentous injury to the knee if it is used as a fulcrum

Failure to reduce

Avascular necrosis of the femoral head

Pearls and Pitfalls

1. If the patient is scheduled to go to the operating room for other injuries the reduction will be relatively simple once general anesthesia is induced.
2. If the patient is able to be stabilized without surgery, then the reduction must be done within 4 hours to avoid avascular necrosis of the hip.
3. If the patient has a concomitant hip fracture that will prevent countertraction on the pelvic girdle, such as a fracture through the pelvic ring or sacroiliac joint, then reduction should not be attempted without orthopedic consultation.
4. Hip dislocations can be dramatic and draw the attention away from other significant injuries. Always suspect pelvic or abdominal injuries in a patient whose mechanism of injury is consistent with multiple system trauma or in patients who are not responding to fluid resuscitation.

References

Rosen P, Dailey R (eds): Emergency Medicine Concepts and Clinical Practice. St. Louis, CV Mosby, 1983.

Tintinalli J, Krome R (eds): Emergency Medicine: A Comprehensive Review Guide. New York, McGraw-Hill Book Company, 1988.

Knee Dislocation Reduction

KEVIN FERGUSON, MD

Knee dislocations of the tibia off the femur represent a true orthopedic emergency because of their high association with neurovascular injury in the affected limb. The popliteal artery and the peroneal nerve are frequently compromised. Anterior dislocations (tibia anterior to femur) are more frequent than posterior dislocations. Because of the frequency of associated neurovascular injury on presentation, a thorough neurovascular examination must be performed prior to any attempts at reduction or manipulation of the extremity and immediately afterward. Any dislocation of the knee must be immediately reduced if associated with neurovascular compromise.

Patellar dislocations are commonly seen as an isolated injury and often spontaneously reduce prior to presentation. They do not carry the same concern for neurovascular injury or difficulty in reduction as do tibial-femur dislocations. The patient with an isolated patellar dislocation typically presents with the lower leg flexed at 20 to 30 degrees and the patella displaced laterally. Medial, superior, or intracondylar patellar dislocations are very rare.

Indications

Any dislocation of the knee with neurovascular compromise and no orthopedic consultation immediately available

Patellar dislocation

Contraindications

More serious injury to be addressed (i.e., hemodynamics instability or airway compromise)

Immediate availability of orthopedic consultation

Equipment

Knee immobilizer

Universal Precautions

1. Wear gloves if any bleeding is present.

Technique

Preparation

1. Explain the procedure to the patient and obtain consent.
2. If the patient has only the isolated orthopedic injury and is stable, some analgesic medication may be given; however, the reduction of the dislocation associated with neurovascular compromise should not suffer prolonged delays while waiting for complete analgesia.

Procedure

Anterior Dislocation (Femur Posterior to Tibia) (Figure 16–19)

1. Position the patient supine with the dislocated leg straight.
2. Have your assistant stand next to the mid femur of the involved leg and grasp the distal femur (not in the popliteal space) with both hands. The assistant applies countertraction to the femur while lifting it upward.
3. Stand at the patient's foot facing the dislocated knee. Grasp the distal lower leg and apply straight traction to the tibia until the femur moves up into position.
4. The reduction may be facilitated by having a third person simultaneously push the proximal tibia downward.
5. Place the knee in a knee immobilizer.
6. Reassess neurovascular function.
7. Obtain a postreduction x-ray film and look at it.
8. Arrange for admission to the hospital.

Posterior Dislocation (Femur Anterior to Tibia) (Figure 16–20)

1. Position the patient supine with the involved leg straight.
2. Have your assistant stand next to the mid femur of the involved leg and grasp the distal femur (not in the popliteal space) to apply countertraction and downward force.
3. Stand at the patient's foot facing the dislocated knee, grasp the distal tibia with your dominant hand, and apply traction away from the knee while placing your nondominant hand under the proximal tibia (but not in the popliteal fossa) to lift the tibia into position.
4. The reduction may be facilitated if three persons participate; one to apply countertraction to the femur, one to apply traction to the tibia, and one to depress the distal femur while lifting the proximal tibia.
5. Place the knee in a knee immobilizer.
6. Reassess neurovascular function.
7. Obtain a postreduction x-ray and look at it.
8. Arrange for admission to the hospital.

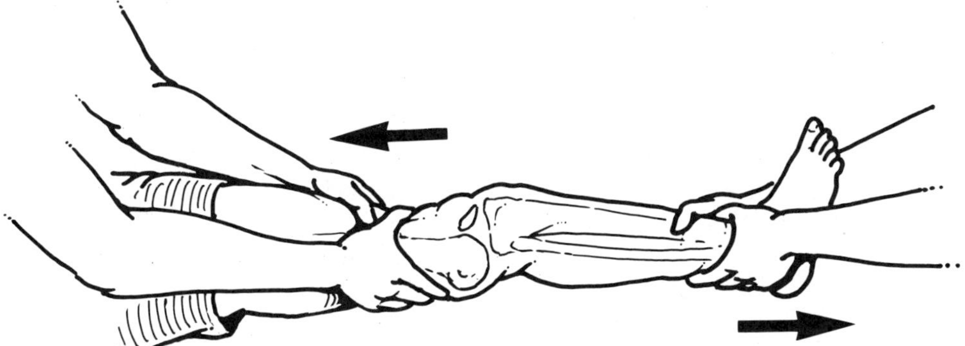

FIGURE 16–19. Reduction of anterior knee dislocation.

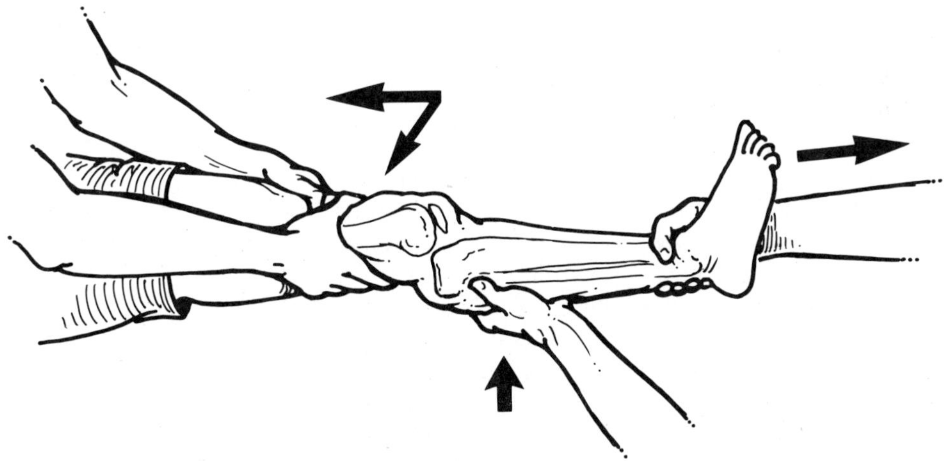

FIGURE 16–20. Reduction of posterior knee dislocation.

Patellar Dislocation (Figure 16–21)

1. Position the patient supine.
2. Stand at the side of the affected knee facing the knee.
3. Grasp the lower tibia with one hand and the patella with your other hand.
4. Flex the knee to 90 degrees, then gently extend the knee to 180 degrees while pushing the patella anteriorly and medially.
5. Obtain a postreduction x-ray and look at it.
6. Place the knee in a knee immobilizer and discharge the patient on crutches with instructions not to bear weight until seen in orthopedic follow-up in 2 to 3 days.

Complications

Failure of reduction (anterior and posterior dislocations are usually not successfully reduced without general anesthesia)

Associated neurovascular and hip injuries (common with anterior and posterior dislocations)

Pearls and Pitfalls

1. Since the presence of this dislocation implies tremendous injury to the ligaments and cartilage of the joint, it is unstable and requires immobilization to maintain reduction and prevent any further injury to the neurovascular structures.
2. If the patient has more serious injuries to be addressed, the extremity should be immobilized and presumed to be compromised.
3. Lateral dislocations may be more easily reduced by flexing the knee to 90 degrees (this relaxes the hamstrings) before applying traction and countertraction.
4. Patients who present with a history of a patellar dislocation that has spontaneously reduced should also be managed with immobilization, several days of no weight bearing and orthopedic referral.
5. Complete ligamentous disruption of the knee occurs with anterior or posterior dislocations and usually requires subsequent surgical repair.
6. Because general anesthesia is usually required for successful reduction, emergency department reduction should be attempted only when there is vascular compromise.
7. Pressure should not be applied to the popliteal space when reducing an anterior or posterior dislocation since this may worsen neurovascular damage.

References

Rosen P, Dailey R (eds): Emergency Medicine Concepts and Clinical Practice. St. Louis, CV Mosby, 1983.

Tintinalli J, Krome R (eds): Emergency Medicine: A Comprehensive Review Guide. New York, McGraw-Hill Book Company, 1988.

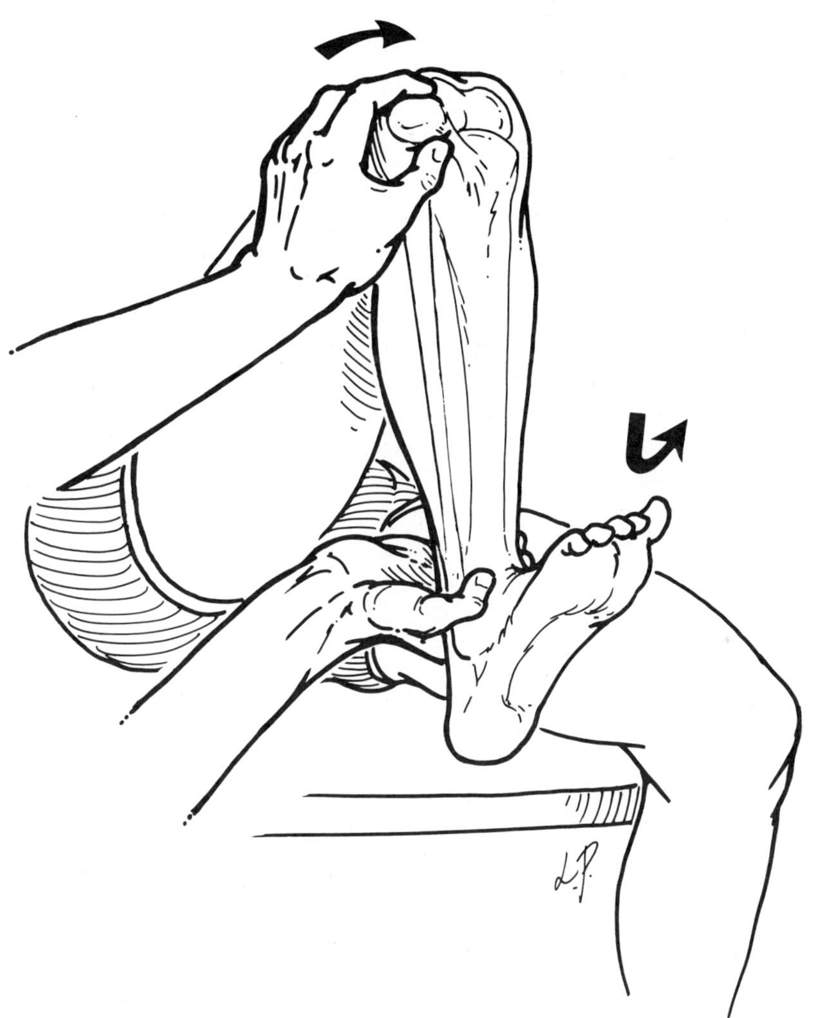

FIGURE 16–21. Reduction of patellar dislocation.

Reduction of Dislocated Mandible

MICHAEL S. JASTREMSKI, MD

Indication

Restoration of normal function. When the temporomandibular joint dislocates, the condyle of the mandible locks anteriorly, causing pain, interfering with speech and swallowing, and preventing complete closure of the mouth.

Contraindications

None

Equipment

Gloves
4 × 4-inch gauze pads

Universal Precautions

1. Wear gloves.
2. Pad thumbs.

Technique

1. Obtain an x-ray film to rule out a fracture if there was physical trauma to the mandible (a dental panorex provides the best view of the mandible). If the dislocation was spontaneous (e.g., with yawning or laughing), an x-ray film is not necessary.

If the mandible is fractured, obtain a maxillofacial surgical consultation and do not attempt to reduce the fracture/dislocation yourself.

---

2. Explain the procedure to the patient and obtain consent.
3. Put on gloves and wrap your thumbs with several gauze pads.
4. Have the patient sit in a chair and stand facing the patient with the patient's knees between your legs.

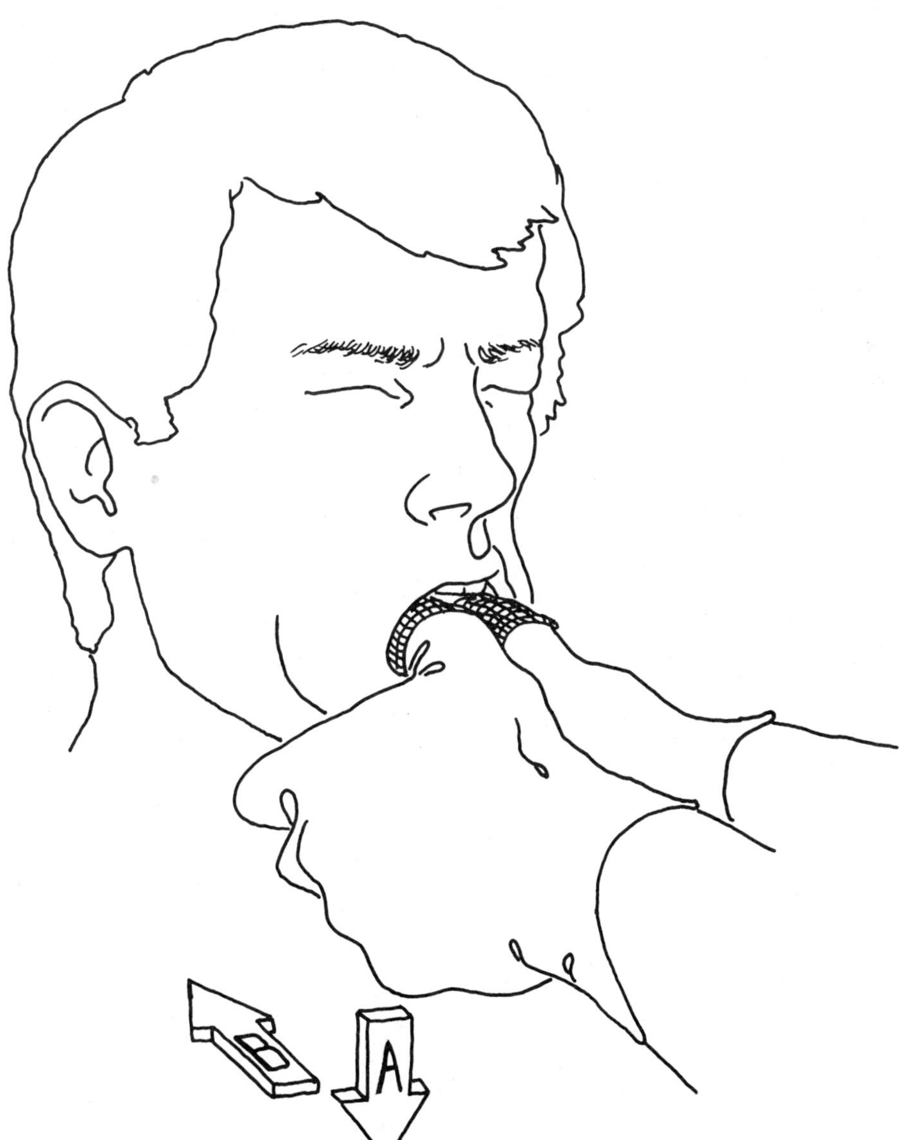

FIGURE 16–22. Reduction of the dislocated mandible.

5. Grasp the patient's mandible with your thumbs on the lower molars and your fingers wrapped under the mandible (see Figure 16–22).
6. Apply pressure to simultaneously open the mouth widely and push the mandible downward. This unlocks the temporomandibular joint (Figures 16–22 and 16–23, arrow A).
7. Then push the chin posteriorly to relocate the condyles in their fossae (Figures 16–22 and 16–23, arrow B).

Complications

Missed fracture

Trauma to your hands when the mandible snaps shut with relocation

Unsuccessful reduction

Pearls and Pitfalls

1. Intravenous sedation and muscle relaxation with a short-acting benzodiazepine will facilitate the procedure.
2. Injection of 1 ml of lidocaine into each mandibular fossa will anesthetize the external pterygoid muscles, which are holding the mandible anteriorly, and allow the other muscles to reduce the dislocation spontaneously.
3. The patient should be instructed to eat a soft diet and to avoid widely opening the mouth for 1 to 2 weeks to help prevent a secondary dislocation until the ligaments have healed.

References

Henny FA: The temporomandibular joint in oral and maxillofacial surgery. In Kruger GO (ed): Textbook of Oral and Maxillofacial Surgery, pp 451–453. St. Louis, CV Mosby, 1984.

Luyk NH, Larsen PE: The diagnosis and treatment of the dislocated mandible. Am J Emerg Med 7:329, 1989.

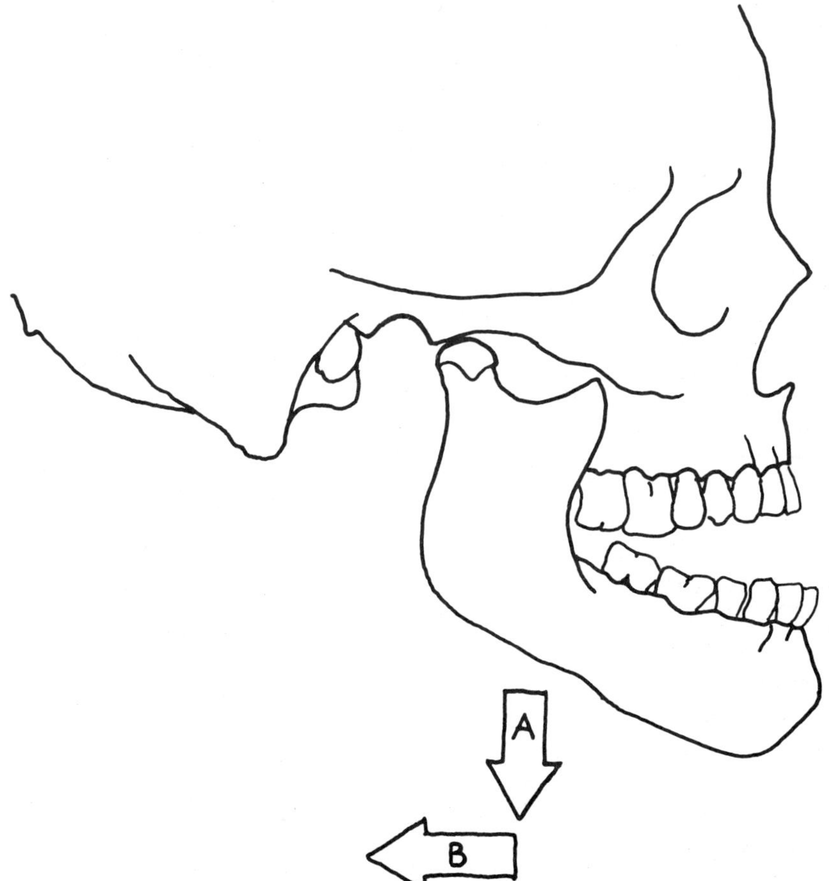

FIGURE 16–23. Reduction of the dislocated mandible.

Reduction of Dislocated Shoulder

GREGORY D. RIEBEL, MD

Indication

Decompression of neuromuscular structures and restoration of normal anatomy and function

Contraindications

None

Equipment

Full-size sheet

Universal Precautions

None

Technique (Hippocratic)

1. Explain procedure, as well as the necessity to relax muscles completely, and obtain consent.
2. Have patient lie supine on a stretcher with the head flat.

3. Wrap sheet around patient: under back, through axilla of affected arm, and across chest (Figure 16–24).
4. Stand at the patient's hip on the affected side, facing the dislocated shoulder (see Figure 16–24).
5. Flex the elbow of the patient's affected arm (to relax biceps).
6. Have an assistant standing near the opposite shoulder, holding the sheet firmly for countertraction (see Figure 16–24).
7. While holding the patient's arm, which is slightly abducted, lean back to provide gradual increasing traction on the flexed arm (reduction often occurs at this point) (see Figure 16–24).
8. Reduction may be assisted by gradual internal and external rotation of the shoulder.
9. Obtain and review a postreduction x-ray film to evaluate reduction and rule out fracture.

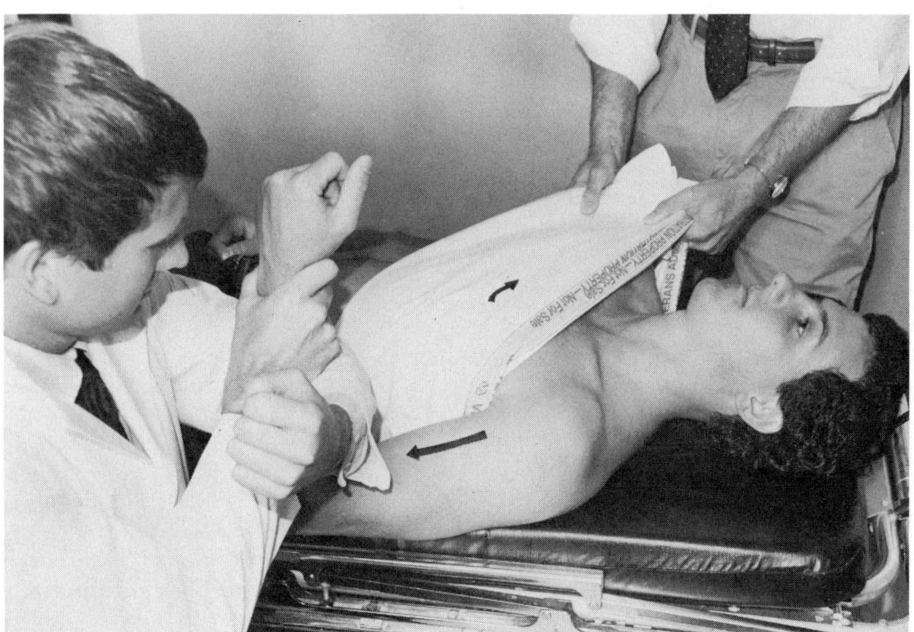

FIGURE 16–24. The hippocratic technique of shoulder reduction.

Technique (Milch)

1. Explain the procedure to the patient and obtain consent.
2. Position patient lying supine on a stretcher with the head somewhat elevated.
3. Stand at the patient's head facing the dislocated shoulder (Figure 16–25).
4. Slowly and gently abduct the patient's arm to an overhead position with elbow flexed, holding the wrist with your right hand and the distal upper arm with your left hand (see Figure 16–25*A*).
5. While applying gradually increasing traction, slowly, externally rotate the arm (see Figure 16–25*A*). Reduction will usually take place at this point, with restoration of normal shoulder contour. The perception of the reduction itself may be subtle.
6. Sometimes the reduction may be facilitated by having an assistant apply thumb pressure directly over the humeral head, pushing laterally (Figure 16–25*B*).
7. Obtain and review a postreduction x-ray film to evaluate reduction and rule out fracture.

Postreduction Treatment

1. The patient should be placed in a shoulder immobilizer or sling and swathe. This will remain in place, except for showers, for 3 weeks.
2. Encourage use of the hand and wrist to decrease swelling.
3. Apply ice on a cloth to the affected shoulder 30 minutes, three times daily for 3 days.
4. When showering, hold affected arm across the chest; external rotation is to be avoided.

Complications

Unsuccessful reduction

Displacement of unrecognized fracture

Neurovascular injury due to traction or excessive pressure in the axilla

Pearls and Pitfalls

1. Intravenous analgesics and/or muscle relaxants may be helpful, especially in anxious patients.
2. The ease and efficacy of reduction techniques decrease the longer the shoulder is dislocated.
3. The key to avoiding complications is slow, gentle reduction.
4. This injury is usually evident on an anteroposterior x-ray film. A transcapular or axillary view may be needed to evaluate the location of the humeral head. Examine the area carefully for fracture of posterior glenoid, humeral head, or tuberosities.

Reference

Extensive experience.

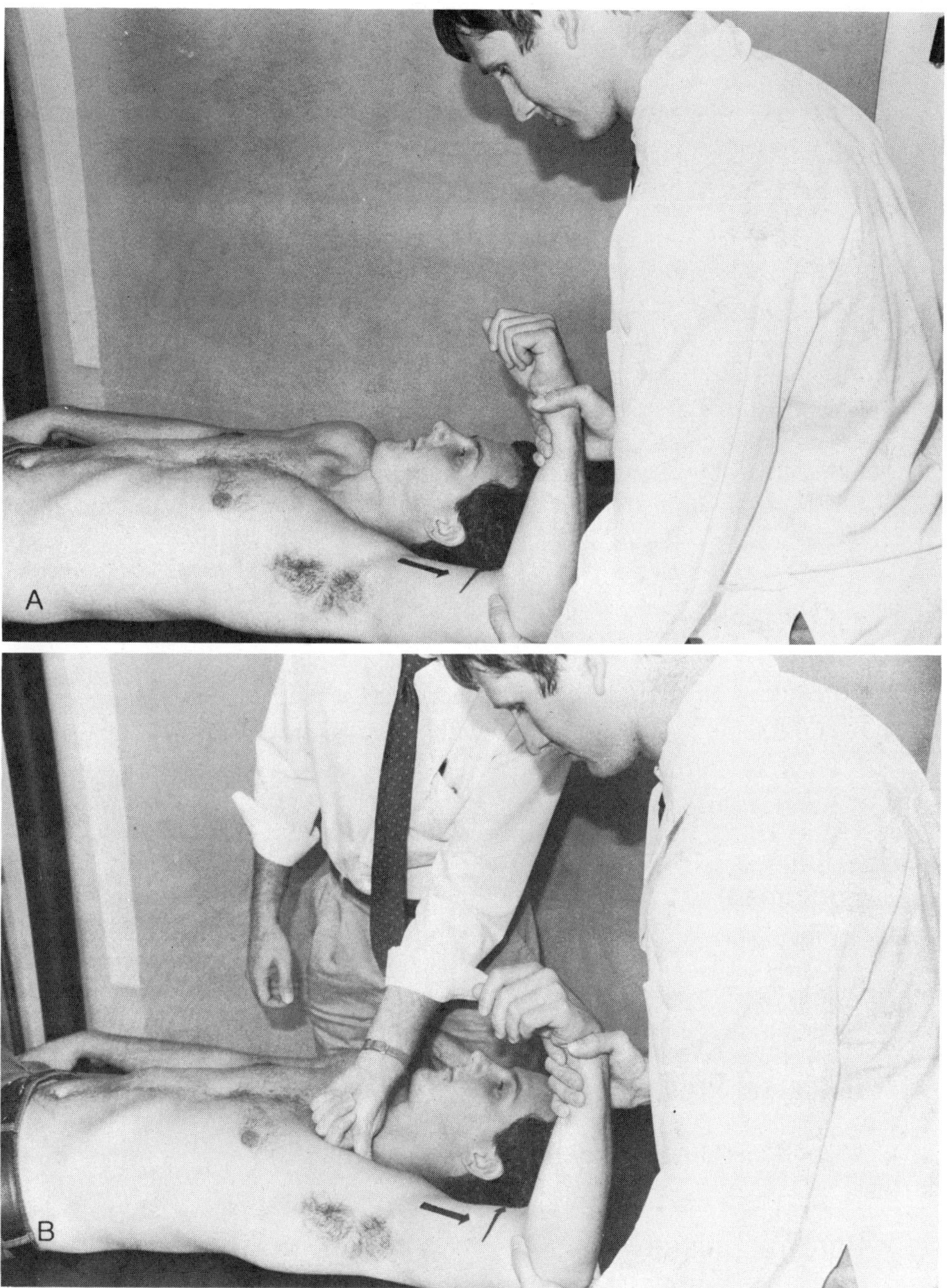

FIGURE 16–25. The Milch technique of shoulder reduction.

Traction Splinting

RICHARD A. CHERRY, NREMTP

Indications

Traction splinting is designed for midshaft and distal femur fractures and for some tibial fractures. Its purpose is to align the fragments, decrease the effects of muscle spasm, relieve pain, prevent damage to vascular or nerve structures, and minimize blood loss by exerting a tension against the supporting muscles. It accomplishes this by applying a steady pull on the distal extremity with an ankle hitch device and simultaneous countertraction to the ischium and groin.

Contraindications

Fractures close to or involving the knee
Hip fractures and hip injuries with gross displacement
Pelvic fractures
Injuries close to the ankle

Equipment

There are two standard types of traction splints used today: the Hare traction splint (ischial ring device) and the Sager traction splint.

Universal Precautions

1. Wear gloves if any bleeding is present.

Hare Technique

The Hare traction splint requires two persons to apply it.

1. Explain the procedure to the patient.
2. Manually stabilize the affected leg above and below the fracture site (Figure 16–26).
3. Remove the shoe and sock and perform distal circulation, sensory, and motor function tests.

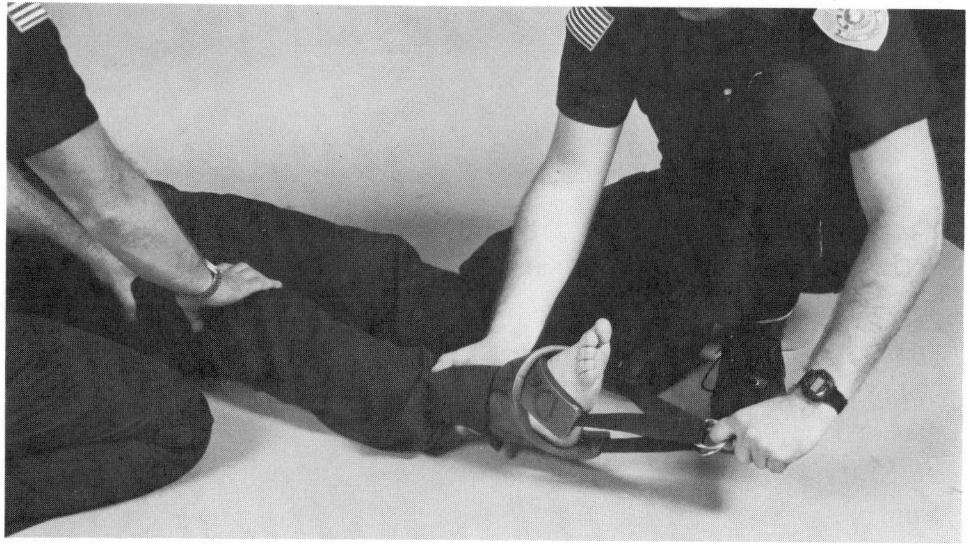

FIGURE 16–26. Hare traction: Step 1.

4. Wrap the ankle hitch and apply manual traction by pulling with both hands and lifting the leg approximately 8 inches off the ground (see Figure 16–26).
5. Place the traction device next to the patient and adjust the length from the ischial tuberosity to 8 to 10 inches beyond the foot. The device telescopes to the proper length and is secured with a locking sleeve device.
6. Extend the heel stand and open the support straps.
7. Slide the splint under the patient and up against the ischial tuberosity (Figure 16–27).

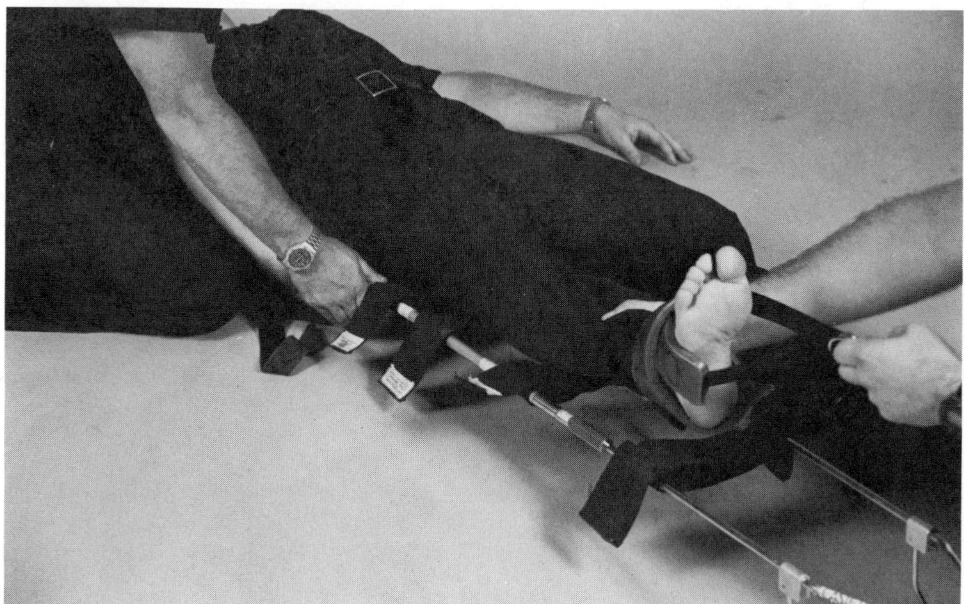

FIGURE 16–27. Hare traction: Step 2.

8. Fasten the ischial strap securely (Figure 16–28).
9. Insert the "S" hook of the mechanical device into the "O" ring of the ankle hitch (Figure 16–29).
10. Apply mechanical traction by turning the ratchet until manual traction is equaled or until muscle spasms are reduced (Figure 16–29).
11. Fasten the leg support straps—two above the knee, two below the knee (Figure 16–30).
12. Reassess distal neurovascular function. Reduce traction if there is perfusion compromise or new neurologic deficit.

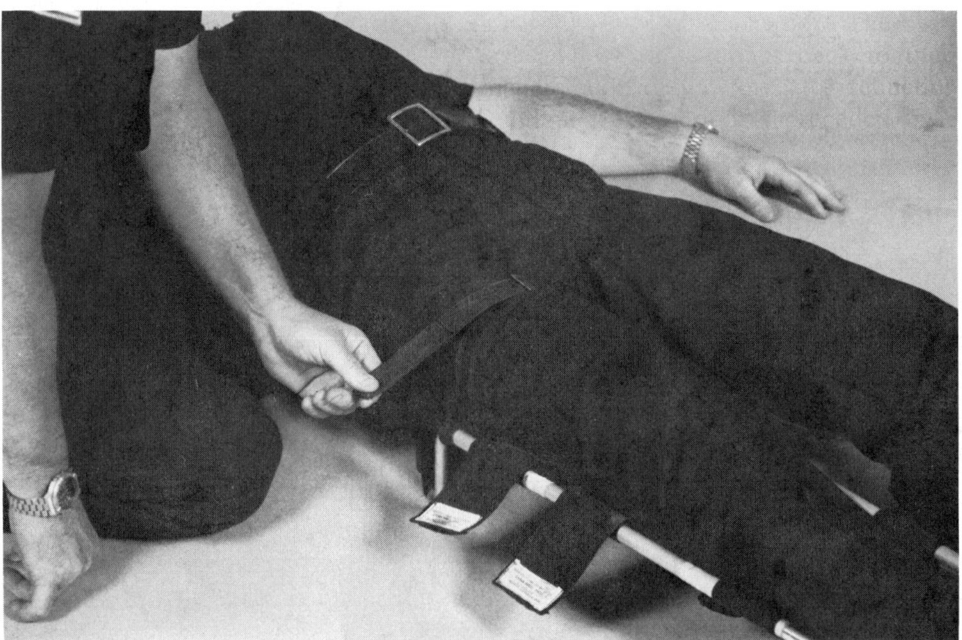

FIGURE 16–28. Hare traction: Step 3.

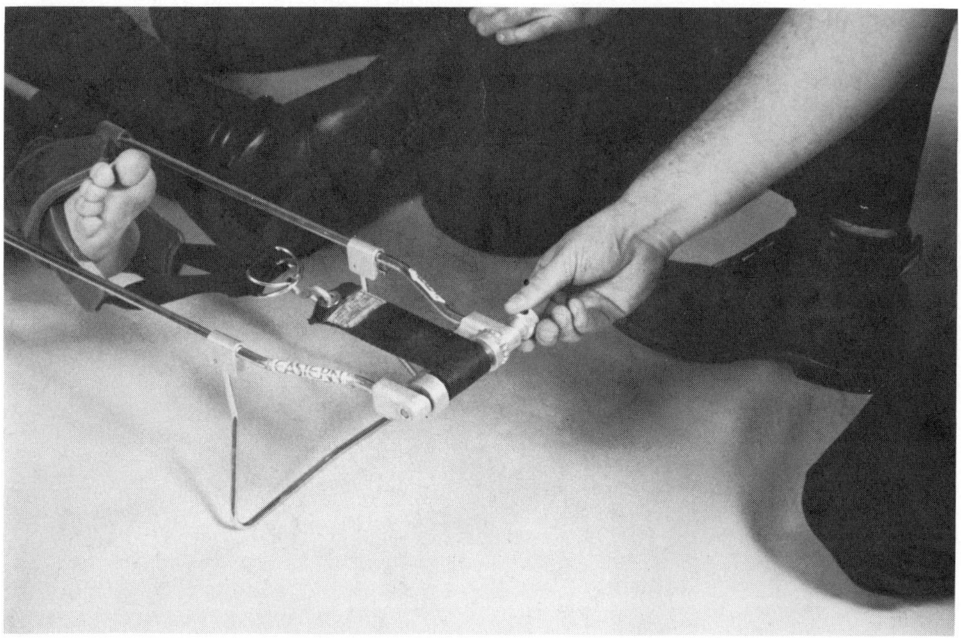

FIGURE 16–29. Hare traction: Step 4.

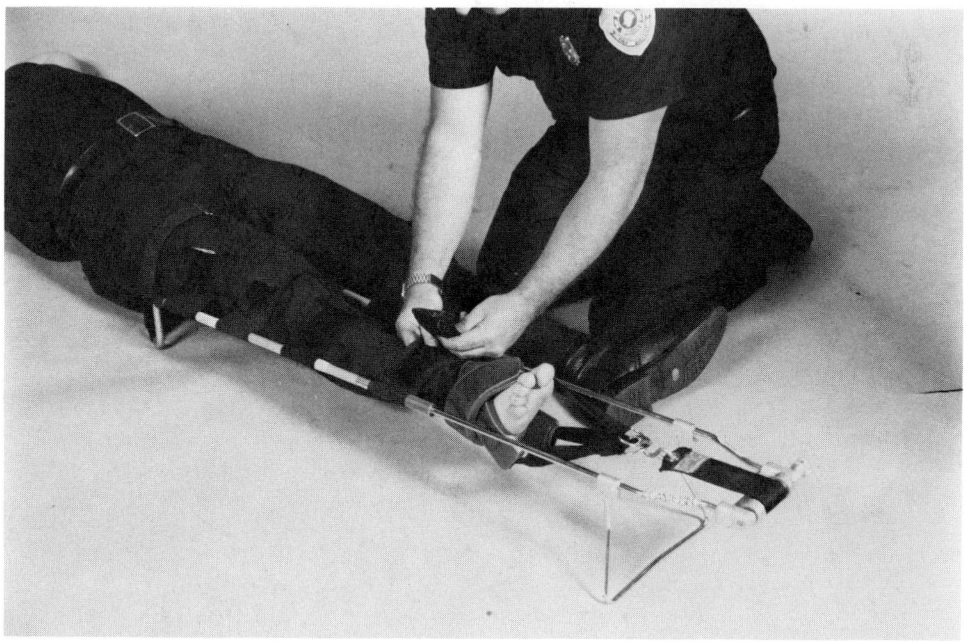

FIGURE 16–30. Hare traction: Step 5.

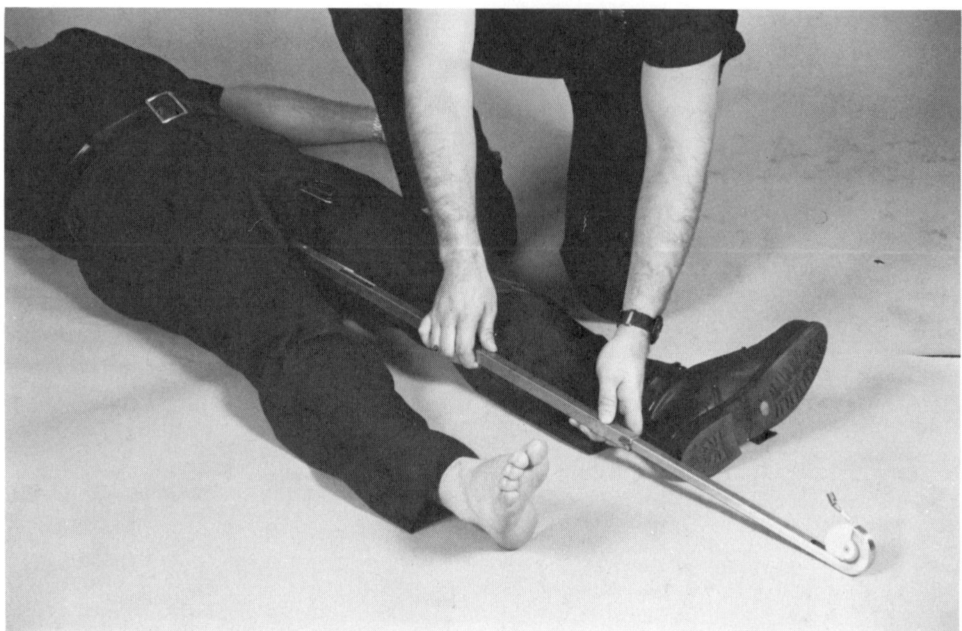

FIGURE 16–31. Sager traction: Step 1.

Sager Technique

The Sager splint requires one person to apply it.

1. Explain the procedure to the patient.
2. Remove the shoe and sock and perform distal circulation, sensory, and motor function tests.

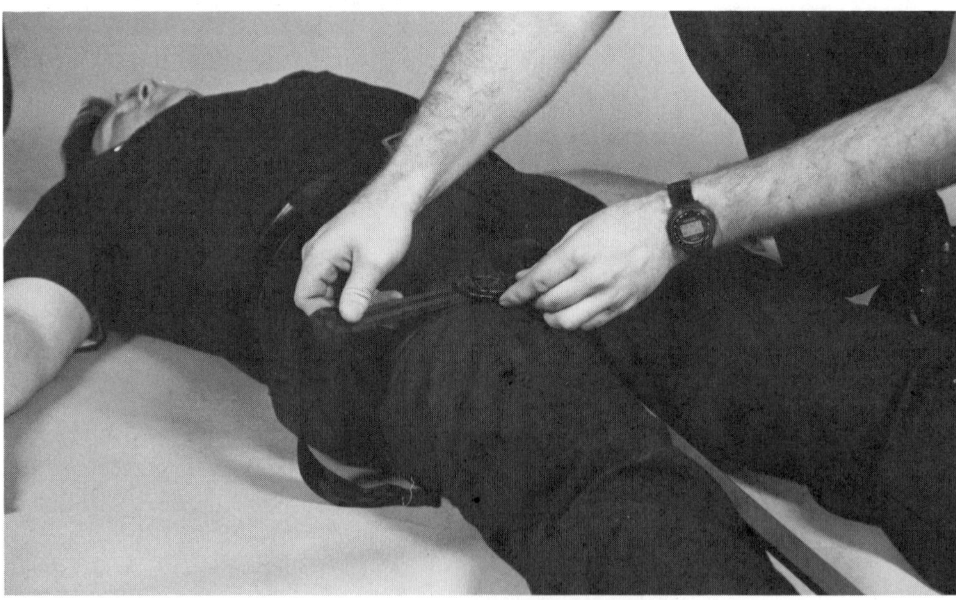

FIGURE 16–32. Sager traction: Step 2.

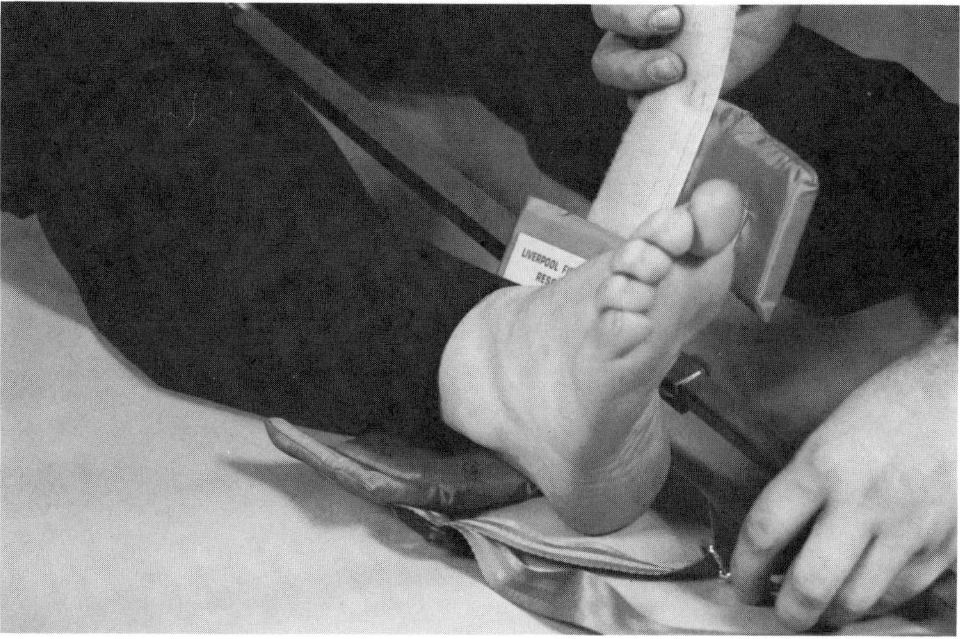

FIGURE 16–33. Sager traction: Step 3.

3. Place the splint medially so that the wheel is at the heel and the perineal cushion is snug against the perineum and ischial tuberosity (Figure 16–31).
4. Tighten the thigh strap (Figure 16–32).
5. Wrap the ankle hitch tightly just above the medial and lateral malleoli. Check pedal pulses before continuing (Figure 16–33).
6. Shorten the loop of the ankle hitch by pulling on the strap threaded through the device.
7. Extend the splint to achieve the desired traction in pounds (10% of body weight) on the calibrated pulley wheel (Figure 16–34).

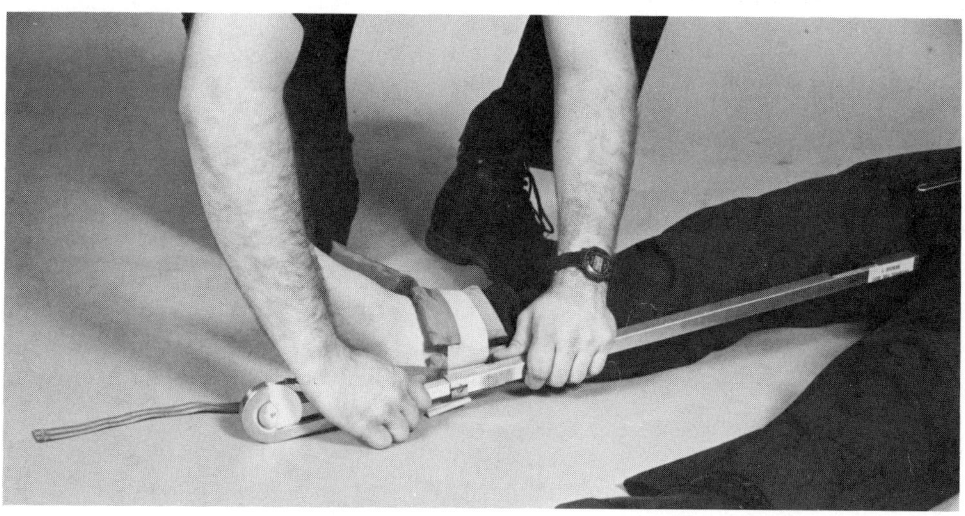

FIGURE 16–34. Sager traction: Step 4.

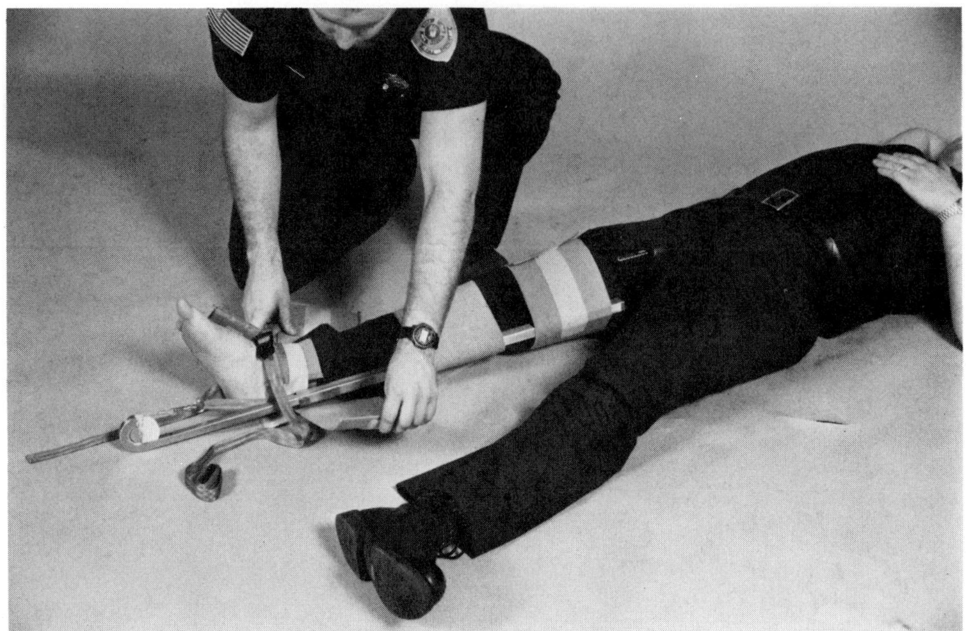

FIGURE 16–35. Sager traction: Step 5.

8. Fasten the leg support straps at the thigh, knee, and lower leg (Figure 16–35).
9. Apply a figure-eight strap around both ankles and secure snugly.

Complications

Hyperseparation of the bone fragments
Dislocation of the knee
Further damage if traction is released during application of the splint
Neurovascular compromise

Pearls and Pitfalls

1. Once the splint is applied, do not let go of the manual traction until it is equaled by mechanical traction.
2. If the ankle hitch is applied too tightly, evidenced by a loss of pulses or edema, loosen it slightly.
3. The Sager splint can be applied medially, laterally, or bilaterally and can also be used for children.
4. While the ischial ring traction devices, such as the Hare splint, can put pressure on the sciatic nerve and angulate the fracture site, the Sager splint does not.

References

Advanced Trauma Life Support Program. Chicago, American College of Surgeons Committee on Trauma, 1989.

Grant HD, Murray RH, Bergeron JD: Brady Emergency Care. Englewood Cliffs, NJ, Prentice-Hall, 1990.

17

Peritoneal Lavage

LUKE YIP, MD

Indications

- Multisystem blunt trauma with
  - Altered mental status
  - Unexplained hypotension
  - Falling hematocrit
  - Unreliable abdominal examination (e.g., fractured ribs, pelvis, spinal column)
  - Paraplegia
- Temperature control
  - Hypothermia
  - Hyperthermia
- Acute pancreatitis (data controversial)
- Selected drug overdoses
- Access for peritoneal dialysis

Contraindications

Absolute

- Existing indication for exploratory laparotomy
  - Physical evidence of abdominal trauma and hemodynamic instability
  - Unequivocal signs of peritoneal irritation
  - Intra-abdominal free air (chest and abdominal x-ray films should be obtained prior to peritoneal lavage)
  - Evisceration of abdominal contents

Relative

Multiple prior laparotomies (especially pelvic)
Morbid obesity
Advanced stage of cirrhosis
Advanced gravid uterus
Stab wounds to the abdomen (selective celiotomy may be indicated)

Equipment

Foley catheter
Nasogastric tube
Surgical shaving kit
Betadine solution
Surgical marker
Sterile surgical drapes/towels
1% lidocaine with epinephrine
Bedside cautery
No. 10 scalpels
Skin retractors
Hemostats
Needle holder
Suture scissors
25-gauge 1 inch, 20-gauge 1½ inch needles
Syringes, 10 ml and 20 ml
Allis clamps
Tissue forceps
4×4-inch gauze pads
Surgical tapes
Lap pads
Peritoneal dialysis catheter setup
1 L warm lactated Ringer's or normal saline intravenous solution (if diagnostic lavage)
1.5% Dineal if therapeutic catheter is placed
Blood transfusion intravenous tubing (if diagnostic lavage)
Y dialysis tubing/drainage set if therapeutic procedure
Sutures: 2–0 Vicryl and 4–0 nylon
Proper surgical attire: cap, gown, mask, gloves, eye shield
Good light source

Universal Precautions

1. Wear gloves, mask, cap, and gown.
2. Use an eye shield.

Technique (Open)

1. Explain procedure to patient and obtain consent if situation permits.
2. Decompress stomach and bladder by insertion of nasogastric tube and Foley catheter.
3. Place patient in the supine position.
4. Shave mid abdomen.
5. Put on cap, gown, mask, eye shield, and gloves. (*Note:* Strict aseptic technique is to be followed from this point.)

6. Scrub and paint abdomen with Betadine solution.
7. Locate the midline extending from the umbilicus to the symphysis pubis. Using a surgical marker, begin just below the umbilicus and mark off approximately 5 cm caudally (Figure 17–1).
8. Place surgical drapes over the abdomen leaving the surgically marked area exposed (Figure 17–2).

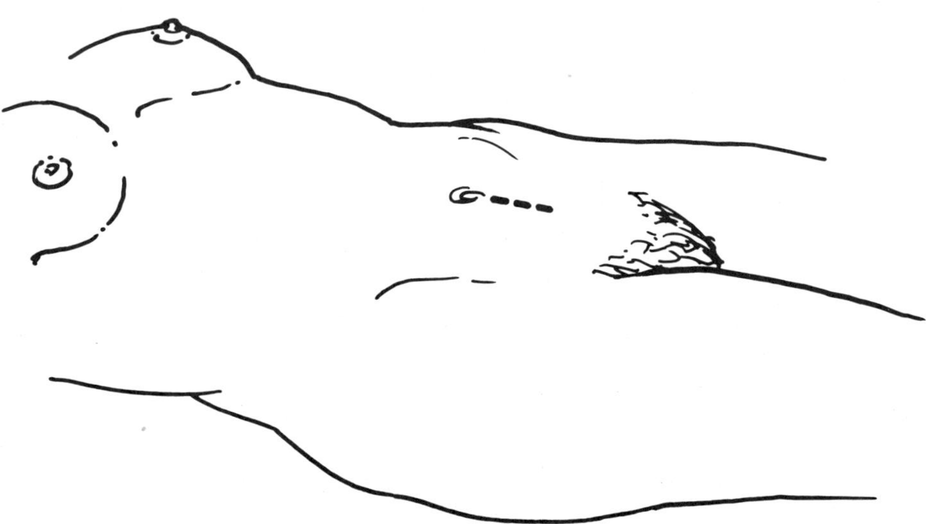

FIGURE 17–1. Site for peritoneal lavage.

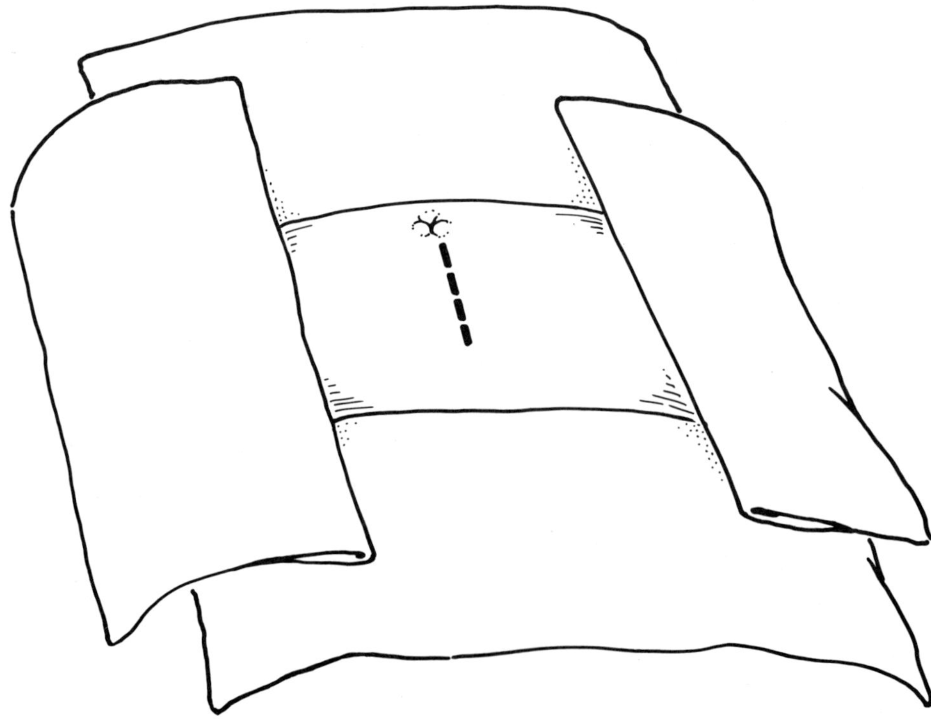

FIGURE 17–2. Peritoneal lavage: Draping and skin incision.

9. Infiltrate local anesthetic (1% lidocaine with epinephrine) into the skin and subcutaneous tissue of the incision site using the 10-ml syringe and 25-gauge needle.
10. Make a 4- to 5-cm horizontal skin incision at the mark using a No. 10 scalpel.
11. Dissect the exposed adipose tissue with a hemostat until the linea alba ("pearly white") of the anterior rectus sheath (Figure 17–3, arrow) is identified. Keep the field dry at all times by cauterizing all bleeding vessels. Use 4 × 4-inch gauze pads to retract the subcutaneous tissue and help keep the field dry during the blunt dissection.
12. Grasp the linea alba on either side of the midline with hemostats and make a 3-cm vertical incision through the fascia.

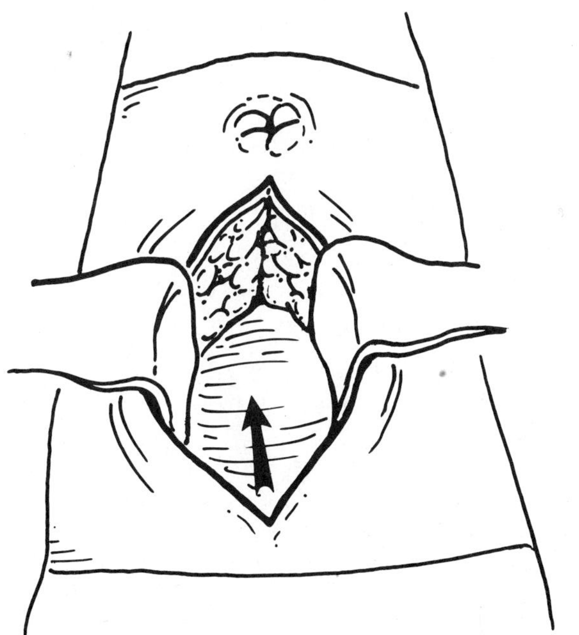

FIGURE 17–3. Peritoneal lavage: Identification of linea alba (→).

13. Expose the posterior rectus sheath by grasping the incised edges of the linea alba with Allis clamps. The assistant can provide better exposure by giving countertraction with the Allis clamps (Figure 17–4).
14. Carefully tent the posterior rectus sheath and the peritoneum by applying hemostats on either side of the midline (Figure 17–5, arrow).
15. Pinch and roll the tented area between the thumb and index fingers. Feel with the fingers to make certain that no portion of the bowel has been grabbed along with the fascia and peritoneum.
16. Make a surgical nick between the hemostats using the No. 10 scalpel.
17. Carefully introduce a dialysis catheter into this small surgical opening. Advance the catheter in the direction of either pelvic gutter (Figure 17–6), without using excessive force if resistance is met.

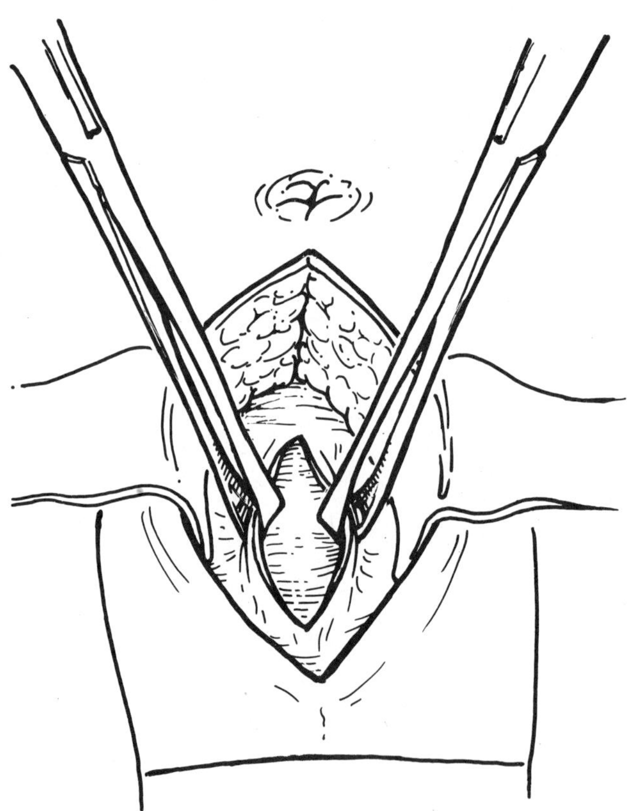

FIGURE 17–4. Peritoneal lavage: Opening linea alba.

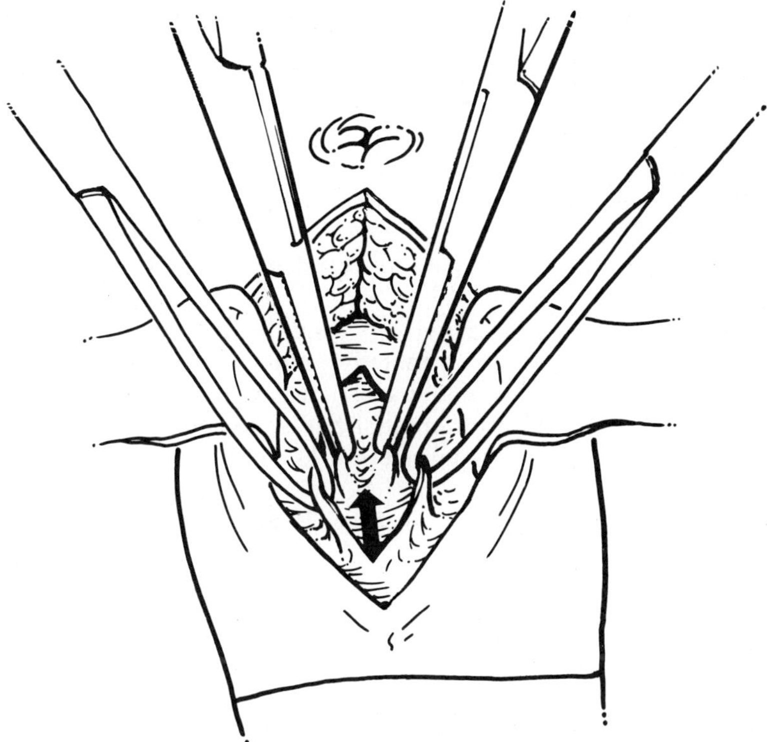

FIGURE 17–5. Peritoneal lavage: Tenting peritoneum.

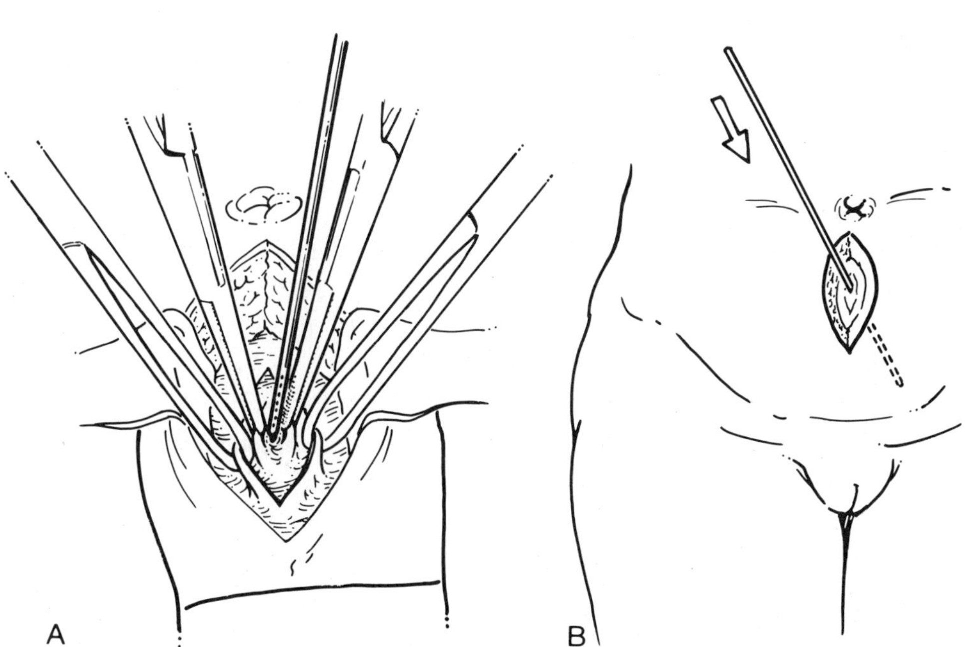

FIGURE 17–6. Peritoneal lavage: Insertion of catheter.

If diagnostic peritoneal lavage:

18. Attach the 20-ml syringe onto the catheter and aspirate. If gross blood ($\geq$10 ml) is noted on aspiration, it is an indication for celiotomy (positive tap) and negates the lavage portion of this procedure.
19. If no gross blood is obtained by aspiration, then attach the catheter to 1 L of warmed lactated Ringer's or normal saline intravenous solution through blood transfusion intravenous tubing. Run in 10 ml/kg (maximum 1 L) of solution. Gently agitate the fluid-filled abdomen and let sit for approximately 5 minutes.
20. Siphon off the fluid by gravity by placing the intravenous fluid bag on the floor. The container must be vented to allow free return of fluid. Remove the catheter after approximately 0.5 L of fluid has been recovered.
21. Send the lavage fluid for differential cell count and amylase.
22. Close the surgical wounds in layers: 2–0 Vicryl for the fascias; 4–0 nylon for the skin.
23. Dress the wound with 4 × 4-inch gauge pads and bandage with surgical tape.

If therapeutic peritoneal catheter placement:

18. Attach 1L of 1.5% dineal to peritoneal catheter and rapidly infuse into the peritoneal cavity.
19. Allow solution to dwell for 5 to 10 minutes.
20. Drain by gravity.
21. Proceed with peritoneal dialysis.
22. Close the surgical wounds in layers: 2–0 Vicryl for the fascias; 4–0 nylon for the skin.
23. Dress the wound with 4 × 4-inch gauze pads and bandage with surgical tape.

Criteria for a positive peritoneal lavage in the trauma patient:

Gross blood
100,000 RBC/mm^3
500 WBC/mm^3
Return of bowel contents
Lavage fluid out a chest tube (indicates ruptured diaphragm)
Amylase, 200 units/dl

Complications

Bowel or bladder perforation (more likely with closed technique)
Local wound infection (cellulitis) at the surgical site
Abdominal hernia from inadequate closure of the fascia at the surgical site
Peritonitis
Hemorrhage due to large vessel injury (aorta, epigastric artery, mesenteric vessels)

Pearls and Pitfalls

1. Negative (false-negative) peritoneal lavage does not rule out intestinal perforations, injuries to the retroperitoneum, diaphragm, or the urinary tract.
2. X-ray films of the chest and abdomen should be performed prior to the peritoneal lavage.
3. The "open technique" is the safest but takes longer.
4. Keep in the midline at all times.
5. Keep a dry operating field; cauterize bleeding vessels.
6. Make sure there is adequate exposure and lighting throughout the procedure.
7. Be absolutely certain that the linea alba ("pearly white") is identified as the landmark for entering the peritoneum.
8. Use a supraumbilical approach (3 cm above the umbilicus) if there is a pelvic fracture.
9. A coagulopathy is not a contraindication and does not influence accuracy.

References

Advanced Trauma Life Support Course Student Manual. Chicago, American College of Surgeons, pp 98–100, 105–107, 1985.

Dunham CM, Cowley RA: Shock Trauma/Critical Care Handbook, pp 201–211. Rockville, MD, Aspen Publishers, 1986.

Moore JB, Moore EE, Markovchick VJ, Rosen P: Diagnostic peritoneal lavage for abdominal trauma: Superiority of the open technique at the infraumbilical ring. J Trauma 21:570–572, 1981.

18 Pulmonary Artery Catheterization

JONATHAN WARREN, MD

Indications

To obtain hemodynamic and oxygen transport data for diagnosis
To guide therapy in patients with cardiorespiratory compromise

Contraindications

Artificial tricuspid or pulmonary valve

Equipment

Cap, mask, and eye shield
Sterile gown and gloves
Sterile drape, full body
Betadine skin prep
6-foot pressure tubing
Three-way stopcock
Needle holder
Suture scissors
3–0 nylon suture on curved needle
Two 10-ml syringes
3-ml syringe
Pressure monitor/flush systems
Oscilloscope and/or strip chart recorder
ECG monitor
25-gauge, 1½-inch needle
Pulse oximeter (use for nonintubated patients only)
Supplemental oxygen (use for nonintubated patients only)
Pulmonary artery catheter with compatible cardiac output computer
Catheter protective sleeve
Betadine ointment
Lidocaine 1% without epinephrine for skin anesthesia
Lidocaine (100 mg) for intravenous administration (stand by)
Sterile 4 × 4-inch gauze pads
Tape
DC defibrillator and crash cart (stand by)

Types of Pulmonary Artery Catheters (Figure 18–1)

Standard—has proximal central venous pressure port, distal pulmonary artery port, and thermodilution cardiac output capabilities

VIP—same as standard catheter but with an additional central venous pressure port

Pace-Port—same as standard catheter but with a right ventricular port through which a temporary pacing wire can be passed for emergency cardiac pacing

Oximetric—same as standard catheter but with a fiberoptic system for the continuous measurement of mixed venous oxygen saturation

REF—same as standard catheter but with a special injection port, ECG electrodes, and a fast-response thermistor for the measurement of right ventricular ejection fraction

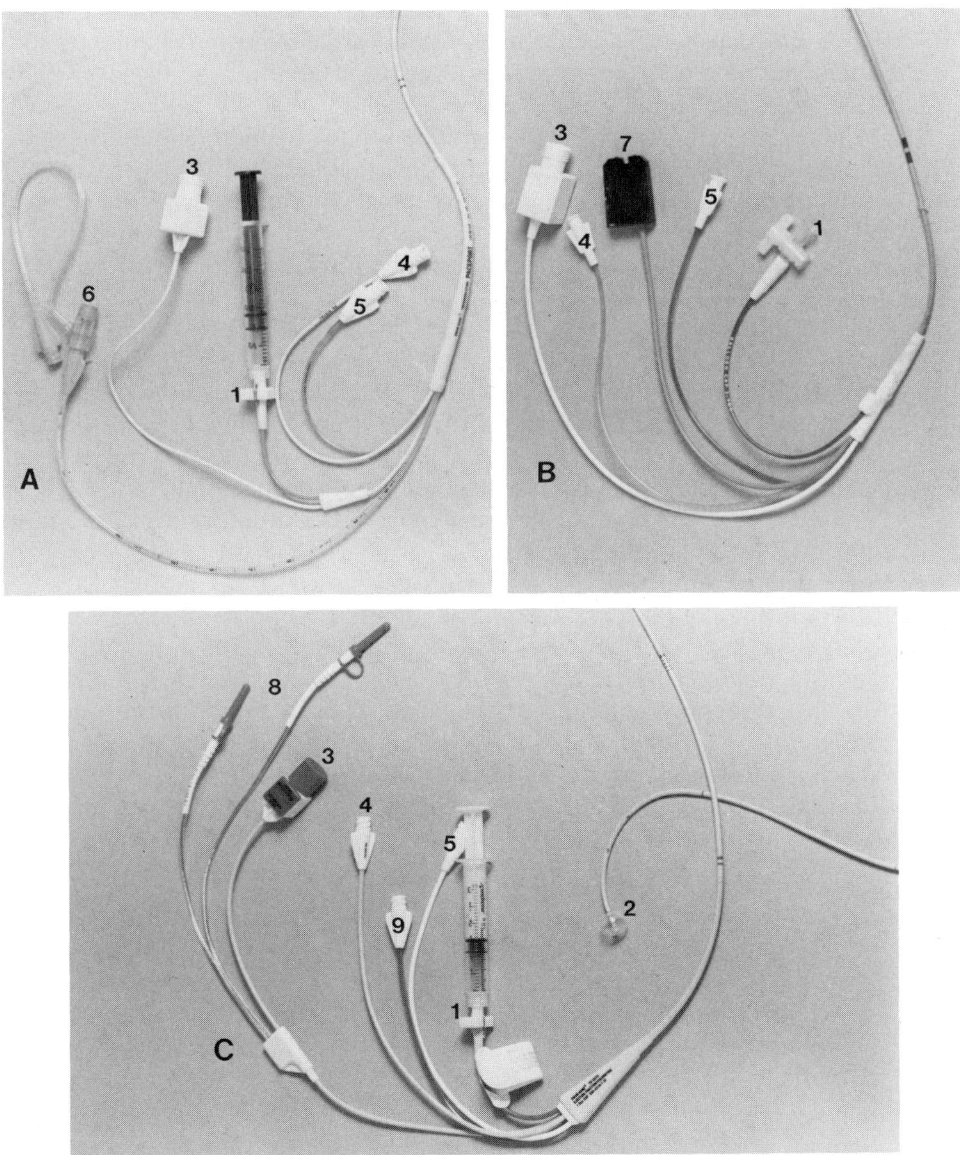

FIGURE 18–1. A, Paceport catheter. **B,** Oximetric catheter. **C,** REF catheter. *1,* Port to balloon; *2,* balloon; *3,* thermistor connection for cardiac output; *4,* distal port for PA and PCW pressures; *5,* CVP port; *6,* right ventricular port for emergency pacing; *7,* optical connector for mixed venous oxygen saturation measurement; *8,* ECG electrodes; *9,* injection port for right ventricular ejection fraction.

Universal Precautions

1. Wear cap, mask, and sterile gloves and gown.
2. Use an eye shield.

Technique

Many pulmonary artery catheter insertion techniques are currently practiced. The following protocol is designed to minimize complications both during and after insertion:

1. If patient status and circumstances allow, explain the procedure to the patient and obtain informed consent.
2. Place patient on continuous ECG monitoring.
3. For nonintubated patients, begin continuous pulse oximetry monitoring and administer supplemental oxygen as indicated to maintain adequate oxygenation, especially during the interval that patient's face is covered by the sterile drape.
4. Position patient supine in bed, and zero the pressure transducer at midaxillary (left atrial) level.
5. Put on cap, mask, eye shield, and sterile gown and gloves.
6. Choose the site for vascular access. Possibilities include the subclavian, internal jugular, femoral, and brachial veins. Vascular access may be obtained de novo (see Chapter 24), through a previously placed introducer sheath, or by a guide wire change of an existing central venous catheter (single or multiple lumen) into a catheter introducer sheath.
7. Prep area of catheter insertion (including introducer or central venous catheter if present) with Betadine.
8. Cover patient with sterile full-body drape.
9. If there is not already a catheter introducer sheath in place, secure vascular access by a de novo insertion or a guide wire change of an existing central venous pressure catheter.
10. Attach a three-way stopcock to the distal port of the pulmonary artery catheter.
11. Attach a 6-foot pressure tubing to this stopcock.
12. Hand the opposite end of the 6-foot pressure tubing for attachment to the

pressure monitor/flush system. Flush tubing and the distal catheter port. Be sure to remove all gas bubbles from the fluid pathway.

13. Use the side port of the three-way stopcock to fill 10-ml syringes with flush solution.
14. Remove air from syringes, and attach one syringe to each of the remaining catheter ports. Flush by hand to remove all air from the fluid pathways. Leave syringes attached to ports.
15. Pass the catheter protective sleeve over the catheter. Do not expand the sleeve.
16. Test-fill the catheter flotation balloon with its full volume of air as recommended by the manufacturer (usually 1.5 ml) using the syringe supplied with the catheter or a 3-ml syringe. Check the balloon for symmetry and air leaks, and ensure that the catheter tip is buried within the balloon (see Figure 1*C*). Deflate balloon. *Note:* The balloon should always be allowed to deflate passively to avoid balloon damage. Never actively aspirate the air from the balloon.
17. Test the catheter thermister for electrical continuity by plugging it into a cardiac output computer and confirming a reading of room temperature. If using an oximetry catheter, also attach the oximetry lead to the box and perform an in vitro calibration.
18. Check for zero position of the transducer by holding the catheter tip at the midaxillary line. Pressure should read zero. If not, re-zero the transducer.
19. Test for transducer signal quality by rapidly oscillating the catheter tip. An oscillating pressure should be visualized on the oscilloscope and/or strip chart recorder. The absence of this indicates an obstruction in the fluid pathway, air in the flush system, a malfunctioning transducer, or an incorrect adjustment in the transducer output gain.
20. Pass the catheter into the introducer sheath until the catheter balloon tip protrudes from the introducer (usually 17 to 20 cm). Inflate the catheter balloon with its full volume of air as recommended by the manufacturer. If resistance to inflation is felt, *do not force.* Try advancing the catheter an additional 1 or 2 cm and attempt inflation once again. If resistance is still present, remove the catheter and inspect it. Evaluate the possibility that the catheter is traveling an incorrect pathway on exit from the introducer (e.g., up the internal jugular vein from the subclavian vein).
21. Begin continuous observation of the ECG and the pressure tracing recorded from the catheter distal port.

22. Advance the catheter, with balloon inflated, observing the catheter tip (by pressure tracing) pass consecutively through the right atrium, right ventricle, and into the pulmonary artery (Figure 18–2). The pulmonary artery is usually reached with the insertion of 40 to 50 cm of catheter, depending on the insertion site, size of the right ventricle, and patient. The length of catheter required to reach this point will be substantially greater if using an antecubital or femoral venous insertion site.
23. With the balloon still inflated, advance the catheter a few centimeters farther until a wedge tracing is observed.
24. Deflate the balloon and observe the reappearance of a pulmonary artery waveform. If a wedge tracing persists, withdraw the catheter slightly until a pulmonary artery tracing is observed.
25. Slowly reinflate the balloon. A wedge tracing should occur at the end of full balloon inflation. If less than full inflation is required, the catheter tip is too distally placed. Deflate the balloon and withdraw the catheter 1 or 2 cm and attempt inflation once again. Repeat procedure until optimal catheter position is achieved.
26. Expand the catheter sleeve and lock it into proper position as described by the manufacturer.
27. Suture the catheter to the skin, leaving a large loop of catheter distal to the suture site.
28. Apply Betadine ointment to puncture and suture sites.
29. Apply sterile dressing.

Complications

Atrial or ventricular dysrhythmias

Right bundle branch block

Pulmonary artery perforation and hemorrhage

Thrombosis (subclavian or internal jugular veins, superior vena cava, pulmonary artery)

Bacterial endocarditis

Cardiac valvular vegetations

Catheter knots; entanglements around cardiac structures

Catheter infection

Air embolism

Pulmonary infarction

Pearls and Pitfalls

1. Pulmonary artery catheters can dislodge previously placed transvenous pacemakers. Therefore, fluoroscopic guidance should be used during catheter introduction under these circumstances.
2. Because right bundle branch block can occur during catheter passage, patients with preexisting left bundle branch block are at risk for developing complete heart block during catheter placement. Therefore, a temporary transvenous pacemaker should be placed in patients with left bundle branch block before the introduction of a pulmonary artery catheter, or a transcutaneous pacemaker should be available at the bedside.

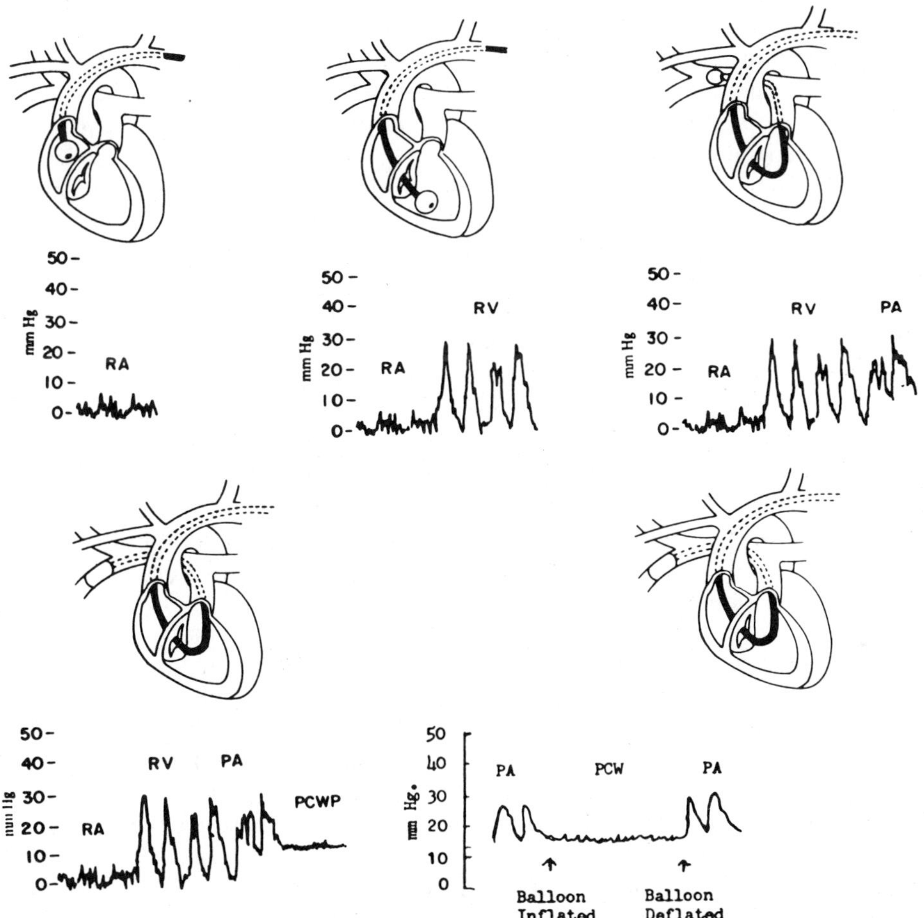

FIGURE 18–2. Hemodynamic aspects of balloon catheter insertions into the pulmonary artery. *RA,* right atrium; *RV,* right ventricle; *PA,* pulmonary artery; *PCWP,* pulmonary capillary wedge pressure.

3. The right subclavian vein is a notoriously poor insertion site for pulmonary artery catheters. The right subclavian vein is usually too short to hold the entire length of an introducer without its distal tip abutting against the medial wall of the superior vena cava. Pulmonary artery catheters passed through these introducers almost always kink as they exit the introducer, resulting in poor function of the catheter. Specifically, pressure waveforms may appear damped, thermistor wires may fracture, and one or more of the catheter lumens may be difficult to infuse through, or may even clot.
4. The pacing wire that can be passed through a Pace-Port pulmonary artery catheter comes in a separate package, which contains detailed instructions on its insertion procedure. These wires are often difficult to pass because they bind in the catheter, especially at sharp curves. Expect to take at least 5 to 10 minutes to pass one of these wires. They tend to be somewhat unreliable, and a standard transvenous pacer is better if the patient is truly pacer dependent.
5. It is not unusual for a catheter introducer placed through the subclavian vein to go up the internal jugular vein. When the pulmonary artery catheter is then passed, it, too, will go up the internal jugular vein, as evidenced by resistance to its advancement and a pressure waveform that goes off the upper scale, and sometimes visible movement of the neck is seen with advancement of the catheter. When faced with this problem, try the following. First, pull the introducer back 5 or 6 cm and then try advancing the catheter. Often it will take the correct route even when the introducer did not. If this fails, then insert the pulmonary artery catheter to 20 to 30 cm and fully withdraw the introducer. Then inflate the balloon on the pulmonary artery catheter and gently pull it back until it is caught on the wall of the subclavian vein. Then advance the catheter with its balloon inflated, and the flow of blood will usually carry the inflated balloon in the correct direction. When the pulmonary artery catheter is properly positioned, then reinsert the introducer by sliding it over the pulmonary artery catheter.
6. Most pulmonary artery catheters sail through the heart to their proper position on the first pass, but not all do. The old adage "if at first you don't succeed, try, try, again" holds true here. If you are not in proper position by 50 to 60 cm, deflate the balloon, pull the catheter back to 20 cm, reinflate the balloon, and readvance. Sooner or later it will get there. Stiffening the catheter by injecting iced sterile saline through it, twisting the catheter as you are advancing it, and having a cooperative patient take a deep breath as you advance the catheter are tricks that sometimes help. Be careful never to insert more than 60 cm of catheter (when coming from the superior vena cava or subclavian veins) or you may tie the catheter in a knot.

References

Insertion Technique

Swan HJC, et al: Catheterization of the heart in man with use of a flow-directed balloon-tipped catheter. N Engl J Med 283:447–451, 1970.

Swan HJC, Ganz W: Guidelines for use of balloon-tipped catheter. Am J Cardiol 34:119, 1974.

Dysrhythmias

Cairns JA, Holder D: Ventricular fibrillation due to passage of a Swan-Ganz catheter. Am J Cardiol 35:589, 1975.

Damen J: Ventricular arrhythmias during insertion and removal of pulmonary artery catheters. Chest 88:190–193, 1985.
Geha DG, et al: Persistent atrial arrhythmias associated with placement of a Swan-Ganz catheter. Anesthesiology 39:651–653, 1973.
Shaw TJI: The Swan-Ganz pulmonary artery catheter: Incidence of complications, with particular reference to ventricular dysrhythimias, and their prevention. Anesthesia 34:651–655, 1979.
Sprung CL, et al: Advanced ventricular arrhythmias during bedside pulmonary artery catheterization. Am J Med 72:203–208, 1982.

Pulmonary Artery Hemorrhage

Golden MS, et al: Fatal pulmonary hemorrhage complicating use of a flow-directed balloon-tipped catheter in a patient receiving anticoagulant therapy. Am J Cardiol 32:865–867, 1973.
Lapin ES, Murray JA: Hemoptysis with flow-directed cardiac catheterization. JAMA 220:1246, 1972.
Paulson DM, et al: Pulmonary hemorrhage associated with balloon flotation catheters. J Thorac Cardiovasc Surg 80:453–458, 1980.

Thrombosis

Chastre J, et al: Thrombosis as a complication of pulmonary-artery catheterization via the internal jugular vein: Prospective evaluation by phlebography. N Engl J Med 306:278–281, 1982.
Goodman DJ, et al: Thromboembolic complications with the indwelling balloon-tipped pulmonary artery catheter. N Engl J Med 291:777, 1974.
Hoar PF, et al: Thrombogenesis associated with Swan-Ganz catheters. Anesthesiology 48:445–447, 1978.

Endocarditis and Valvular Vegetations

Becker AE, et al: Bland thrombosis and infection in relation to intracardiac catheter. Circulation 46:200–203, 1972.
Ford SE, Manley PN: Indwelling cardiac catheters: An autopsy study of associated endocardial lesions. Arch Pathol Lab Med 106:311–317, 1982.
Green JF, Cummings KC: Aseptic thrombotic endocardial vegetations: A complication of indwelling pulmonary artery catheters. JAMA 225:1525–1527, 1973.
Green JF, et al: Local complications associated with indwelling Swan-Ganz catheters: Autopsy study of 36 cases. Am J Cardiol 52:1108–1111, 1983.
Pace NL, Horton W: Indwelling pulmonary artery catheters: Their relationship to aseptic thrombotic endocardial vegetations. JAMA 233:893–894, 1974.
Rowley KM, et al: Right-sided infective endocarditis as a consequence of flow-directed pulmonary artery catheterization: A clinicopathological study of 55 autopsied patients. N Engl J Med 311:1152–1156, 1984.

Knots and Tangles

Daum S, Schapira M: Intracardiac knot formation in a Swan-Ganz catheter. Anesth Analg 52:862–863, 1973.
Lipp H, et al: Intracardiac knotting of a flow-directed balloon catheter. N Engl J Med 284:220, 1971.
Meister SG, et al: Knotting of a flow-directed catheter about a cardiac structure. Cathet Cardiovasc Diagn 3:171–175, 1971.
Schwartz KV, Garcia FG: Entanglement of Swan-Ganz catheter around an intracardiac structure. JAMA 237:1198, 1977.
Smith WR, Glauser FL: Ruptured chordae of the tricuspid valve: The consequence of flow-directed Swan-Ganz catheterization. Chest 70:790–792, 1976.

19

Resuscitation

Emergency External Pacing

MICHAEL S. JASTREMSKI, MD

Indication

Symptomatic bradydysrhythmias

Contraindications

None, if the clinical situation indicates the need for pacing

Equipment

External pacing machine (Figure 19–1)
Two special external pacing electrodes (are specific for each brand of external pacer)

Universal Precautions

None

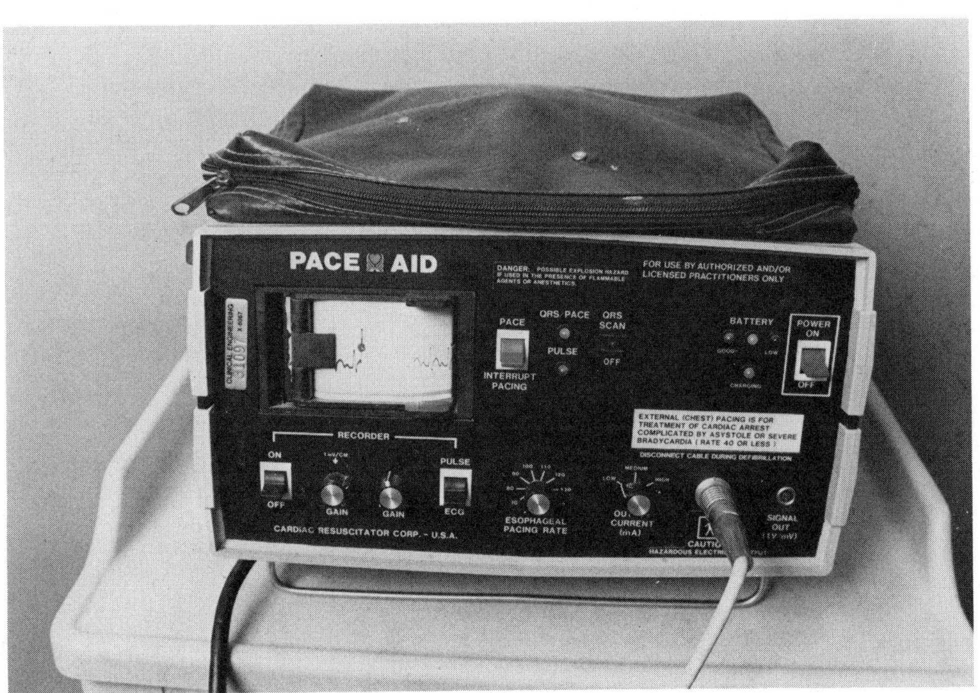

FIGURE 19–1. External pacer.

Technique

1. If the patient's condition and circumstances allow, explain the procedure to the patient and obtain informed consent. Be sure to warn the patient that he may experience some mildly unpleasant contractions of the chest wall musculature and/or feel the electrical discharge of each pacing stimulus.
2. Apply one special large pacing electrode to the patient's back in the left hemithorax below the scapula. Apply the other electrode over the apex of the heart on the anterior chest wall (Figure 19–2).
3. Attach the electrodes to the external pacing machine using the cable supplied with the machine that meshes with that company's electrodes.
4. Set the external pacer to maximal sensitivity (some models are fixed-rate pacers that do not sense), minimal pacing output, and a rate greater than the patient's intrinsic rate.
5. Turn on the pacer.
6. Increase the pacing output until capture occurs consistently.
7. Arrange for expeditious placement of a transvenous pacer under fluoroscopic guidance or insert a balloon-tipped transvenous pacer if fluoroscopy is not available.

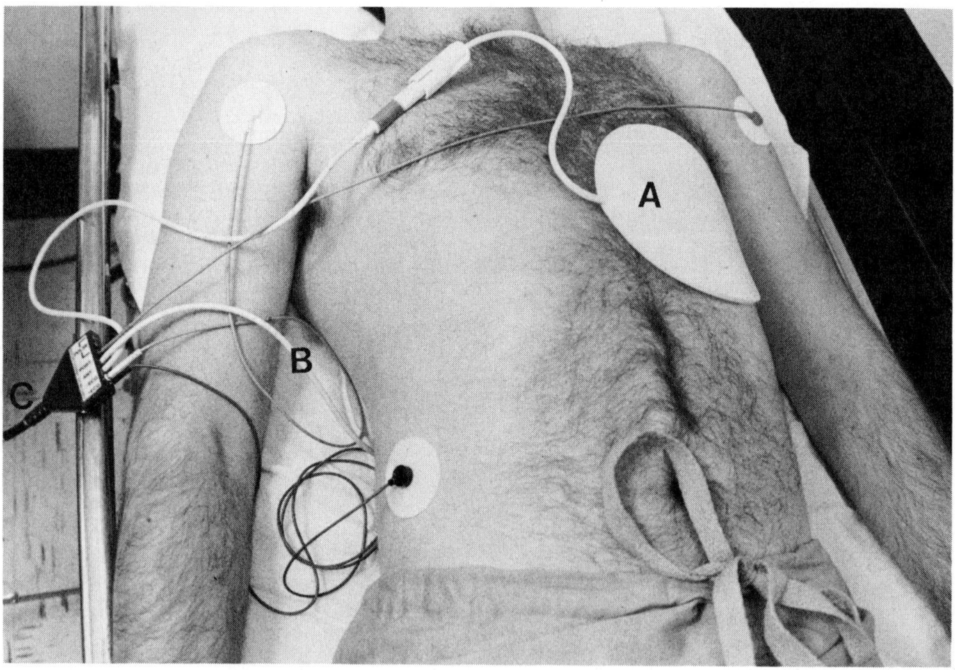

FIGURE 19–2. *A,* Anterior pacing electrode; *B,* cable to posterior electrode; *C,* cable to pacer.

Complications

Failure to pace
Pain
Skin irritation
Failure to sense
Dysrhythmias

Pearls and Pitfalls

1. External pacing is the quickest means to establish emergency pacing.
2. Spend some time learning how the external pacing machine available in your institution works *before* you need to use it on a patient.

Reference

Extensive experience.

Transthoracic Pacing

GARY JOHNSON, MD

Indications

Cardiac arrest due to asystole
Failure of external pacing in the above setting

Contraindications

None

Equipment

The needle, pacing wire, and adapter to connect the wire to the pulse generator usually come as a prepackaged kit (Figure 19–3).

- Pacing wire
- Long (e.g., 12 cm) needle of appropriate diameter (16–18 gauge) to allow pacing wire to pass through the needle
- 5-ml syringe
- Antiseptic solution
- Sterile drapes
- 4 × 4-inch gauze pads
- Electrical pulse generator
- Cardiac monitor
- Sterile gown
- Sterile gloves
- Mask and eye shield

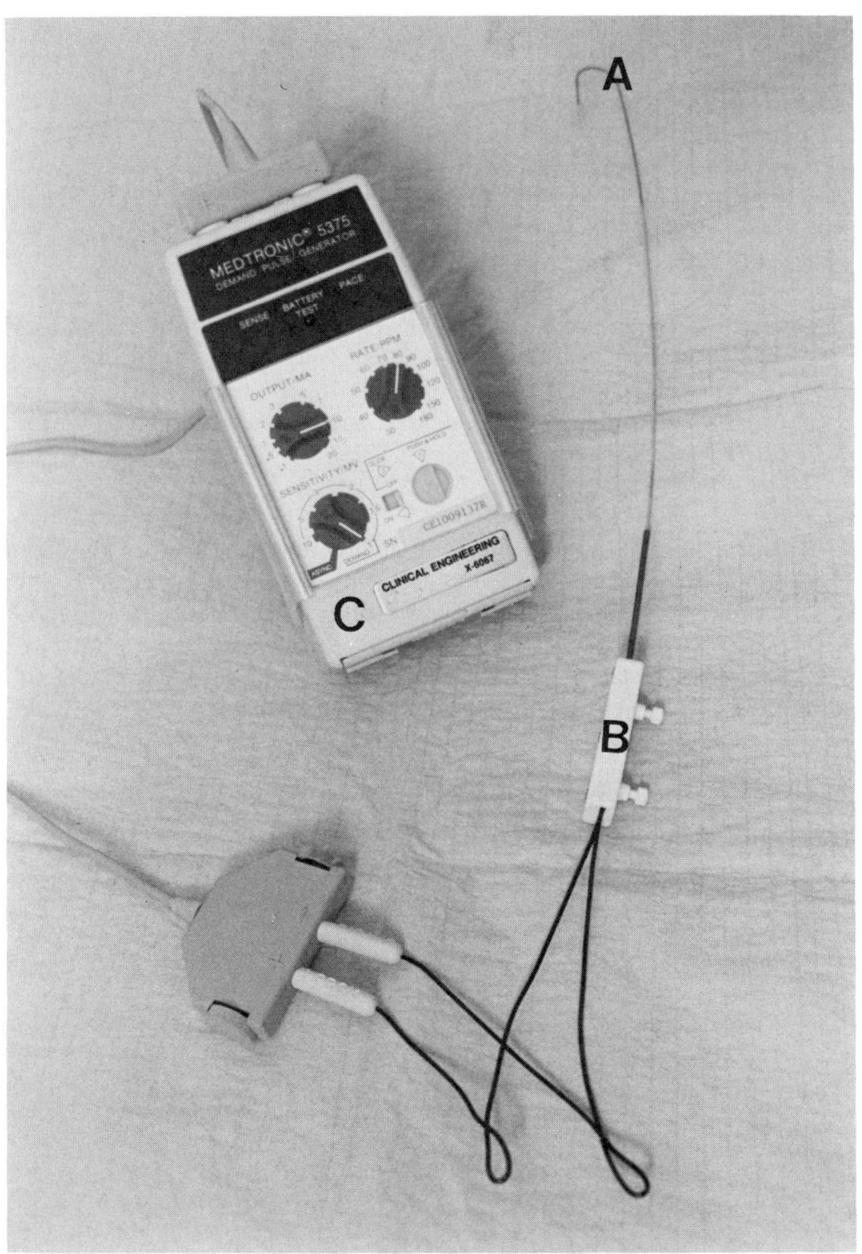

FIGURE 19–3. *A,* Pacing wire; *B,* connector; *C,* pulse generator.

Universal Precautions

1. Wear gown, mask, and sterile gloves.
2. Use an eye shield.

Technique

Choose one of two techniques:

A. *Parasternal technique.* Puncture site is at the fifth intercostal space at the left border of the sternum. Advance needle medially, dorsally, and cephalad at 60 degrees to the skin. This should direct the needle toward the left second intercostal space (Figure 19–4).
B. *Subxiphoid technique.* Puncture site is at the left xiphocostal junction aimed toward the left shoulder with the needle at 30 degrees to the skin (Figure 19–5).
   1. Position the patient supine on a stretcher and stand at the patient's right side facing his left shoulder. The patient should be connected to a cardiac monitor.
   2. Put on mask, eye shield, gown, and sterile gloves.
   3. Prep the area with Betadine and drape it with sterile towels.
   4. Enter the skin at the chosen puncture site and advance the needle as directed above while continuously aspirating with the 5-ml syringe. The cardiac ventricular muscles should offer some resistance to the needle. Intraventricular placement is indicated by aspiration of clotting blood (aspirated blood can be placed in a tube without anticoagulant to see if it clots).

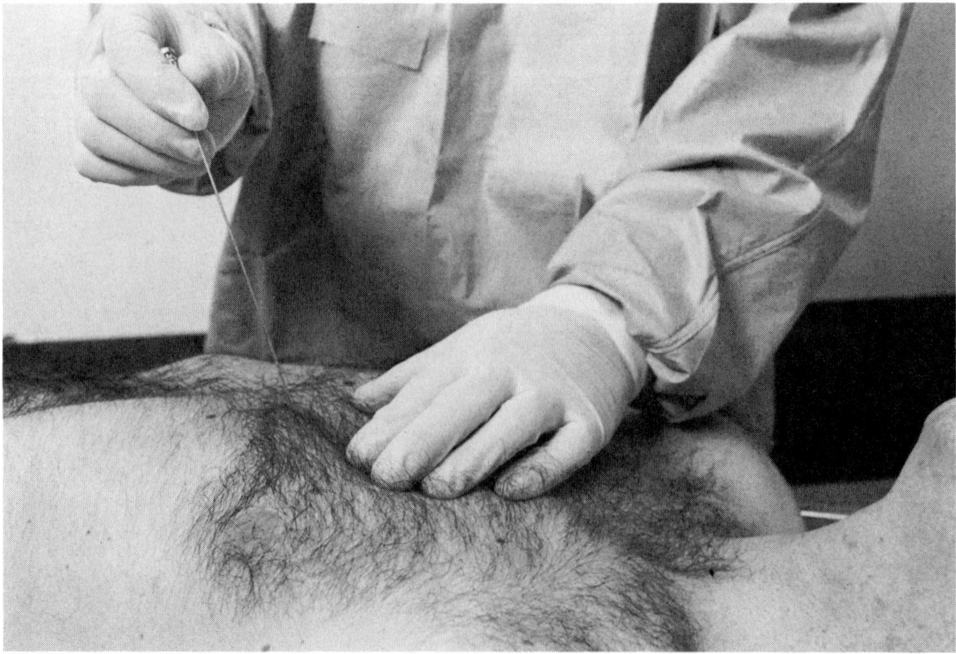

FIGURE 19–4. Parasternal approach for transthoracic pacing.

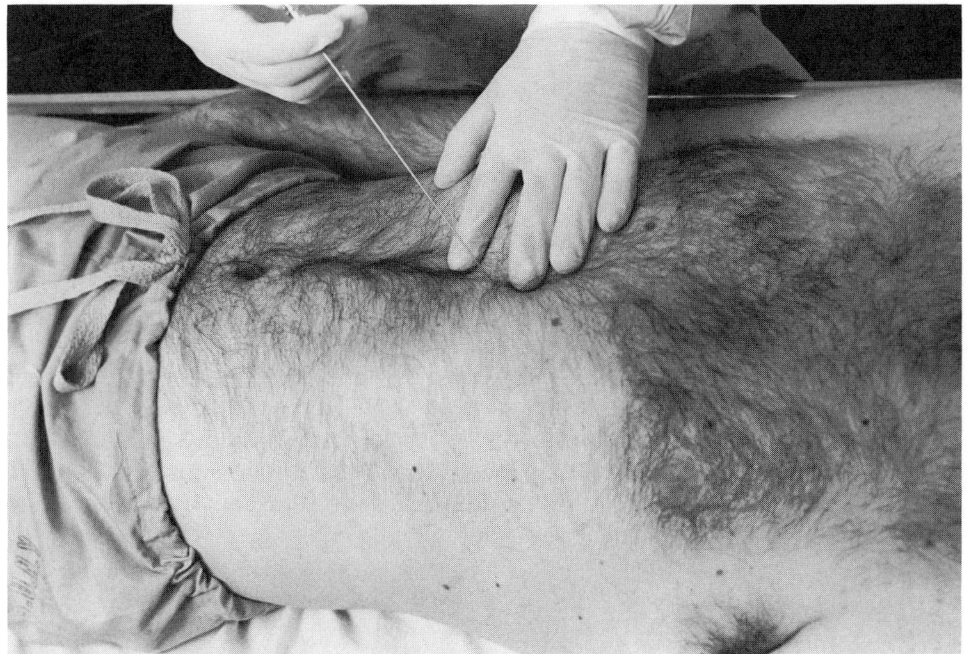

FIGURE 19–5. Subxiphoid approach for transthoracic pacing.

5. Remove the syringe and feed the pacing wire through the needle until resistance is met.
6. Remove the needle while holding the wire to secure its position.
7. Attach the electrical pulse generator to the wire and set the pacer to demand pacing, minimal output (amperes), and a rate of 100. Turn on the pulse generator and increase the output until electrical capture occurs or the maximal output is reached.
8. If electrical capture is achieved, check for pulses to indicate mechanical capture. If mechanical capture is present, continue with resuscitation and prepare to insert a transvenous pacemaker (see page 323).
9. If electrical capture does not occur, turn the generator off. Turn or slowly withdraw the pacing wire, then turn the generator back on and check the monitor for capture. You may need to try several positions before achieving electrical capture.
10. If electrical but not mechanical capture occurs, treat the patient for possible causes of electrical mechanical dissociation (i.e., hypovolemia, tension pneumothorax, or pericardial tamponade).

Complications

Infection

Visceral puncture (atrium, lung, pulmonary artery, inferior vena cava, liver, internal mammary artery)

Coronary artery puncture

Cardiac tamponade

Pearls and Pitfalls

1. The fifth intercostal left sternal border technique is most likely to have success and the least likely to have complications. However, individual variation in anatomy is significant. Therefore, try an alternative method if you have no success with the above technique.
2. Always reposition the needle by pulling the needle toward the skin and then redirecting and inserting it again. If you move the needle laterally, the bevel of the needle acts as a scalpel and lacerates the involved tissue.
3. Y connectors are available that allow the pacing wire to be passed through a side port. Therefore, the syringe would not need to be removed.
4. Pacing in asystolic arrest has not been shown to be beneficial. However, it is reasonable to presume that a patient who has recently become asystolic may benefit from cardiac pacing if the pacemaker is placed immediately. It is not clear whether transthoracic or external pacing should be used first in this setting. Obviously, only those procedures that an emergency care provider feels comfortable with should be performed.

References

Brown CG, Gurley TH, Hutchins GM, MacKenzie J, White JD: Injuries associated with percutaneous placement of transthoracic pacemakers. Ann Emerg Med 14:223–228, 1985.

Brown CG, Hutchins GM, Gurley HT, White JD, MacKenzie EJ: Placement accuracy of percutaneous transthoracic pacemakers. Am J Emerg Med 3:193–198, 1985.

Temporary Transvenous Pacing

MICHAEL S. JASTREMSKI, MD

Indications

Symptomatic bradydysrhythmias
Overdrive pacing of tachydysrhythmias (i.e., torsades)

Contraindications

Recent administration of thrombolytic agents (relative). Try external pacing first.
Cardiac arrest (relative). Try external pacing if you want to try pacing at all. It is unlikely that the pacer will go into the right ventricle without any flow to carry the balloon or intrinsic cardiac activity to indicate the position of the pacer tip. In addition, there is no evidence to indicate that pacing changes the outcome of asystole.

Equipment

Balloon-tipped flow-guided pacing catheter (Figure 19–6)
Cable to connect pacing catheter to generator (pacer) box
Materials for central venous access (see Chapter 24)
ECG machine
Gown, cap, mask, eye shield
Sterile gloves
4 × 4-inch gauze pads
3–0 nylon suture on needle
Suture holder
Scissors
Betadine
3-ml syringe
Sterile drapes

Universal Precautions

1. Wear gown, cap, mask, and sterile gloves.
2. Use an eye shield.

Technique

1. If the patient's condition and circumstances allow, explain the procedure to the patient and obtain informed consent.
2. Attach the limb leads of the ECG machine to the patient.
3. Put on cap, mask, eye shield, gown, and sterile gloves.
4. Obtain central vascular access (subclavian, internal jugular, or femoral) and place an introducer of an appropriate size to accept the pacing catheter (see pages 421, 426, and 448).
5. If there is already an introducer in place, prep skin and introducer with Betadine and widely drape.
6. Stand at the patient's side facing the introducer.
7. Check the balloon in the pacing catheter to ensure that it inflates properly without a leak using the 3-ml syringe filled with the volume of air recommended for the brand of catheter you are using.
8. Using the connector that is supplied with the pacing catheter, attach the distal pacing electrode to the V lead of the ECG machine and set the ECG machine to record lead V_1. The distal tip of the pacer is now a unipolar exploring electrode.
9. Advance the pacing catheter through the introducer until 15 to 20 cm of catheter has been inserted.
10. Inflate the catheter balloon with the recommended volume of air.

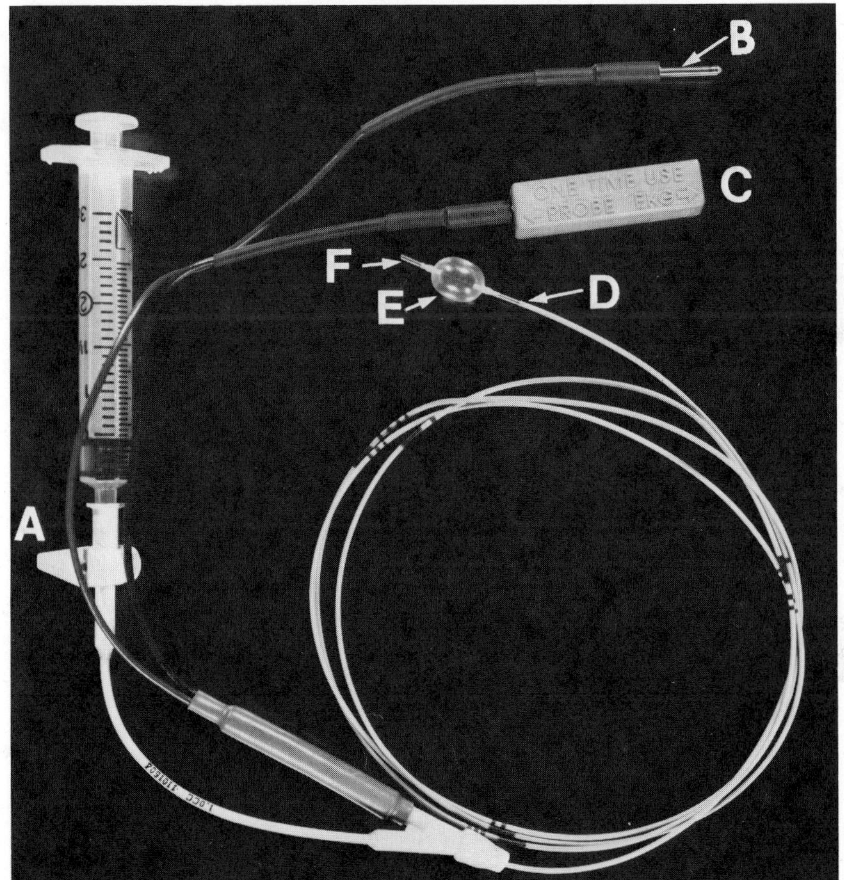

FIGURE 19–6. Temporary transvenous pacing balloon-tipped pacing catheter. *A,* Proximal balloon port; *B,* proximal electrode lead; *C,* distal electrode lead; *D,* proximal electrode; *E,* balloon; *F,* distal electrode.

11. Smoothly advance the catheter while observing the intracavity tracing (Figure 19–7*A* and *B*) to determine the position of the distal electrode.
12. When the intracavity tracing indicates endocardial contact (Figure 19–7*B*, tracing H), disconnect the catheter from the ECG machine and connect it to the pacer box. The distal catheter electrode is attached to the negative terminal of the pacer box and the proximal catheter electrode is attached to the positive terminal.
13. Set pacer box to maximal sensitivity, lowest milliamperes, and a rate greater than the patient's intrinsic rate.

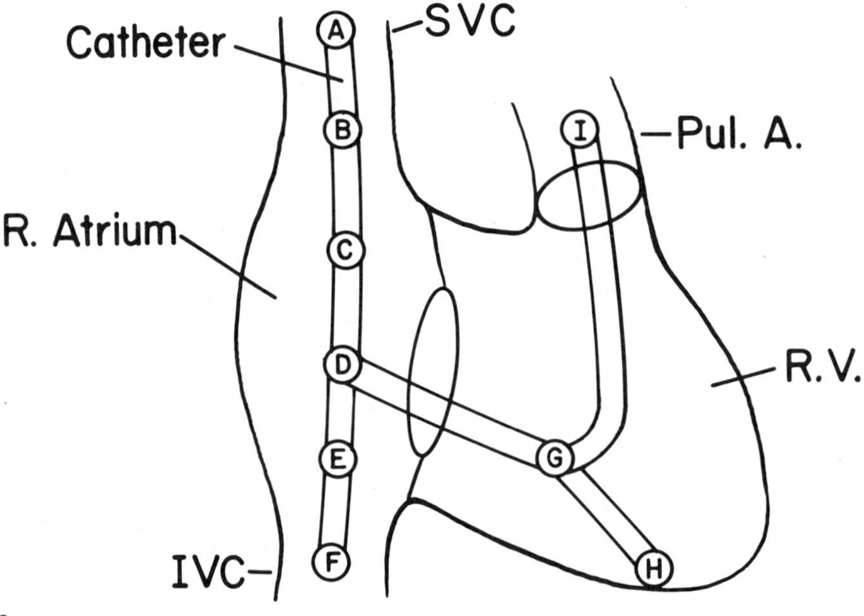

FIGURE 19–7. Intracavitary ECG tracings from a transvenous pacer. Locations shown in *A* demonstrate the ECG tracing with the corresponding letter shown in *B*. (**B,** Reprinted by permission of the New England Journal of Medicine, 287:651, 1972.)

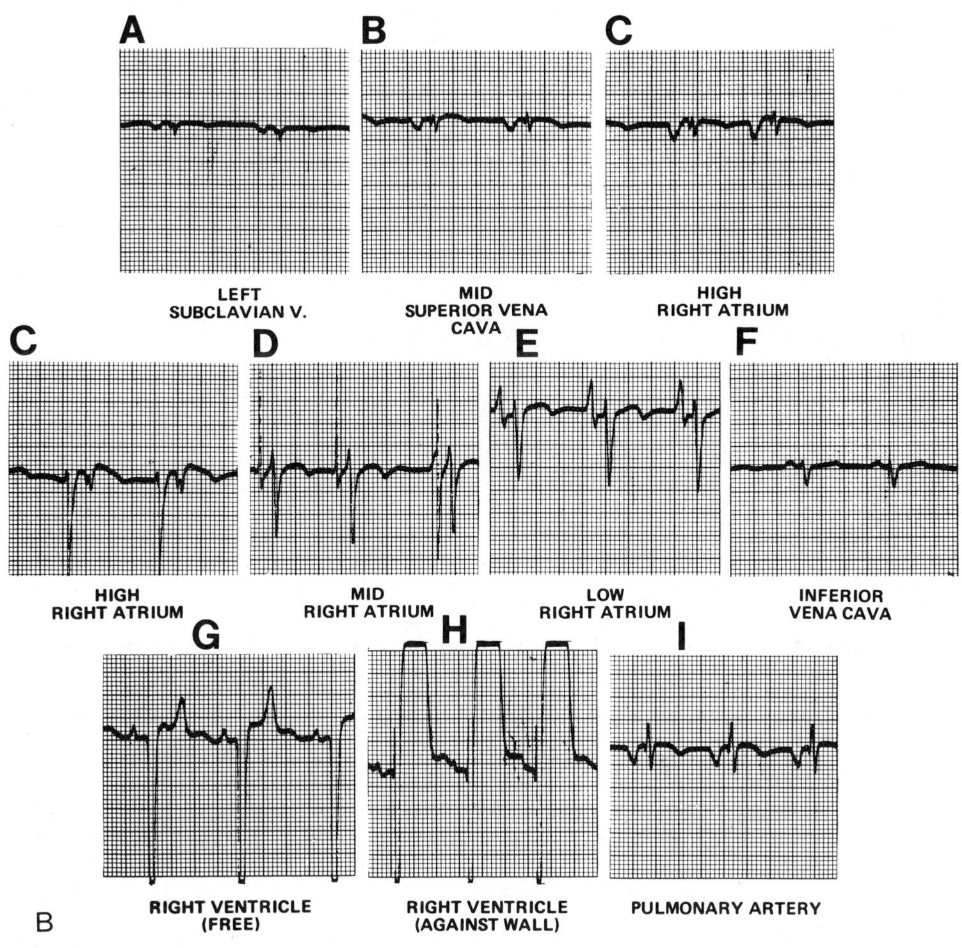

FIGURE 19–7 *Continued*

14. Turn on the pacer during one of the patient's intrinsic QRS complexes.
15. Increase the milliamperes of the pacing stimulus until capture consistently occurs. With a good pacer position this pacing threshold should be 1 mA or less.
16. When the pacing threshold has been determined, set the pacer at maximal sensitivity, the desired rate, and a milliampere two to three times the pacing threshold.
17. Suture the pacing catheter in place. First, place a loose skin suture 1 to 2 cm away from the proximal end of the introducer, leaving both ends of the suture material equal in length. Make a loop in the pacing catheter. Make several circles around the point in the catheter loop where the cross occurs with each end of the suture material. Tie the suture around the cross of the catheter loop. With this suturing technique, it is nearly impossible to dislodge the pacing catheter since any traction on the catheter can only pull on the loop, but not on the portion of the catheter going into the patient (Figure 19–8).
18. Apply a sterile dressing.
19. Obtain a chest x-ray film and look at it.

Complications

All the complications of central venous access
Failure to pace
Failure to sense
Perforation of the heart
Ventricular tachydysrhythmias

Pearls and Pitfalls

1. Catheters passed from the femoral vein tend to naturally go to the apex of the right ventricle, which is the optimal position for pacing. Thus, the success rate for placing balloon-tipped pacing catheters may be better if the femoral route is used.
2. In very unstable patients with low cardiac outputs, placement of balloon-tipped floating pacer catheters may be very prolonged and difficult. A better approach in these patients may be immediate external pacing (see page 314) followed by fluoroscopically guided placement of a stiff pacing wire.
3. Atropine (0.5 mg IV every 5 minutes to a maximum of 2 mg) or isoproterenol (continuous IV infusion of 2 to 20 μg/min titrated to heart rate) can be used as chemical pacemakers to improve perfusion until an electrical pacer can be placed. However, not all patients with symptomatic bradycardia will respond to these drugs.
4. If sensing failure occurs, this can be fixed by passing a wire suture through the skin on the chest wall and attaching the positive terminal of the pacer box to this. The proximal pacer electrode is left unattached and should be wrapped in a rubber glove to insulate it.

Reference

Bing OHL, McDowell JW, Hartman J, Messer JV: Pacemaker placement by electrocardiographic monitoring. N Engl J Med 287:651, 1972.

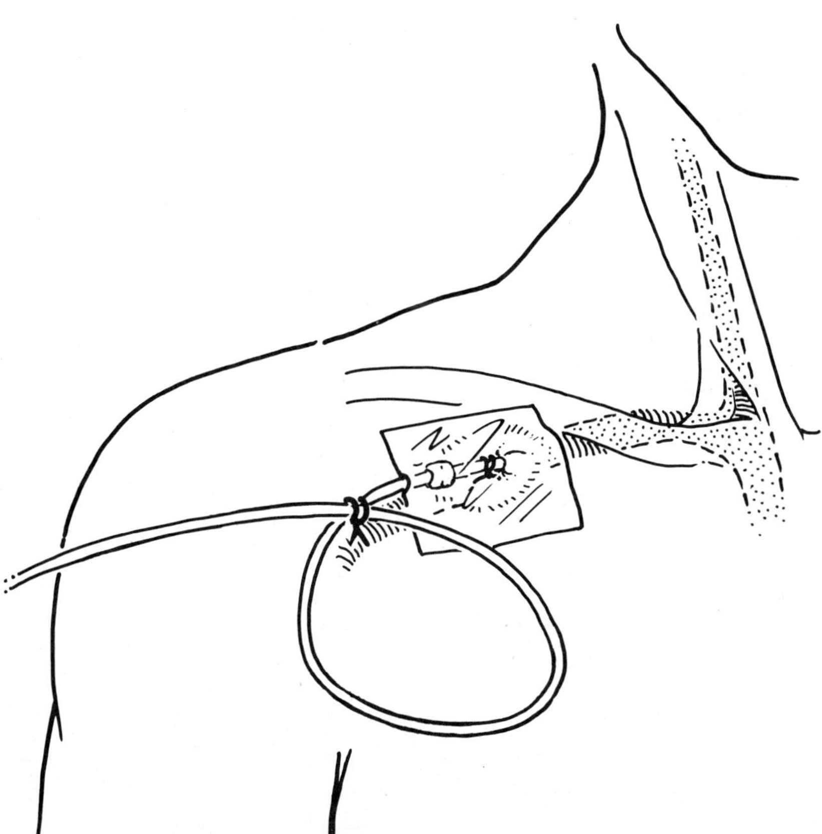

FIGURE 19–8. Technique for securing a transvenous pacer.

Defibrillation

CONNIE WALLECK, RN

Indications

Ventricular fibrillation
Ventricular tachycardia with pulselessness
Ventricular tachycardia in a patient with a pulse but no response to lidocaine bolus (synchronized cardioversion preferred)

Equipment

Defibrillator with external paddles (Figure 19–9)
Electrode paste
ECG machine or ECG capability with defibrillator
Emergency cart and medications

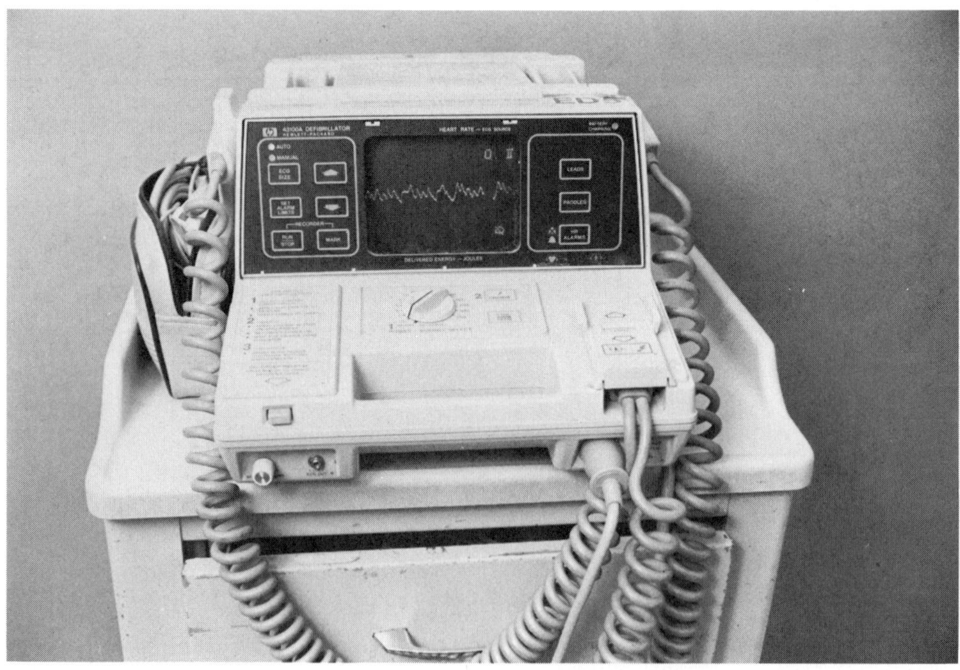

FIGURE 19–9. Defibrillator.

Universal Precautions

1. Avoid electrical injury to any of the rescuers.

Technique

1. Clinically confirm the diagnosis of cardiac arrest, identify the need for defibrillation, and call for help.
2. Initiate basic life support while awaiting defibrillation equipment.
3. Turn on defibrillator.
4. Select energy level to be delivered (begin at 200 joules initially; if unsuccessful, repeat immediately at 200 to 300 joules; remainder of defibrillation attempts should be made at 360 joules). (If patient weighs less than 50 kg, deliver 2 joules/kg.)
5. Apply electrode paste generously to both paddles (or use 3-inch defibrillator pads).
6. Press charge button on defibrillator.
7. Place sternum paddle on chest to right of sternum at second intercostal space (Figure 19–10).
8. Place apex paddle on chest along midaxillary line at fifth intercostal space (see Figure 19–10).
9. Call out loudly "clear the patient," and make a visual check to ensure that neither yourself nor any other persons are in contact with the bed or patient.
10. Apply 25 pounds of pressure downward with the paddles.
11. Depress both paddle switches simultaneously (see Figure 19–10).

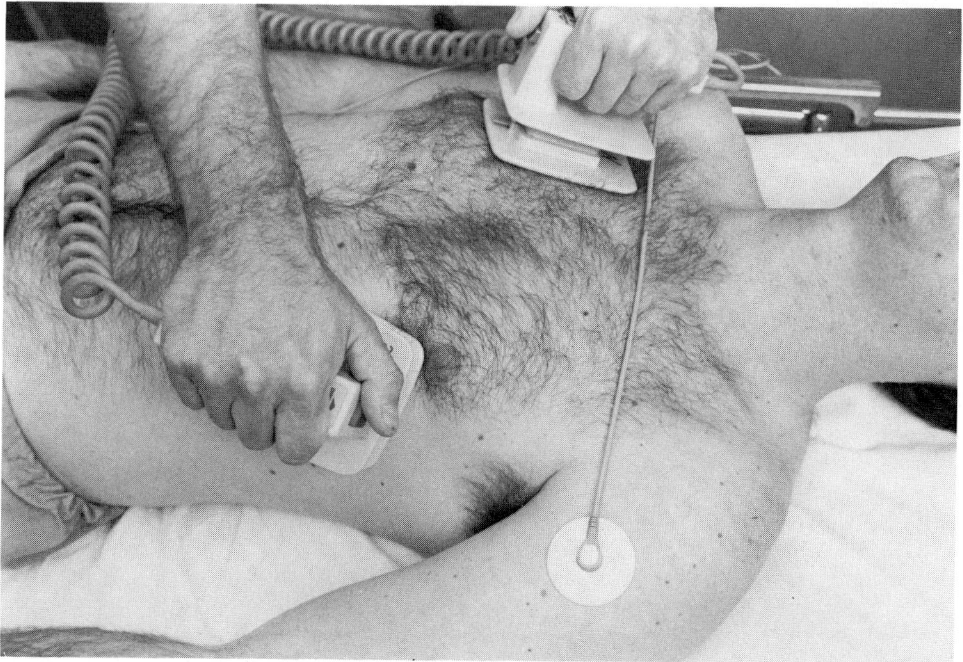

FIGURE 19–10. Paddle position for defibrillation.

12. Maintain paddle to skin contact.
13. Observe monitor for restoration of functional cardiac rhythm.
14. Check carotid pulse after each defibrillation.
15. If ventricular fibrillation or tachycardia persists, continue cardiopulmonary resuscitation, recharge defibrillator, and repeat procedure. This step may be repeated twice, resulting in a total of three defibrillations initially.
16. Continue resuscitation following the American Heart Association's Advanced Cardiac Life Support guidelines.

Complications

Skin burns

Shock to clinical personnel who do not "clear the patient"

Arcing of current over the chest wall between paddles

Failure to achieve a rhythm

Dysrhythmias

Cardiac arrest (when converting ventricular tachycardia with a pulse)

Equipment malfunction

Pearls and Pitfalls

1. It is important to wipe off excess defibrillator paste from paddles and skin between defibrillations to prevent slipping of the paddles and bridging of the electrical current.
2. Always wait for the defibrillator to fully charge and indicate the correct energy level before attempting to defibrillate the patient or the procedure will be unsuccessful.
3. Some defibrillators must be plugged in before they will work. Always check to see if this is necessary.
4. Remember to support patient with cardiopulmonary resuscitation between defibrillations.
5. Make sure the machine is not in the synchronize mode since the paddles will not discharge during ventricular fibrillation if in the synchronize mode.
6. Spend some time learning how the defibrillator available to you works *before* you have to use it in a cardiac arrest.

Reference

Extensive experience.

Emergency Thoracotomy

KEVIN FERGUSON, MD

Few procedures in emergency medicine have sparked as passionate and at times ego-driven debate as the performance of thoracotomy. The literature demonstrates some clear indications for the performance of emergency department thoracotomy and, in these circumstances, transport to the operating room prior to resuscitation and thoracotomy is contraindicated. The procedure is, however, filled with pitfalls and complications, and even in the best hands the survival to discharge without neurologic sequelae is low. Although many surgeons believe only surgeons should perform the procedure, there have been published studies on the outcome of emergency department thoracotomy by emergency-trained physicians with survival rates comparable to those performed by surgeons. The procedure ought to be performed by the most experienced physician immediately available. The preference is always to perform the procedure in the operating room when possible, but thoracotomy is part of the resuscitation of trauma victims in the emergency setting; with some injuries there is simply no way to resuscitate a patient without open thoracotomy. The argument for the training of emergency physicians in this technique is the reality that surgical personnel will not always be available to perform the procedure in time to make a difference, while there is always an emergency physician in house. The reason the emergency physician must learn and maintain this skill is precisely for the few cases in which a patient presents to a facility for whom the delay in treatment will be lethal.

Until the operating room team is ready to accept the patient and until the patient has been hemodynamically resuscitated the patient should remain in the emergency department and surgical personnel should prepare the operating room for the patient or come to the emergency department to assist in the resuscitation. There is little benefit by transporting a patient with no vital signs to an operating room that is not prepared for the case. By the same token there is no benefit in doing cardiorrhaphy in the emergency department once the patient has been resuscitated and the operating room is prepared to accept the patient.

Indications

1. Cardiac arrest following penetrating chest trauma. The most treatable lesions in traumatic cardiac arrest following penetrating chest trauma are tension pneumothorax and pericardial tamponade, and these should be the first things sought in the open thoracotomy. Other treatable lesions include great vessel injury, bronchial injury, and cardiac lacerations. Greatest salvage rate is in patients who had vital signs on arrival in the emergency department.

2. Traumatic cardiac tamponade. Operating room thoracotomy is preferred if the patient is not in cardiac arrest. The patient awaiting the arrival of the surgical team may get short-term relief with pericardiocentesis. However, experience has been that the pericardium is filled with mostly clotted blood and palliation with pericardiocentesis is unlikely to succeed. Open thoracotomy and pericardiotomy is the indicated procedure; and if the patient's condition deteriorates despite aggressive fluid resuscitation while awaiting the operating room, the procedure should be performed in the emergency department.
3. Massive intra-abdominal hemorrhage and deteriorating vital signs despite adequate volume replacement and MAST suit tamponade. The bleeding in this case is presumed to be aortic, and only proximal occlusion offers control of the bleeding and the maintenance of diastolic pressure to maintain cerebral and coronary blood flow while the patient is transferred to the operating room. The survival to discharge rates for these patients are very low, and therefore many authors have argued against thoracotomy to control abdominal aortic bleeding. This is a complicated, surgical procedure best done by a thoracic or trauma surgeon, but it is appropriate for the emergency department physician to institute it if the patient is agonal.

Contraindications

Presence of vital signs
Immediate availability of operating room and necessary personnel

---

Thoracotomy and aortic clamping should be done only when the patient can be transferred to the operating room within 20 minutes.
These patients will need definitive surgical repair and, therefore, the emergency physician must have adequate, prompt surgical and anesthesia backup to even consider this procedure.
Endotracheal intubation must be performed before the procedure.

Equipment

Nos. 10 and 11 scalpel blades
Scalpel handle
Mayo scissors, curved
Metzenbaum scissors
10½-inch Masson needle holder
Mayo Hegan needle holder
Sternum osteotome and hammer
Rib retractor
6-inch tissue forceps
10-inch tissue forceps
5½-inch Crile forceps
6¼-inch Crile forceps
Gown, mask, eye shield
Sterile gloves
Betadine
Satinsky clamp
8-inch Mayo Pean forceps, curved
Three DeBakey tangential occlusion clamps
Yankauer suction, with finger control
Backhaus towel clips
Teflon pledgets
Thirty 4 × 4-inch gauze pads
2–0 silk suture

This procedure will cause exposure to large amounts of blood. Universal precautions with mask, gown, sterile gloves, and an eye shield should be observed at all times by all personnel present during the procedure.

Technique

1. Position the patient supine with the left scapula elevated on a rolled towel or sand bag to elevate the left chest off of the table (Figure 19–11).
2. Put on mask, eye shield, gown, and sterile gloves.
3. Stand on the patient's left side, facing the chest.
4. As thorough a skin preparation as is practical should be done.

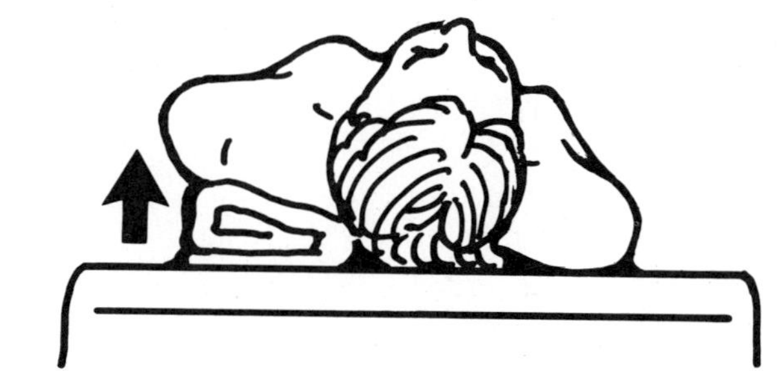

FIGURE 19–11. Patient position for emergency thoracotomy.

5. A left anterolateral thoracotomy is the preferred incision in the emergency department. This incision provides the easiest access to approach and repair cardiac wounds, cross-clamp the aorta, and perform open cardiac massage. If necessary, the incision can be extended into the right chest by dividing the sternum. The incision is made in the fifth intercostal space from the left parasternal border to the posterior axillary line. In women, the incision is made below, along the inferior mammary crease (Figure 19–12). The incision should penetrate the skin, subcutaneous tissue, and pectoral muscles in as few strokes of the scalpel (preferably two) as possible.
6. Using blunt scissors, cut the intercostal muscles and pleura and enter the chest cavity (Figure 19–13). Insert the rib spreader and spread the ribs forcefully; if necessary, the costochondral joints may be dislocated and the ribs may be fractured to gain adequate exposure. Adequate exposure is the key to approaching and identifying the injury(s). At this time, be prepared for a large gush of blood in the event of massive hemothorax. If this is found, the blood must be scooped out manually, since there will be large clots and the suction will not be sufficient.
7. Visualize the heart and pericardium, and note any cardiac activity. If cardiac arrest has not occurred at this point, the sources of any rapid bleeding should be sought and controlled with a finger, hemostat, or suture ligature. If cardiac arrest has occurred, the pericardium is opened first and internal cardiac massage is started. If the pericardium is full of blood, it will be taut and dark maroon. Using a tissue forceps, elevate the pericardium and make a small stab incision *anterior to the phrenic nerve.* Insert the curved Mayo scissors and carry the incision superiorly while being *careful not to injure the phrenic nerve.* The heart should then be delivered from the pericardium and the blood carefully removed and the heart inspected for any injury and/or dysrhythmia. Cardiac activity may spontaneously restart when the tamponade is relieved or may require epinephrine and other Advanced Cardiac Life Support resuscitation. Remember, in trauma, as a rule, hypotension is due to hypovolemia and bradycardia is due to hypoxia.

Complications

Severing of the internal mammary artery on entering the chest
Costosternal dislocation and rib fractures
Pulmonary lacerations
Phrenic nerve injury
Infection

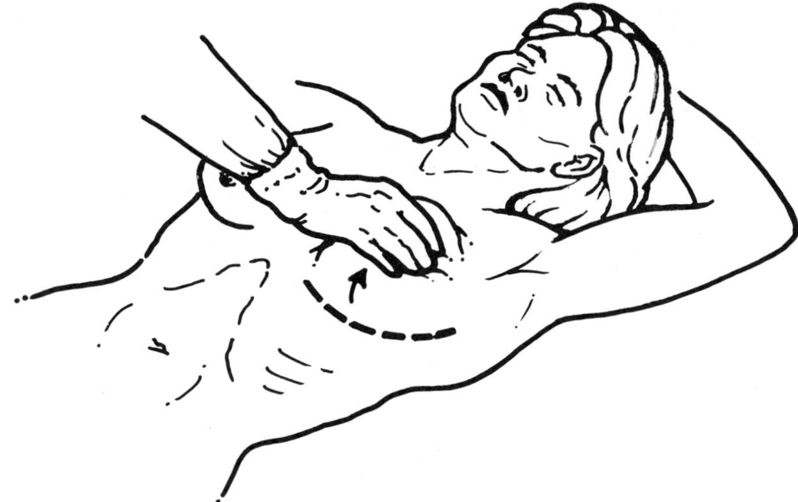

FIGURE 19–12. The dashes indicate the incision line.

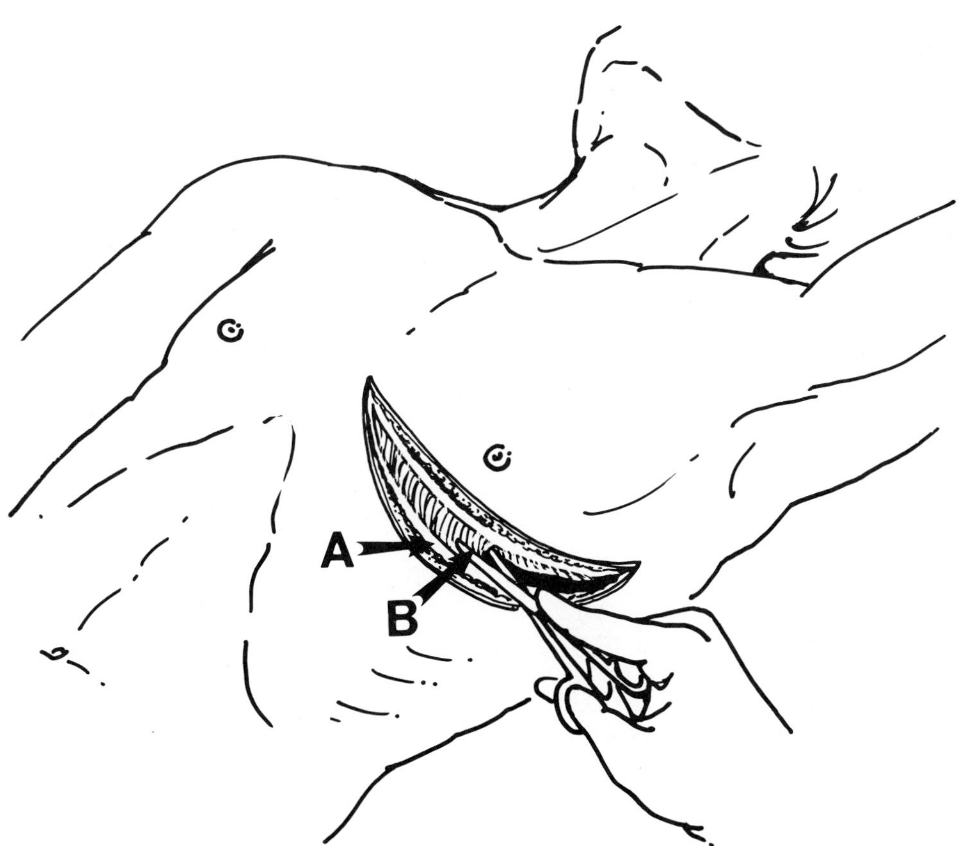

FIGURE 19–13. *A*, Rib; *B*, pleura.

Pearls and Pitfalls

Anesthetic agents must be available in the emergency department since the patient may regain consciousness following successful resuscitation.

---

1. Preparation for a thoracotomy depends on the stability of the patient. The patient must, however, be intubated and ventilated with 100% oxygen under positive pressure. At the same time the patient is intubated, large-bore intravenous lines, a Foley catheter, and nasogastric tubes should be inserted and volume resuscitation begun.
2. Despite the usual lack of adequate surgical prep and scrub, these patients have had a remarkably low incidence of postoperative infection. Therefore, the scrub should be as brief as possible, given the dire condition of the patients undergoing this operation. All nonessential personnel should avoid the operative field.
3. Simultaneous activation of the trauma system and immediate surgical backup by a thoracic or trauma surgeon is essential whenever the option of thoracotomy is being proposed.
4. Indications for abandoning the resuscitation include irreparable massive cardiac injury; total exsanguination and the finding of an empty, flaccid heart; lack of vital signs or cardiac rhythm after 15 minutes of resuscitative effort; and no sustained systolic blood pressure of 60 mm Hg for 30 minutes. These conditions herald either a futile resuscitative effort or severe cerebral anoxia from which a neurologically viable patient is not a likely outcome.

VENTRICULAR REPAIR

After the pericardium is opened the heart is inspected for injury and cardiac activity. If the heart has no activity and a ventricular injury is discovered, there are two possible approaches. If the repair can be done quickly, it may be preferable to attempt the repair first, since suturing a beating heart is difficult. Alternatively, the instigation of open cardiac massage and resumption of cardiac activity may begin first.

If the pericardiotomy and fluid resuscitation return cardiac activity, the patient's vital signs improve, and the operating room is ready to receive the patient, control the bleeding with simple digital pressure on, *but not in,* the injury, and transport the patient to the operating room for the repair while maintaining digital control of the bleeding.

If ventricular repair is to be done in the emergency department and the heart is beating, some find that placing an apical traction stitch (Beck's stitch) for control of the heart is useful. The nondominant hand is used to hold the stitch placed through the apex of the heart between the third finger and thumb, and the index finger is used to maintain tamponade on the injury. The other hand is used to place the suture. Great care must be taken when tying or pulling on the sutures since the muscle is delicate and stitches may pull through the tissue. The apex is the chosen site for the traction suture given its relatively avascular state and the distance from any of the major coronary arteries. Most authors prefer a nonabsorbable 2–0 silk suture with a curved cutting needle.

When examining a cardiac laceration the depth and the proximity of any coronary arteries are important. A laceration that has not penetrated into the underlying chamber is less likely to cause exsanguinating hemorrhage than one that does. Lacerations near coronary arteries must be closely examined to ensure that coronary arteries are not inadvertently ligated.

In general the sutures should be placed 5 to 6 mm from the wound edge and the suture pulled just tight enough to stop the bleeding. The style of suture placed depends on the severity and location of the injury and on the mechanism of injury.

For small linear lacerations or punctures a simple interrupted suture is usually all that is necessary. Longer simple lacerations may be closed by several interrupted sutures, by a horizontal mattress stitch, or by a simple running stitch. The attraction of the latter is it can be done while maintaining pressure on the bleeding site with a finger (Figure 19–14).

If the injury is close to a major coronary vessel, a horizontal mattress suture can be passed beneath the artery and tied without ligating the vessel; large injuries are also best repaired with this technique.

Technique

1. The sutures should pass down deep into the myocardium, but violation of the endocardium is to be avoided. To avoid possible injury to the coronary vessel, begin the stitch on the side of the artery away from the laceration and be sure the needle has passed beyond the laceration before exiting the epicardium.
2. Make the next puncture of the epicardium 1 cm away from and parallel to the laceration without tying the suture. Be sure the needle passes beyond the coronary artery before bringing the needle to the surface.
3. Tie the usual surgeon's knot, and draw it down just tight enough to stop the bleeding. Avoid cutting into the myocardium (Figure 19–15).
4. If sutures are to be placed near devitalized myocardium or pulled through the cardiac tissue, pass them through Teflon pledgets to keep them from cutting into the muscle.

Complications

Coronary artery injury/ligation
Air embolism
Infection

Pearls and Pitfalls

The operating room is the most appropriate place to perform cardiac and vascular repairs. If cardiac rhythm and adequate perfusion can be restored, the patient should be transported to the operating room suite whenever the surgical team is ready and a transfer of patient care is possible.

With large ventricular wounds in which there is massive blood loss from ventricular contraction some authors have recommended elective fibrillation of the heart using defibrillation paddles at 20 joules of DC countercurrent in an anterior to posterior direction. While the heart is fibrillating the large defect is repaired; then the heart is defibrillated and the minor repairs are performed using traction on the Beck's suture.

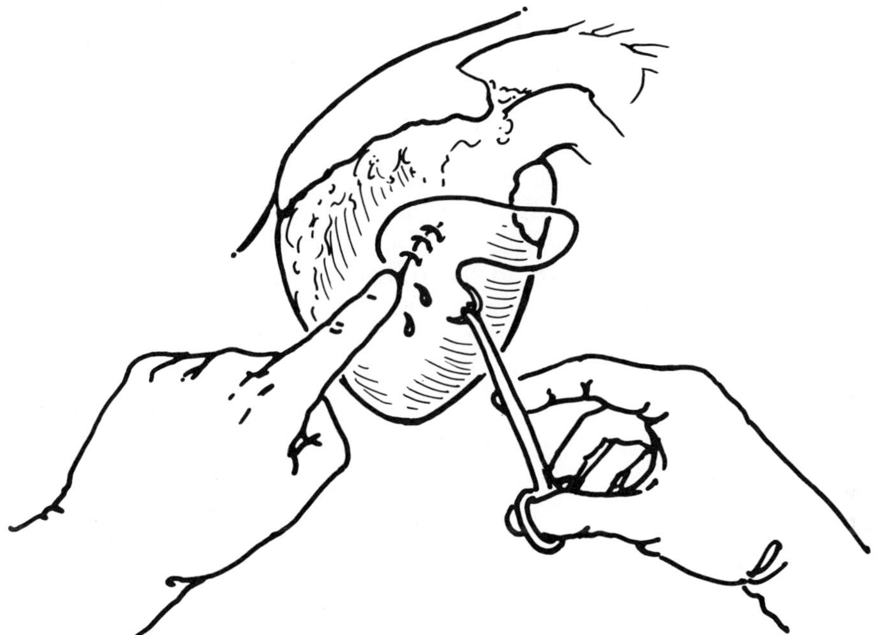

FIGURE 19–14. Repair of a cardiac laceration.

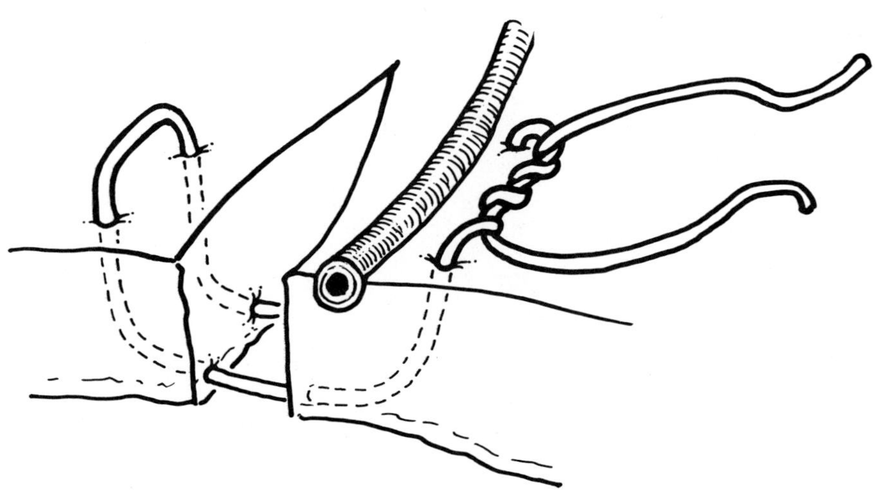

FIGURE 19–15. Myocardial suture.

ATRIAL REPAIR

Atrial wounds of the heart do not always merit closure in the emergency department. If there are other more serious injuries, consideration should be given to placing an atraumatic vascular occlusion clamp across the wound and moving to the other repairs. This repair may be left to the operating room. Wounds near the atrial caval junction may be tamponaded using a 12 to 14 F Foley catheter. The catheter is passed through the wound into the heart. Then the balloon is inflated, and the catheter pulled back to occlude the cardiac wound. A Kelly clamp is placed on the end of the Foley catheter and allowed to hang from the chest to provide adequate traction. When a marginal atrial injury is found, this can be simply suture-ligated as a bleeding vessel would. If atrial repair is undertaken, it is important not to penetrate the endocardium since the exposure of the suture of the relatively slow moving blood in the atria will lead to mural thrombosis.

VASCULAR INJURY

Most nonaortic vascular injuries can simply be clamped or suture-ligated until surgery. Injuries to the aorta or major branches of the brachiocephalic system should be controlled with a vascular tangential partial occluding clamp to avoid cerebral ischemia and left to the thoracic surgeon to repair.

Injury to coronary arteries can be controlled with digital pressure, but emergency department ligation followed by operative bypass may be preferable if there is a surgical pump room quickly available.

ATRIAL CANNULATION

If no cardiac repairs are needed or when they are complete if the patient remains hypotensive the right atrium of the heart can be cannulated for massive volume replacement directly into the heart. The cannula should be the size of intravenous tubing, and this is best obtained by cutting the "plug" tip off sterile extension tubing.

Technique

1. An assistant using two hemostats with the tips pointing toward each other grasps the atrial appendage and lifts up the anterior wall (Figure 19–16).
2. A pursestring suture is placed between the hemostats but not drawn or tied (Figure 19–17).
3. A partial occluder vascular clamp is placed between the pursestring circle and the proximal atria to avoid air being sucked into the heart when the incision is made (Figure 19–18).

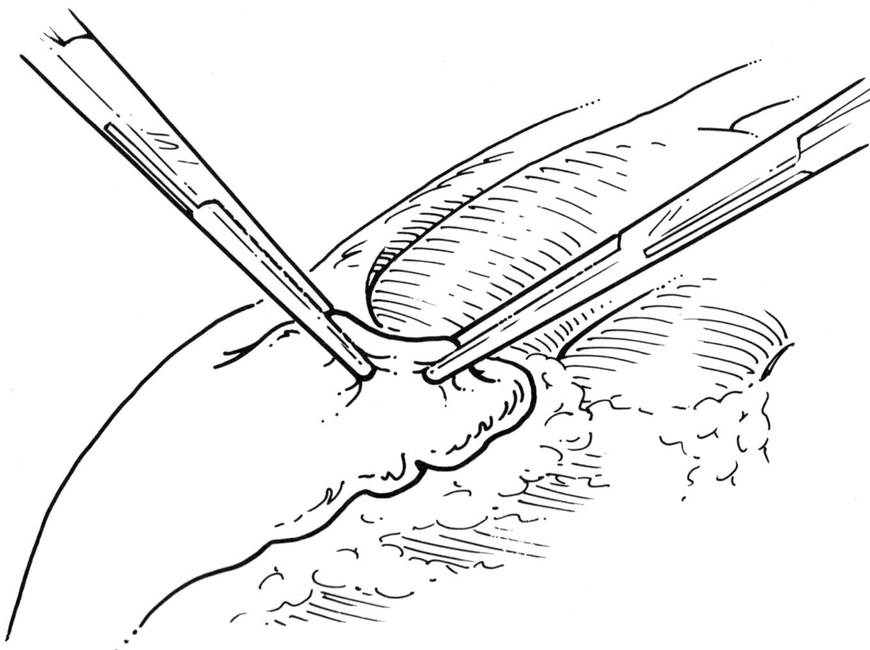

FIGURE 19–16. Atrial cannulation: Step 1.

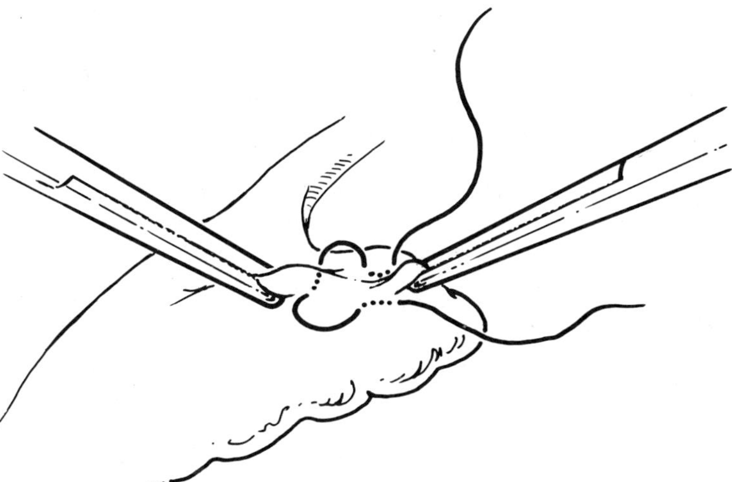

FIGURE 19–17. Atrial cannulation: Step 2.

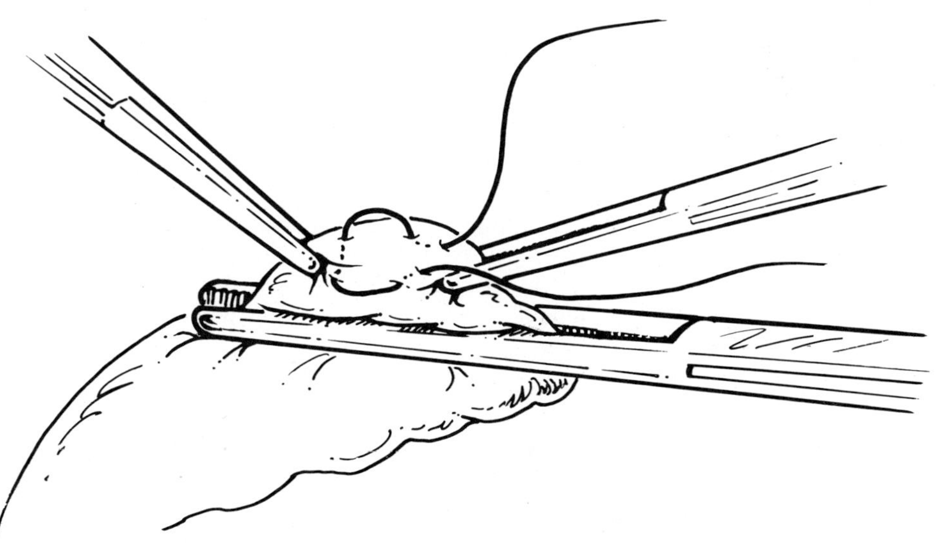

FIGURE 19–18. Atrial cannulation: Step 3.

4. A stab incision is then made with a No. 11 scalpel inside the pursestring suture, and the extension tubing is inserted into the chamber (Figure 19–19). The air and blood in the pocket between the clamp and the insertion site are expressed out, and the suture is then drawn tight and a knot placed on the epicardium. The suture is passed around the tubing several times, and a second knot is placed on the tubing (Figure 19–20).
5. Remove the partial occluder clamp.

It is imperative that all the air is flushed out of the extension tubing before the line is inserted into the heart to avoid air embolism. This is preferably done with blood since even small bubbles can be easily seen.

Complications

Air embolism
Infection
Bleeding

Pearls and Pitfalls

1. The atrial catheter should be attached to an infusate of both blood and normal saline warmed to 40°C. I prefer to mix the unit of blood with warmed 0.9% normal saline to decrease the viscosity of the blood, as well as prevent the refrigerated blood from cooling the heart and making resumption of cardiac rhythm more difficult.
2. When any patient receives massive transfusion of banked blood there is the risk of hypothermia, and instillation directly into the heart increases the risk of cardiac hypothermia and dysrhythmias.
3. The line should be placed in the right atrium since this allows oxygenation of the blood and subsequent filling of the left side of the heart with oxygen-rich blood.

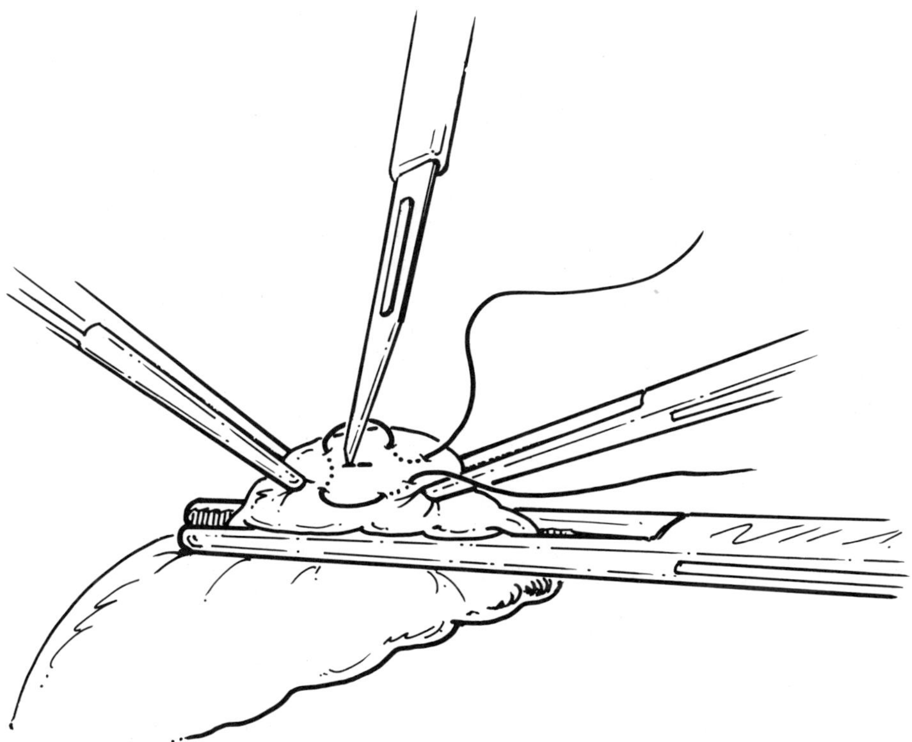

FIGURE 19–19. Atrial cannulation: Step 4.

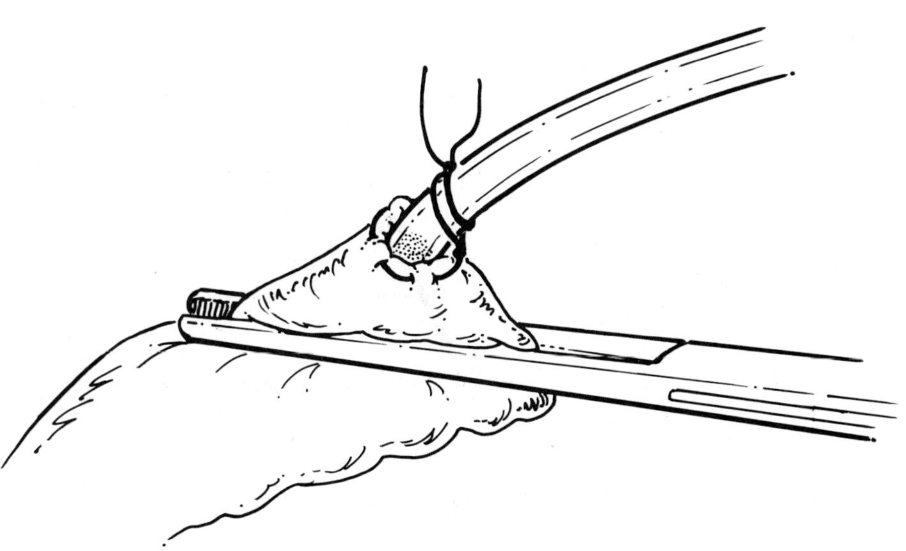

FIGURE 19–20. Atrial cannulation: Step 5.

OPEN CARDIAC MASSAGE

Technique

1. The most effective technique of open cardiac massage is with two hands. A one-handed technique is less efficient and more likely to injure the myocardium.
2. The heart is held such that the palm of the right hand is posterior to the heart with the apex between the thenar and hypothenar prominences. The left hand is placed over the heart and right hand (Figure 19–21).
3. The heart is compressed beginning at the apex and toward the aortic root. Pressure is smooth but forceful. The rate is the same as for closed-chest cardiopulmonary resuscitation; however, be certain the heart is able to fill between contractions.

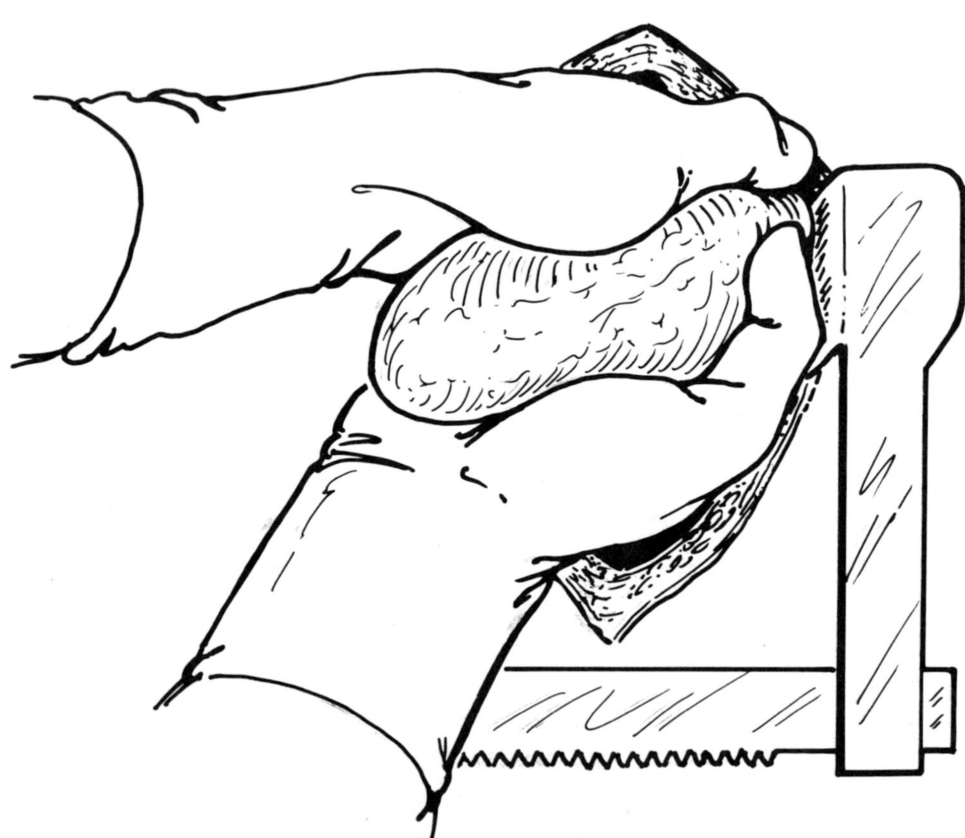

FIGURE 19–21. Open cardiac massage.

THORACIC AORTA CLAMPING

Cross clamping the aorta can increase cerebral and coronary artery perfusion in the severely hypovolemic patient. However, the procedure is fraught with complications and in no case should the clamp time exceed 30 minutes. When volume resuscitation has returned the blood pressure to above 130 mm Hg, the clamp should be removed and aggressive fluid replacement used to treat the shock. In such a volume-depleted patient the aorta is particularly difficult to separate from the esophagus, which runs immediately anterior and medial to the aorta. The easiest way to differentiate the two is to place a nasogastric tube and palpate for its presence prior to clamping. The aorta must never be clamped proximal to the takeoff of the brachiocephalic branches. If any of these vessels are injured, they must be selectively clamped and repaired.

Technique

1. The aorta is easiest to locate by palpating the thoracic vertebrae; the aorta is the structure most immediately anterior to the vertebrae. The aorta and the esophagus both lie beyond the reflection of the pleura.
2. The pleura should be incised longitudinally and the aorta dissected away from the esophagus by blunt dissection with a Kelly hemostat or your finger.
3. Once the aorta is isolated a DeBakey clamp can be gently placed across it to the point where flow is occluded, or it may be compressed manually.

Clamping the aorta will cause severe afterload on the left ventricle. The blood pressure must be monitored no less frequently than every 5 minutes. Clamping the aorta can lead to left-sided heart failure, bowel infarction, renal failure, and spinal cord ischemia.

Complications

Esophageal injury
Paralysis
Ischemia

Pearls and Pitfalls

1. The most common problem is failure to isolate the aorta in a timely manner. It is not easy to identify the aorta if there is no pulse, and it is difficult to dissect away from the esophagus once it is located. Often the best approach is simply to maintain manual pressure on the aorta until the operating room can accept the patient.
2. Inadvertent injury to the esophagus and resultant mediastinitis presents as a postoperative complication; if the aorta cannot be isolated, it cannot be clamped!

References

Flynn TC, Ward RE, Miller PW: Emergency department thoracotomy. Ann Emerg Med 11:413, 1982.
Ordog GJ: Emergency thoracotomy. Am J Emerg Med 5:312, 1987.

Intraosseous Infusions

RICHARD CANTOR, MD

Indication

Establishment of venous access in the critically ill infant or child.

Cannulation of small peripheral vessels in these patients is often impossible in the emergency setting. The bone marrow compartment provides a rich vascular network for the transportation of fluids and drugs from the marrow cavity to the central circulation.

Contraindications

Local trauma or infection
Availability of intravenous access

Equipment

Sterile gloves
Betadine pads (or alcohol)
Intraosseous needles (Cook Critical Care, Illinois sternal needle) or an 18- or 20-gauge spinal needle
Intravenous solution and tubing

Universal Precautions

1. Wear sterile gloves.

Technique

1. This is a lifesaving technique in critical situations. It is not possible to explain the procedure to the parents or obtain consent.
2. Position the patient supine with the leg straight.
3. Stand at the knee on the side you will use facing the patient's knee.
4. Site selection: At present the most commonly used sites are the proximal tibia and the distal tibia. The proximal tibia has the advantage of easy

palpability and a paucity of adipose tissue covering its surface. It is not available for use in children older than 5 years of age. The distal tibia contains the same anatomic advantages of the proximal site and, in addition, may be used in older children and adults. Both sites are demonstrated in Figure 19–22.

a. Proximal tibia. Palpate the tibial tuberosity and grasp the medial aspect of the tibia with the thumb. Insert the needle through the anteromedial surface of the tibia 1 or 2 cm distal from the tibial tuberosity with the needle directed caudad (away from the epiphysis) (Figure 19–23).
b. Distal tibia. The optimal location is on the medial surface of the tibia proximal to the medial malleolus (Figure 19–24).

5. Put on gloves.
6. Prepare the skin surface over the chosen site with alcohol or Betadine.
7. Insert the needle. Apply a rotary motion with downward pressure to the intraosseous needle to penetrate the bone. There will be a decrease in resistance, which indicates penetration of the cortex of the bone. Do not advance the needle any farther after this point. The needle should now be firmly fixed in the bone.
8. Attach a 5-ml syringe of normal saline and slowly flush the needle. A slight amount of resistance will normally be felt. Carefully inspect the insertion site for leakage or extravasation of fluid into the subcutaneous space. If this occurs, remove the needle and do not attempt any further insertions at this site. (In some cases it is possible to aspirate marrow contents. The absence of this does not preclude the appropriate placement of the needle.)
9. Once appropriate placement is ascertained, attach the intravenous tubing to the needle. Any and all resuscitative medications may be delivered by this route.

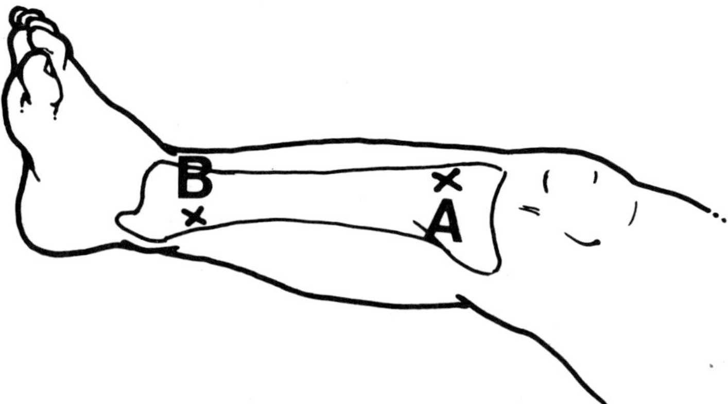

FIGURE 19–22. *A,* Proximal site; *B,* distal site.

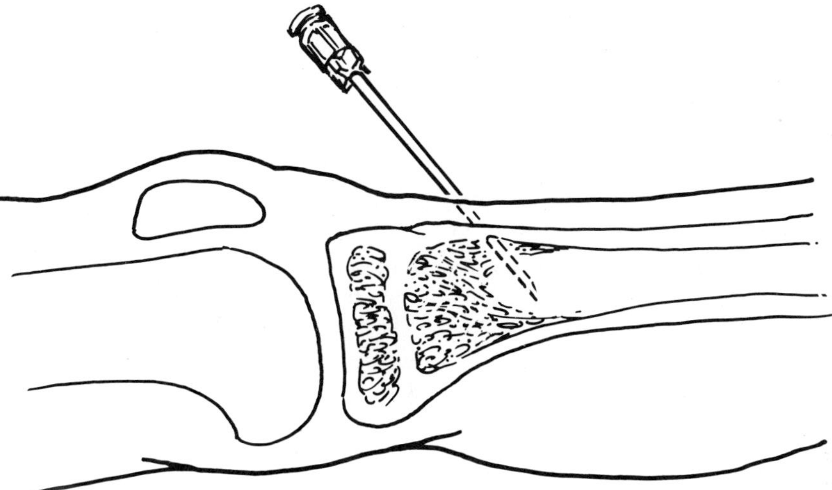

FIGURE 19–23. Intraosseous infusion: proximal tibia

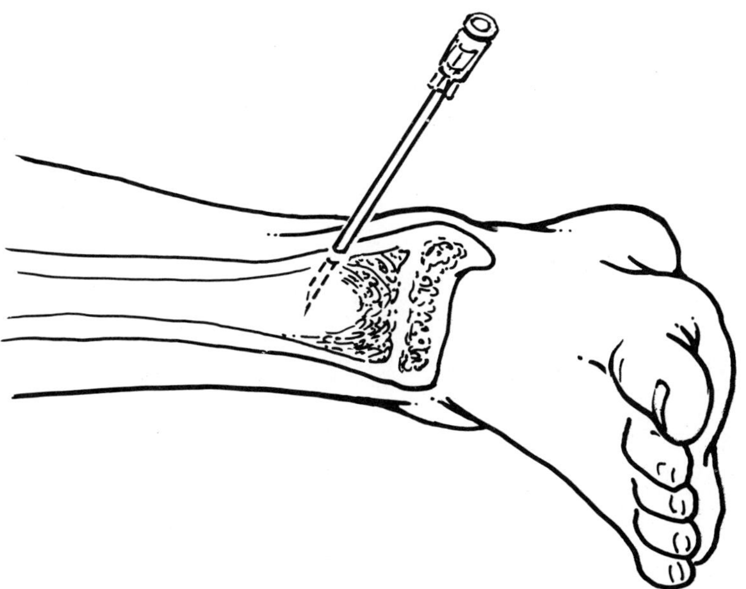

FIGURE 19–24. Intraosseous infusion: distal tibia.

Complications

1. Improper placement. Pitfalls associated with insertion include complete penetration through the other side of the periosteum, extravasation of fluid around the puncture site, and total misplacement out of the marrow cavity.
2. The potential for osteomyelitis is rare. The intraosseous infusion should be discontinued as soon as venous access is obtained.

Pearls and Pitfalls

1. The distal tibia may be used in adults if all other options for intravenous access fail.
2. A raw chicken or turkey thigh provides an excellent training simulator and can be cooked and eaten after you are finished practicing.
3. Damage to the proximal epiphyseal plate may be avoided by appropriate caudal angulation of the needle prior to insertion.

References

Gleser PW, Losck JD: Intraosseous needles: New and improved. Pediatr Emerg Care 4:135, 1988.
Spivey WH: Intraosseous infusions. J Pediatr 5:639–643, 1987.
Wagner MB, McCabe JB: A comparison of four techniques to establish intraosseous infusion. Pediatr Emerg Care 4:87, 1988.

Pericardiocentesis

MICHAEL S. JASTREMSKI, MD

Indications

Drainage of fluid from the pericardial sac to relieve cardiac tamponade
Removal of fluid from the pericardial sac for diagnosis
Injection of chemotherapeutic agents in malignant effusions

Contraindications

Emergency thoracotomy with open drainage of the pericardium is the preferred technique to relieve cardiac tamponade in the setting of electromechanical dissociation caused by penetrating chest trauma.

Equipment

Betadine prep
Sterile drapes
ECG machine
Double alligator clip (sterile)
Local anesthetic
10-ml syringe
50-ml syringe
25-gauge, 1-inch needle
18-gauge, 3-inch spinal needle
20-gauge, 1½-inch needle
Sterile gloves
Gown, mask, cap
Eye shield
4 × 4-inch gauze pads
Bandaid

Universal Precautions

1. Wear cap, gown, mask, and sterile gloves.
2. Use an eye shield.

Technique

1. Explain the procedure to the patient and obtain consent if circumstances allow.
2. Connect the limb leads of the ECG to the patient.
3. Put on cap, mask, eye shield, gown, and sterile gloves.
4. Prep the anterior chest and upper abdomen with Betadine.
5. Drape.
6. Stand on the patient's right side at his or her waist.
7. Locate the site of puncture by palpating the tip of the xiphoid and moving your finger left to the lower costal margin. The puncture site will be below the costal margin at this point.
8. Using the 10-ml syringe and 25-gauge needle, infiltrate the skin with local anesthesia. Then change to the 20-gauge, 1½-inch needle and infiltrate the deeper tissues with local anesthesia.
9. Using the sterile double alligator clip, attach the V_1 lead of the ECG machine to the 18-gauge spinal needle. Attach the 50-ml syringe to the spinal needle.
10. Turn on the ECG machine and run a V_1 rhythm strip continuously during the procedure.
11. Insert the spinal needle at the site of skin anesthesia and advance it toward the patient's left shoulder maintaining it at an angle of 30 degrees to the patient (Figure 19–25).
12. As you advance the needle, maintain negative pressure with the syringe and watch the ECG tracing.

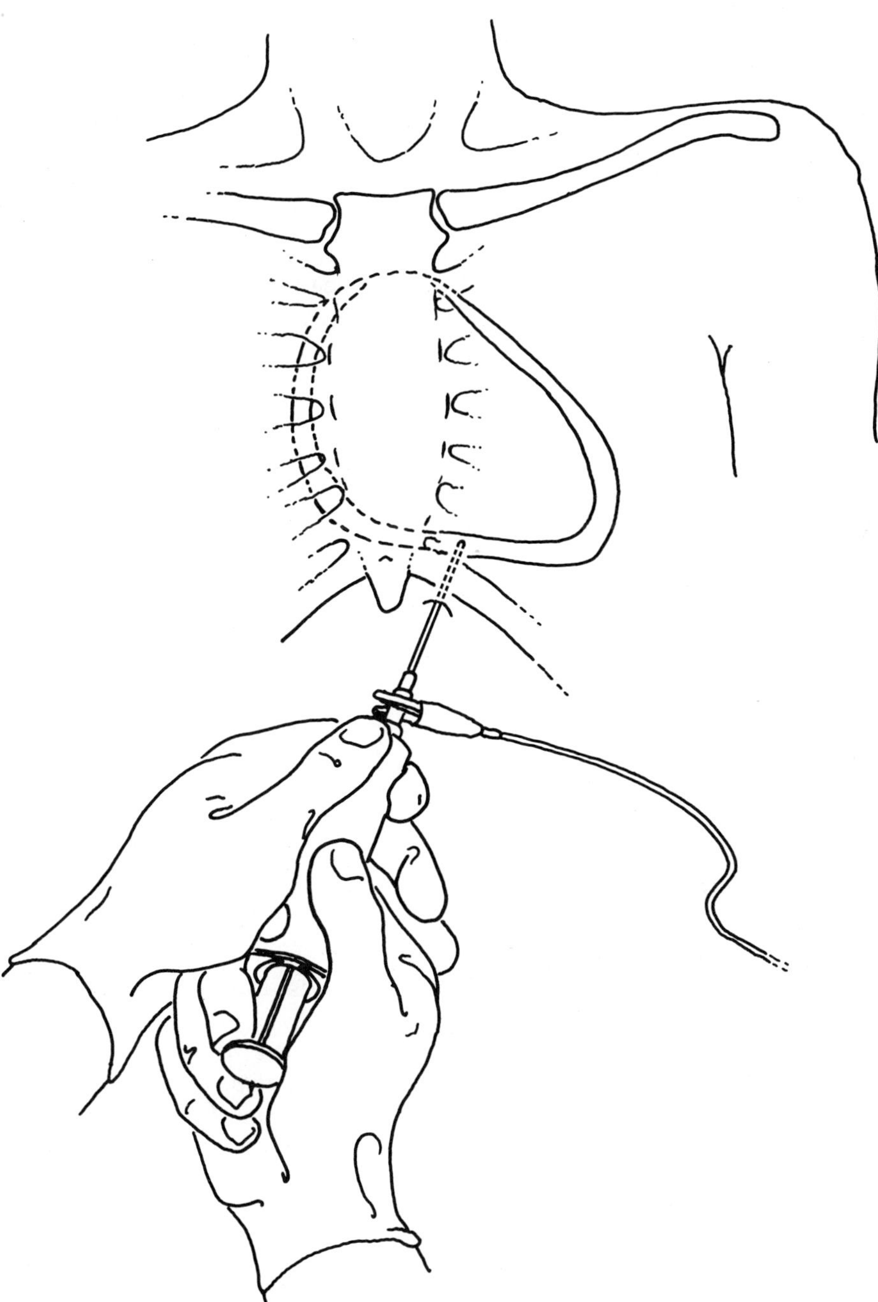

FIGURE 19–25. Pericardiocentesis.

13. You will feel a "pop" as the needle penetrates the pericardium. If fluid is aspirated, remove as much of it as possible. If no fluid returns, slowly advance the needle while maintaining negative pressure until the ECG shows ST-segment elevation, indicating epicardial contact (Figure 19–26). When the ECG shows epicardial contact, withdraw the needle while still maintaining negative pressure.
14. If neither fluid return nor epicardial contact is achieved, withdraw the needle to just under the skin and try advancing it again at a 45-degree angle, aiming to the medial side of the shoulder. Continue withdrawing and readvancing the needle at slightly different angles and aiming points until either the fluid is removed and the patient's hemodynamic status improves or epicardial contact is achieved.
15. Withdraw as much fluid as possible and send samples for culture and laboratory analysis, if indicated by the clinical setting.
16. Remove the needle and put pressure on the wound until any bleeding has stopped.
17. Apply a Bandaid to the puncture site.
18. Obtain and look at a chest x-ray film.

Complications

Pneumothorax
Hemorrhage
Myocardial laceration or perforation
Injury to a coronary artery
Dysrhythmias
Infection
Puncture of abdominal organs (stomach, spleen, colon)

Pearls and Pitfalls

1. Think of cardiac tamponade when there is the clinical triad of hypotension, distended neck veins, and muffled heart sounds. Low voltage on the ECG and a paradoxic pulse are other clinical clues.
2. Patients with trauma, uremia, malignancy, tuberculosis, and myxedema may have associated pericardial effusions with cardiac tamponade.
3. The echocardiogram is the best diagnostic test for pericardial fluid.
4. The chest x-ray film may *not* display cardiac enlargement in acute cardiac tamponade.
5. The characteristic hemodynamic findings of cardiac tamponade found in pulmonary artery catheterization are a low cardiac output, elevation and equalization of end-diastolic pressure (especially right ventricular end-diastolic pressure), and a square root sign in the right ventricular pressure waveform.

Reference

Extensive experience.

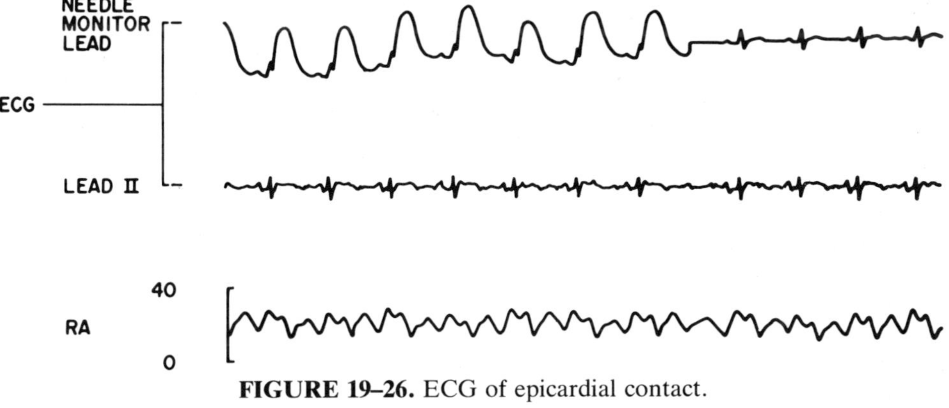

FIGURE 19–26. ECG of epicardial contact.

Pneumatic Antishock Garment

RICHARD A. CHERRY, NREMT-P

Indications

Hypovolemic or vasogenic shock

The pneumatic antishock garment (also known as Military Anti-Shock Trousers [MAST]) raises systolic blood pressure by creating an artificial vasoconstriction under the suit and reducing blood flow to the lower extremities. This increases peripheral vascular resistance and improves perfusion to the major organs during hypovolemic and vasogenic shock when systolic pressures fall below 90 mm Hg. The suit also stabilizes pelvic and lower extremity fractures and tamponades internal and external bleeding.

Contraindications

Absolute

Pulmonary edema
Left ventricular dysfunction
Known diaphragmatic rupture

Relative

The following are all relative contraindications in which the garment should be used either cautiously or with the leg compartments inflated only:

Impaled objects
Intrathoracic hemorrhage
Tension pneumothorax
Pericardial tamponade
Head injuries with increased intracranial pressure
Second or third trimester of pregnancy
Abdominal eviscerations
Lumbar fracture

Equipment

Pneumatic antishock garment
Foot pump and connecting tubing

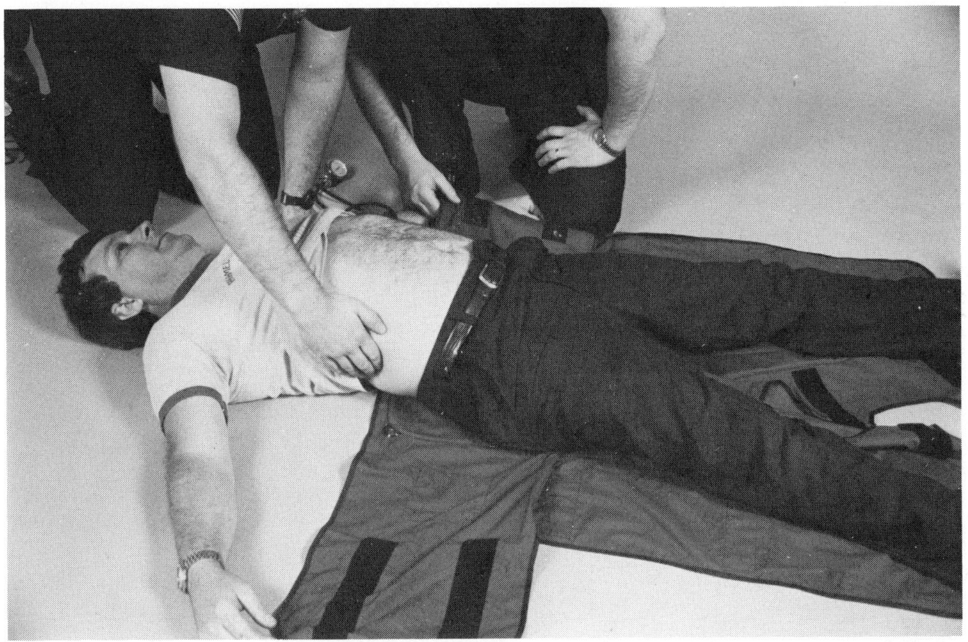

FIGURE 19–27. MAST application: Step 1.

Universal Precautions

1. Wear gloves.

Inflation Technique

1. Explain the procedure to the patient.
2. Check vital signs and confirm indications for use of the garment.
3. Put on gloves.
4. Remove the patient's clothing, including shoes and socks. If this is not feasible, simply remove any sharp objects that may perforate the garment.
5. Unfold the garment and lay it flat.
6. Log roll the patient onto the garment or slip it under the patient.
7. Position the upper edge of the garment just below the rib cage (Figure 19–27).
8. Wrap each leg section (Figure 19–28) and the abdominal section and fasten the Velcro connections firmly (Figure 19–29).
9. Attach the pump tubes to the garment. The longest tube goes to the abdominal section. The two shorter tubes go to the leg sections (Figure 19–30).
10. Open the stopcock valves. The valves are open when the handles or indicator lines are parallel to the tubing.
11. Unless contraindicated, inflate all sections of the garment with the foot pump simultaneously.
12. Inflate the garment until air exhausts through the relief valves or until the Velcro begins to tear open (Figure 19–31).
13. Close the stopcock valves. The valves are closed when the handles or indicator lines are perpendicular to the tubing.
14. Recheck vital signs and distal pulses.

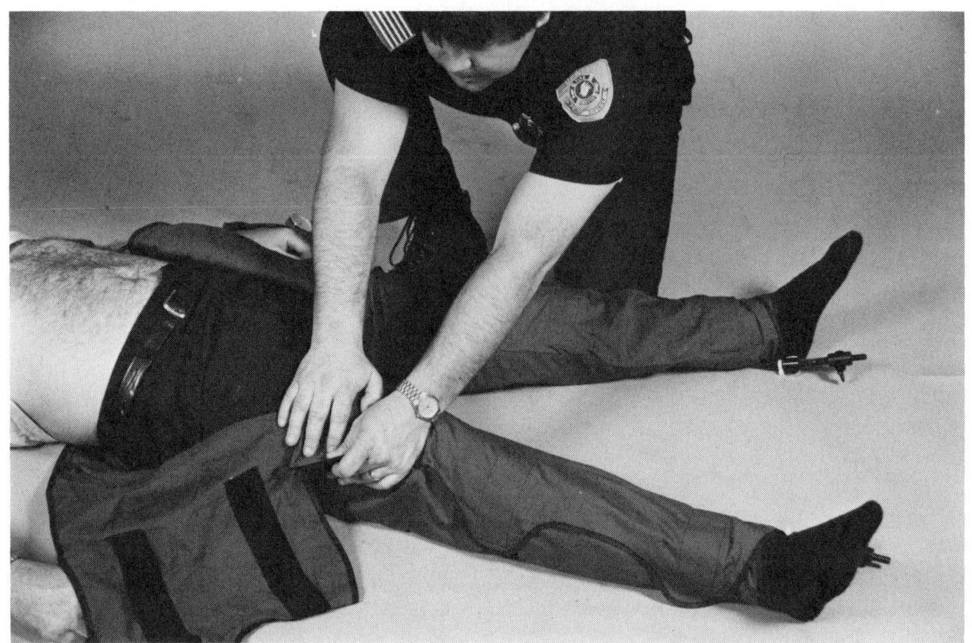

FIGURE 19–28. MAST application: Step 2.

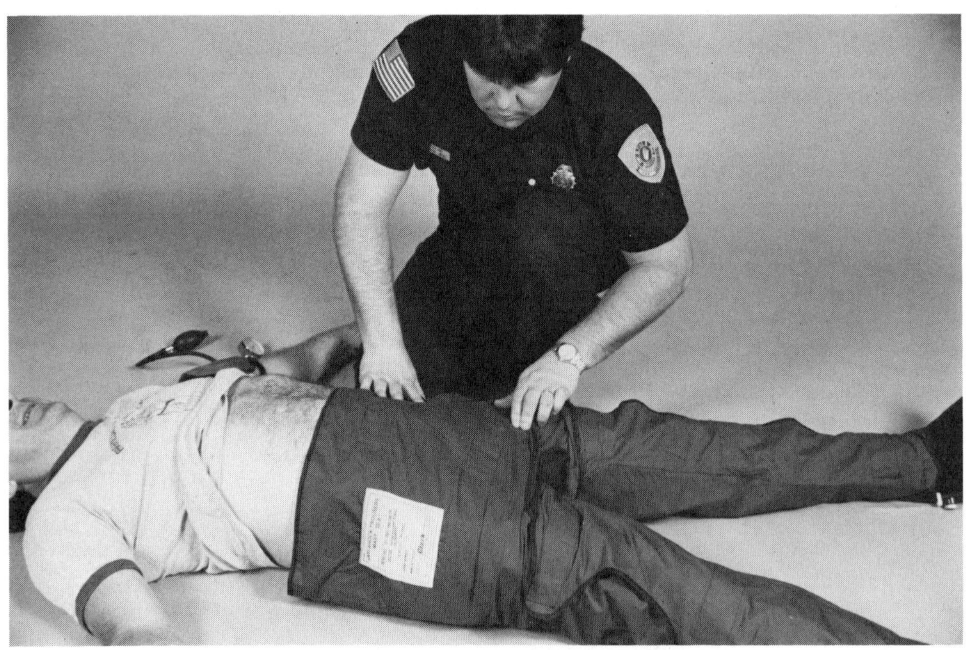

FIGURE 19–29. MAST application: Step 3.

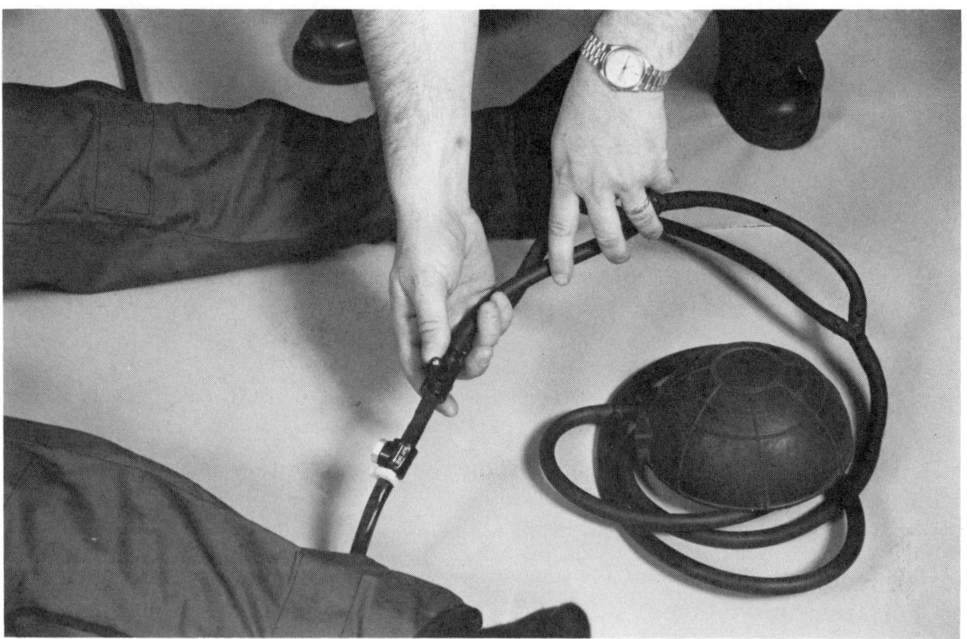

FIGURE 19–30. MAST application: Step 4.

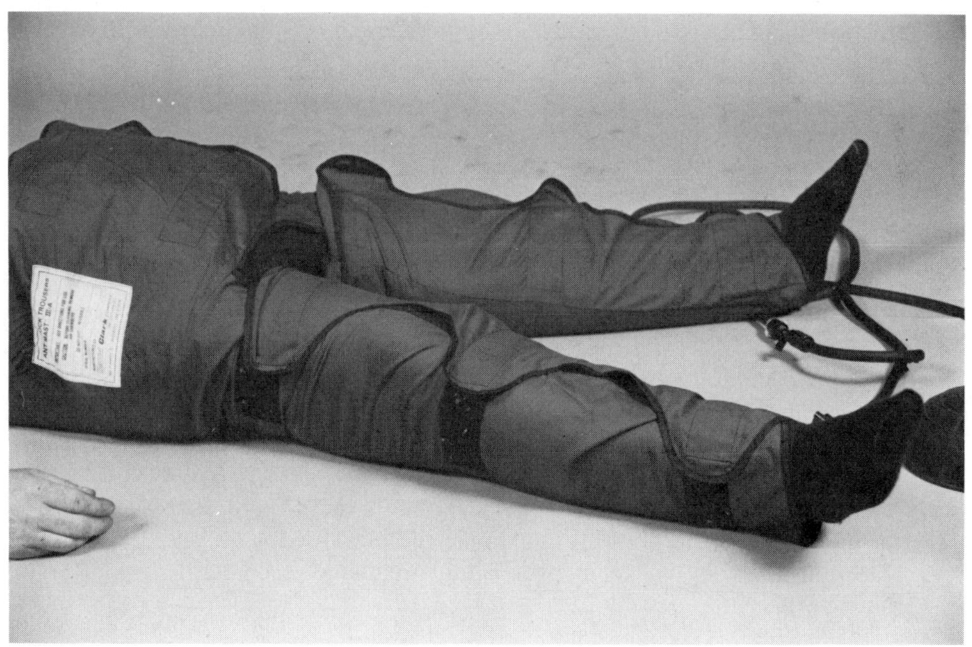

FIGURE 19–31. MAST application: Step 5.

Deflation Technique

1. Reestablish fluid volume and normal blood pressure with multiple large-bore intravenous lines.
2. Monitor vital signs closely during deflation procedure.
3. Slowly open the abdominal valve while monitoring blood pressure.
4. If the blood pressure drops 5 mm Hg or more at any time during the deflation procedure, stop and infuse fluids until normal pressure is restored.
5. If the blood pressure suddenly drops 10 mm Hg or more, stop the procedure and reinflate the garment until more fluid can be given or until surgical intervention can be arranged.
6. After the abdominal section is completely emptied, repeat this procedure with each leg individually.

Complications

A 50% decrease in diaphragm movement with respiratory insufficiency after inflation of abdominal section

Increased intrathoracic pressure and hemorrhage

Decreased perfusion under the garment

Compartment syndrome, ischemia, and anaerobic metabolism in the lower extremities during prolonged use (>2 hours)

Metabolic acidosis after deflation following prolonged use

Damage to the abdominal contents

Regurgitation and aspiration

Distraction of lumbar spine fracture with worsening of spinal cord injury

Pearls and Pitfalls

1. The antishock garment is not a substitute for volume replacement.
2. Inflation pressures may increase during air transport or when the garment is applied in a cold environment and the patient is brought into a warm emergency department.
3. If the garment has inflation pressure gauges, always monitor the patient's blood pressure, not the garment pressure.
4. Fasten the Velcro connections carefully to maximize inflation capabilities.
5. The garment is not recommended in cardiogenic shock or cardiac arrest.
6. Use of the garment may be beneficial in raising collapsed peripheral veins for cannulation.
7. A rapid technique is to inflate the sections by mouth with large volumes of air and then use the pump to maximize the pressure.
8. The value of this device in prehospital medicine is currently a matter of controversy.

References

American College of Surgeons Committee on Trauma: Advanced Trauma Life Support Program. Chicago, American College of Surgeons, 1989.

Bledsoe B: Atlas of Paramedic Skills. Englewood Cliffs, NJ, Prentice-Hall, 1986.

Grant HD, Murray RH, Bergeron JD: Brady Emergency Care. Englewood Cliffs, NJ, Prentice-Hall, 1990.

Mattox KL, McSwain N: Controversy: Medical anti-shock trousers. Prehosp Disaster Med 43:39, 1989.

Synchronized Cardioversion

SAMMY F. SURIANI, RPA-C, EMT-P

Indication

To convert cardiac dysrhythmias to a sinus mechanism

Dysrhythmias considered for cardioversion include unstable ventricular tachycardia and unstable supraventricular tachycardias (atrial flutter or fibrillation, paroxysmal atrial tachycardia). "Unstable" refers to hemodynamic compromise, hypotension, congestive heart failure, chest pain suggesting myocardial ischemia, or evidence of cerebral ischemia. Synchronized cardioversion may also be useful on a less urgent basis in the stable patient with the same dysrhythmias that do not respond to conventional drug therapy.

Contraindications

Nonsustained dysrhythmias (i.e., runs of the dysrhythmia briefly interrupting sinus rhythm). Drug therapy is necessary in this situation.

Digitalis toxicity (relative, since there is a high incidence of complications of cardioversion in this setting, but if the patient is "going out" then you have to cardiovert)

Equipment

Cardiac monitor, DC defibrillator/cardioverter

Supplemental oxygen

Intravenous lifeline with 5% dextrose and water

Conductive gel

Midazolam

"Crash cart" containing intubation equipment and resuscitation medications per Advanced Cardiac Life Support protocols

Universal Precautions

1. Take care to ensure that none of the medical personnel is electrocuted.

Techniques

1. Attach the patient to the cardiac monitor; identify the rhythm and correlate with the clinical presentation. Determine the need for cardioversion based on the clinical status.
2. Explain the procedure to the patient and obtain consent if circumstances permit.
3. Place the patient in the supine position with intravenous lifeline and supplemental oxygen in place and "crash cart" at bedside.
4. If patient is conscious, administer midazolam, 1 to 2 mg initially followed by increments of 1 mg every 5 minutes until adequate sedation is achieved. A state of drowsiness with subsequent amnesia is preferred prior to cardioversion. The patient should be as relaxed as possible.
5. Activate the synchronization mode of the cardioverter. Increase the ECG size on the screen to ensure a high enough R wave amplitude so that the synchronization circuit will sense a regular recurrent R wave. Achievement of this is usually signified by a flashing of the synch button with each passing QRS complex or a bright light on each R wave on the monitor screen. Choose the lead that best shows the R wave for monitoring. Be certain the monitor screen is clear of artifact before proceeding (Figure 19–32).
6. Generously apply conductive gel to cover the paddles.

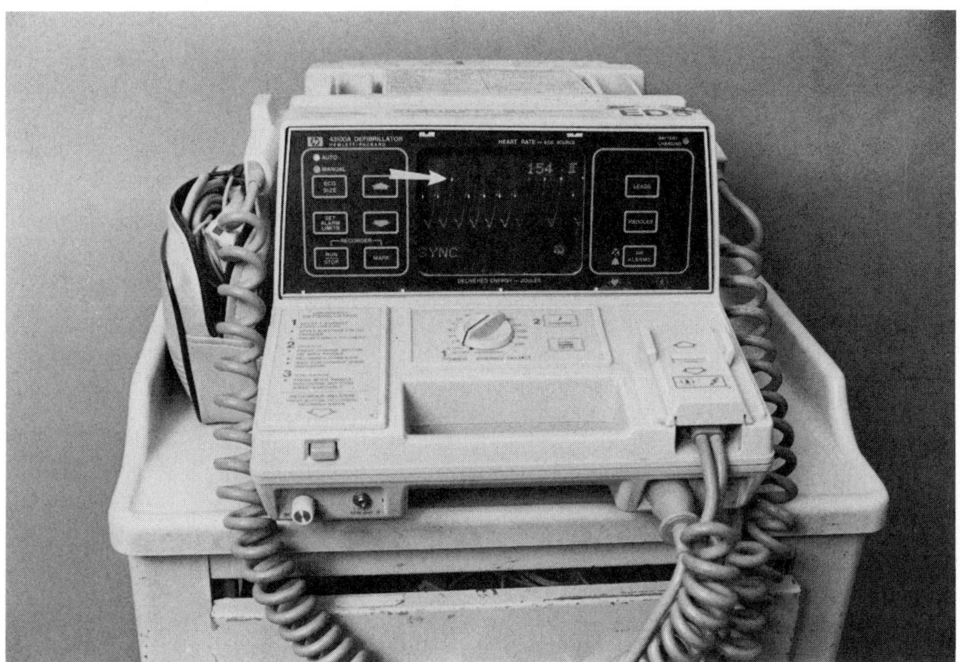

FIGURE 19–32. Synchronized defibrillator: arrow indicates light on R wave.

TABLE 19–1. Cardioverter Energy Output for Specific Dysrhythmias

Rhythm	Initial Energy Level (Joules)
Atrial fibrillation	200
Atrial flutter	50
Supraventricular tachycardia	75
Ventricular tachycardia	50

7. Select the desired energy output on the dial labeled "energy select." Begin at the lowest practical energy for the specific dysrhythmia (Table 19–1). Use lower energy in patients taking digitalis.
8. Apply the paddles to the chest in the anterolateral position (Figure 19–33). Paddles are usually marked "sternum" and "apex" for easy identification. Place the "apex" paddle in the left fourth to fifth intercostal space, midaxillary line. Place the "sternum" paddle to the right of the sternal margin in the second to third intercostal space. Use 20 to 25 pounds of contact pressure to minimize transthoracic impedance and to ensure firm paddle contact.
9. Ensure patient's skin does not come in contact with any metal and that all bystanders remove themselves from the stretcher prior to cardioversion.
10. Reconfirm the rhythm and announce "all clear." Be sure to clear yourself of contact with the patient or the stretcher.
11. Simultaneously depress the discharge buttons on the paddles to discharge current. There is often a few moments' delay before current is discharged, so it is important to maintain constant contact with the chest wall.
12. If normal sinus rhythm is obtained, the operator should stop. Palpate the pulse. If the patient's clinical status permits, wait at least 3 minutes before

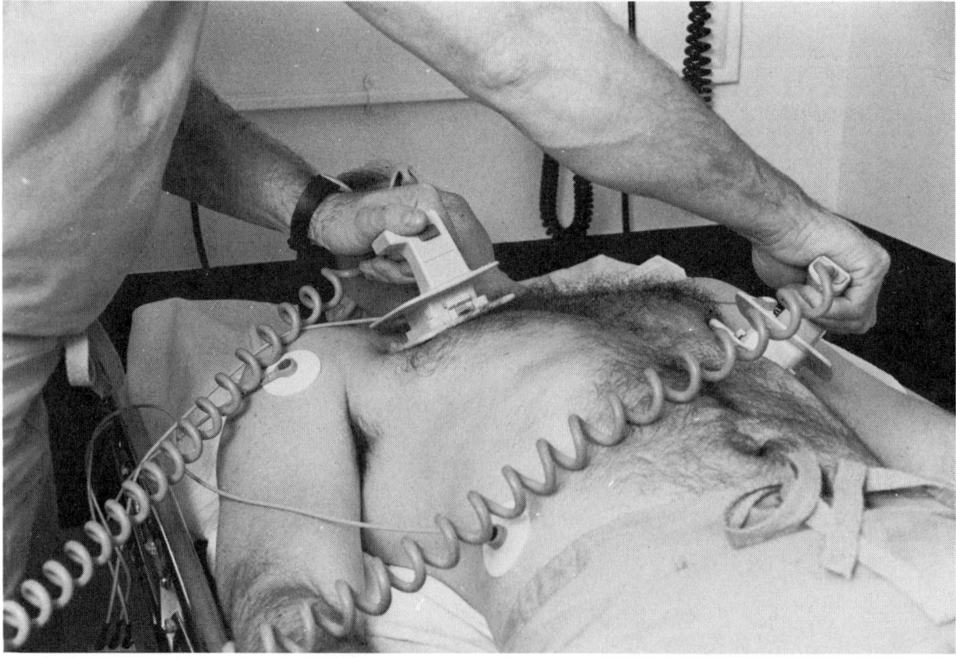

FIGURE 19–33. Paddle position for synchronized cardioversion.

repeat cardioversion at the next higher energy setting should the dysrhythmia persist. If ventricular fibrillation, pulseless ventricular tachycardia, or asystole results, shut the synchronizer off and defibrillate immediately.

13. Begin appropriate antidysrhythmic drug therapy to prevent recurrence of the dysrhythmia.

Complications

Failure to activate synchronizer switch resulting in asynchronous current discharge possibly leading to "R on T" phenomenon and causing ventricular fibrillation

Electrocution of self and others

Cardioversion to a lethal rhythm (ventricular fibrillation, pulseless ventricular tachycardia, asystole)

Superficial skin burns

Slight muscle discomfort

Transient bradycardia immediately following shock

Unfamiliarity with equipment function

Pearls and Pitfalls

1. The presence of myocardial infarction is not a contraindication to cardioversion.
2. The synchronizer may inadvertently interpret artifact as R waves; make certain monitor is clear of artifact before proceeding.
3. History or suspicion of digitalis toxicity is a relative contraindication to the use of emergency cardioversion; low energies must be used in this setting.
4. Antidysrhythmic medication should always be given following successful conversion of ventricular tachycardia.
5. Take care to prevent conductive gel from running together since this may cause current to be diverted over the skin surface and away from the heart.
6. An increase in serum enzyme levels may occur following cardioversion and is usually the consequence of skeletal muscle injury rather than myocardial damage.
7. Complications are directly proportional to shock strength. Therefore, initially use the lowest practical energy setting.
8. It is prudent to familiarize yourself with the operation of the cardioverter available to you *before* you have to use it on a patient.

References

Gazak S: Direct current electrical cardioversion. In Roberts JR, Hedges JR (eds): Clinical Procedures in Emergency Medicine, pp 151–159. Philadelphia, WB Saunders, 1985.

Jaffe AS, et al (eds): Electrical therapy in the malignant arrhythmias. In: Textbook of Advanced Cardiac Life Support, pp 89–96; 241–244. Chicago, American Heart Association, 1987.

Pancoast P, Hamilton GC: Electrical intervention in cardiopulmonary resuscitation: Cardioversion. In Tintinalli JE (ed): Emergency Medicine. Clinics of North America: Symposium of Resuscitation, vol 1, No. 3, pp 535–539. Philadelphia, WB Saunders, 1983.

20

Sexual Assault Examination

CELESTE MADDEN, MD

Indication

Involuntary sexual contact

Contraindications

None. Remember that these victims may have other life-threatening injuries that require attention first.

Equipment

- Pelvic tray
- Gloves
- Crime kit
- *Chlamydia* culture media
- Gonorrhea transport media
- Papanicolaou smear fixative
- Microscope/slides
- Camera
- Wood's lamp
- 8 F pediatric feeding tube
- Dacron microculturette swabs for pediatric specimens

Universal Precautions

1. Wear gloves.

Technique

1. Obtain history with a supportive patient advocate of the patient's choice or a supportive hospital staff member. Explain the procedure to the patient and obtain consent.
2. Complete the physical examination documenting findings of trauma and sexually transmitted diseases, paying particular attention to areas of assault identified in the history.
3. Obtain photographs documenting injuries.
4. Coordinate collection of specimens, including the following:
   a. Crime kit evidence if there was contact with a male perpetrator within 48 hours or if material corroborating patient's history is found during the physical examination
   b. Saline wash(es) to determine presence of sperm in vagina or rectum
   c. Tests for sexually transmitted diseases, including *Neisseria gonorrhoeae* cultures from throat, genitalia, and rectum; *Chlamydia trachomatis* cultures from genitalia and rectum; and serology for syphilis
5. Collect serum pregnancy test in pubertal female victims.
6. Counsel pubertal female victims about risk of pregnancy and options for interruption of pregnancy.
7. Counsel victims about risk of human immunodeficiency virus infection and arrange for testing at approved facility and at appropriate interval following sexual contact.
8. Contact law enforcement agency to initiate or cooperate with criminal investigation.
9. Notify Child Protective Services when parents have failed to protect their child from abuse.
10. Arrange follow up medical examination to
    a. Treat injuries and document sexually transmitted diseases
    b. Reassess for pregnancy and incubating sexually transmitted diseases, including convalescent syphilis and acquired immunodeficiency syndrome serology.
11. Arrange referrals for patient (family) psychosocial counseling.

Complications

Patient psychosocial damage caused by insensitive approach of staff members

Failure to diagnose significant internal injuries, pregnancy, or sexually transmitted diseases

Loss of potential evidence caused by incomplete collection or mishandling of crime kit

Pearls and Pitfalls

1. Photographs should never replace the accurate description of traumatic physical findings in the medical record.
2. A standardized crime kit with instructions and documentation of the "chain of evidence" must be used.
3. A standardized medical record form will encourage documentation of important medical and legal patient information (Figure 20–1).
4. Avoid use of lubricant during physical examination until sexually transmitted disease cultures are obtained.
5. Obtain consent for photography, except in child abuse cases when it is not required.
6. To accurately describe the anatomic location when describing traumatic or infectious genital or rectal lesions, superimpose the face of a clock on the area and note the position (lithotomy, knee-chest) the patient was examined in.
7. Proceed to an examination with the victim under anesthesia when a prepubertal victim has active vaginal bleeding or when there is a strong suspicion of an injury penetrating the vaginal vault or in any victim whose injuries require better visualization than an examination of an awake patient affords.
8. Specifically during pediatric examinations:
   a. Organize specimen collection from least- to most-threatening (venipuncture) procedure.
   b. Avoid touching the sensitive hymenal membrane with swabs when collecting vaginal specimens.
   c. Avoid use of rapid diagnostic tests for *Chlamydia*. The culture remains the only legally admissible documentation of infection.
9. Before pregnancy interruption medications are used, explain side effects, risks, and efficacy to the patient.
10. Criminal investigations must be carried out in all cases of child abuse.
11. Baseline laboratory tests for hepatitis B surface antigen and human immunodeficiency virus may also be indicated.

Reference

Extensive experience.

EMERGENCY DEPARTMENT

SUSPECTED ABUSE FORM

DATE: ______________ PATIENT NAME: ______________ HOSPITAL # ______________

PERSONNEL INVOLVED IN ER:

NURSING: ______________ LAW ENFORCEMENT: ______________

PEDIATRICS: ______________ CPS: ______________

SOCIAL SERVICES: ______________ OTHER: ______________

DATE OF ALLEGED ASSAULT: ______________ GYNECOLOGY: ______________

History Obtained (delineate histories obtained from child, parent, or neighbor—if obtained separately):

FIGURE 20–1. Sexual abuse record.

Illustration continued on following page

EMERGENCY DEPARTMENT

SUSPECTED ABUSE FORM
PAGE 2

DATE:__________ PATIENT NAME:________________ HOSPITAL #______________

SPECIFIC HISTORICAL EVENTS:

1. DID THE ACT INVOLVE:

   COITUS? __________ FELLATIO? __________

   RECTAL PENETRATION?________ HAND-GENITAL CONTACT?__________

   CUNNILINGUS? __________

2. DID EJACULATION OCCUR?______________ WHEN? ______________

   BODY SITE INVOLVED________________

3. WAS THERE LOSS OF CONSCIOUSNESS?__________ HOW? ______________

4. ARE THERE BRUISES EVIDENT?________________ (describe on next page)

5. SINCE THE INCIDENT, HAS THE PATIENT:

   CHANGED UNDERWEAR?__________ BATHED?__________

   EATEN/RINSED MOUTH? __________ DOUCHED?__________

   URINATED/DEFECATED?__________

6. IS PATIENT MENARCHAL?__________ WHAT AGE ONSET?________

   LMP________ CYCLE LENGTH________

   LAST INTERCOURSE__________ METHOD OF CONTRACEPTION USED________

7. DOES THE PATIENT USE CONTRACEPTION?______ WHAT METHOD? ____________

8. LIST ANY SIGNIFICANT PMH OR MEDICATIONS.

   ____

   ____

9. IS THE FAMILY UNIT ALREADY KNOWN TO CHILDREN'S DIVISION?__________

FIGURE 20–1 *Continued*

EMERGENCY DEPARTMENT

SUSPECTED ABUSE FORM
PAGE 3

DATE:________ PATIENT NAME:______________________________HOSPITAL #__________

Physical Examination:

Temp.__________ Pulse__________ RR__________ BP__________ WT__________

General (include emotional state, condition of body/clothing):

Body Surface (if bruises, lacerations present, give history of etiology):

Wood's Lamp Exam ____________________

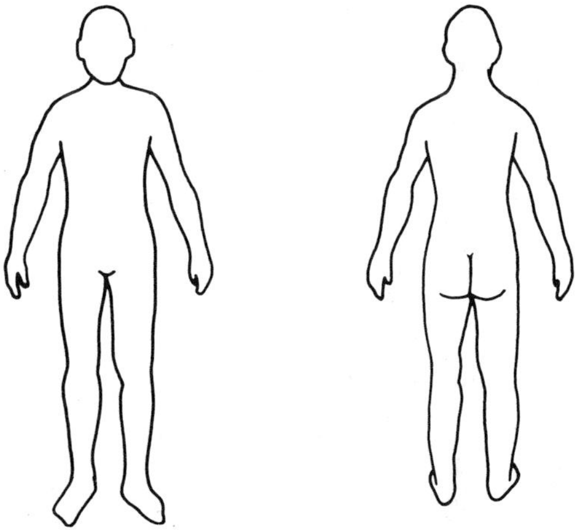

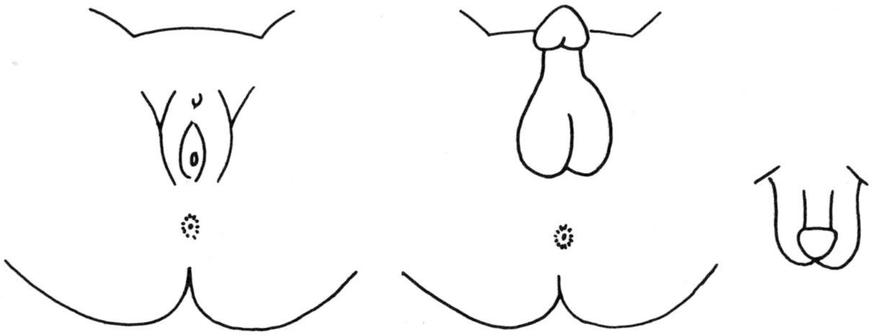

FIGURE 20–1 *Continued*

Form continued on following page

EMERGENCY DEPARTMENT

SUSPECTED ABUSE FORM
PAGE 4

DATE: ____________ PATIENT NAME: ____________ HOSPITAL # ____________

LABORATORY SPECIMENS (Check if Obtained)

_____ throat Cx (for G.C.)
_____ vaginal/cervical Cx (for G.C.)
_____ urethral Cx (for G.C.)
_____ rectal Cx (for G.C.)
_____ throat Cx (for chlamydia)
_____ vaginal/cervical Cx (for chlamydia)
_____ urethral Cx (for chlamydia)
_____ rectal Cx (for chlamydia)

_____ clotting functions
_____ VDRL
_____ Pap smear
_____ urine pregnancy test
_____ serum pregnancy test
_____ urinalysis
_____ urine culture
_____ stool hematest
_____ herpes culture (site: ____________)

EVIDENTIARY MATERIAL (Label each carefully-check if obtained)

*_____ photos
*_____ clothing (list) ____________
*_____ fingernail scrapings
*_____ pubic hair (w/standards)
*_____ scalp hair (w/standards)
*_____ patient saliva on filter paper
*_____ patient blood for typing (purple top)
*_____ air dried slides for sperm and acid phosphatase
  _____ labia _____ vagina/cervix _____ rectum _____ throat
*_____ dry swab for sperm and acid phosphatase
  _____ labia _____ vagina/cervix _____ rectum _____ throat

_____ moist swab in 0.5cc saline
  _____ labia
  _____ vagina/cervix
  _____ rectum
_____ skeletal series
_____ CT scan
_____ bone scan

* These Specimens Go to Crime Lab

Specimens given to: ____________
Badge # ____________
Date/Time ____________

FIGURE 20–1 *Continued*

EMERGENCY DEPARTMENT

SUSPECTED ABUSE FORM
PAGE 5

DATE: ____________ PATIENT NAME: ____________ HOSPITAL # ____________

IMPRESSION:

____

____

____

THERAPY IN ER:

____

____

CPS HOTLINE CALLED? Y N ; BY WHOM? ____________; ON ____________

FORM 2221 FILED? Y N ; BY WHOM? ____________; ON ____________

PATIENT DISCHARGED TO: ____________ WITH ____________

FOLLOWUP:

1. Pediatrician ____________ When? ____________
2. Social Services ____________
3. CPS ____________
4. GYN ____________
5. Rape Crisis ____________
6. Psychologic evaluation/therapy ____________

ADDITIONAL HISTORY (Continued from Page 1-Use if necessary)

____

____

____

____

____

____

____

DATE ____________ PHYSICIAN(S) SIGNATURE ____________

FIGURE 20–1 *Continued*

21

Slit Lamp Examination

DENISE GAVULA, DO

Indications

Detailed examination of the eye with a microscope for visualization of the anterior surface of the eye, anterior chamber, lens, and anterior section of the vitreous humor

Intraocular pressure measurement (measurement device is not on all slit lamps)

Contraindications

None

Equipment

Slit lamp
Fluorescein
Local anesthetic

Universal Precautions

None

Technique

Preparation (See Figure 21–1 for location of controls.)

1. Explain the procedure to the patient.
2. The patient should be seated comfortably on a chair with his or her chin in the scooped chin rest (*A*) and forehead against the bar (*B*) above the chin rest.

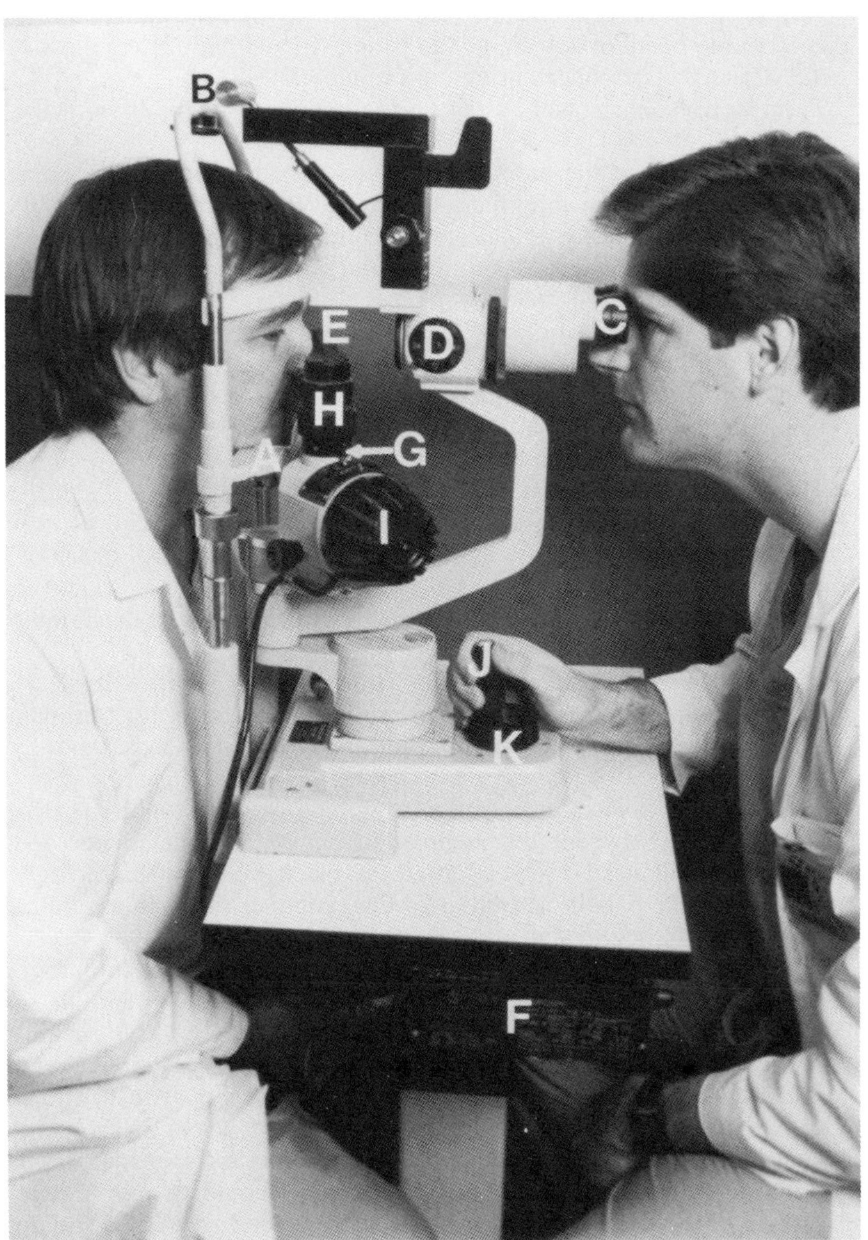

FIGURE 21–1. The slit lamp.

3. The examiner should set the eye pieces of the microscope (*C*) so that they are in the correct position for his or her eyes when seated behind the slit lamp and adjusted to correct for his or her refractive error. Microscopy of the eye should be limited to magnification no greater than 25×, with optimal magnification at 10× to 16× (*D*).
4. Adjust the height of the chin rest so that the eyes of the patient are brought level to the beam of light (*E*). The patient should be instructed not to look directly at the examiner during the examination.
5. Turn on the main power switch on the underside of the base of the table (*F*).
6. The switch (*G*) at the base of the light source can be used to change the color of the light to white, blue, or green. White light is used for all of the examination except for enhancement of the fluorescein stain for which blue light is used. For increased contrast of red objects such as the fundus choose the green light.
7. The angle of the light source can be changed by rotating the source on its base (*H*). The farther away the light is rotated from the microscope, which creates a larger angle, the narrower will be the beam or slit of light. The height of the beam can also be altered by turning the dial (*I*) just behind the switch that is used to change the color of the light.
8. The handle or joystick (*J*) on the table allows movement of the microscope in four directions: toward and away from the patient, providing a mechanism for fine focusing, and from left to right to scan across the structure being examined.
9. The ring at the base of the handle (*K*) is for fine up and down movement of the visualized field.
10. The examination of the eye begins with the most anterior structures and should continue in the following order: lids and lid margins, lacrimal ducts, conjunctiva, sclera, cornea, anterior chamber, iris, lens, and anterior vitreous.
11. The nontransparent tissues can be examined with the white light adjusted at any angle between the illumination device and the microscope. The brightness will need to be adjusted. If the light is too bright, it will be dazzling to the patient as well as to the examiner, and visualization of the structures will be difficult.
12. Examination of the most anterior transparent structure, the cornea, requires adjustment of the light source so that reflection off the mirror-like surfaces of the cornea and the lens is avoided. The angle between the illuminating beam and the microscope should be as large as possible, creating a narrow slit of light. The sharply focused structure of the eye as seen with this slit of light can now be examined. Examination of layers of the cornea for identification of foreign bodies, corneal abrasions, or opacities is best achieved with a narrow slit. This slit of light should be moved across the surface of the cornea, varying the depth if needed to identify the depth of injury or penetration.
13. Movement of the joystick (*J*) toward the patient will change the depth of focus of this slit of light and bring into sharp view the next deeper layer that you wish to visualize. Examination of the anterior chamber will be possible only if the angle between the illumination device and the microscope is no greater than 45 degrees and the slit is wide. The presence of cells and/or exudate will appear as small reflective particles and a cloudy beam, respectively, in the anterior chamber, like a beam of light shining in

a movie theater. Each structure as visualized should be described in the patient's chart following completion of the examination.

14. Turn off the power source after completion of the examination.
15. *The chin rest, head rest, and other areas of patient contact should be cleaned after each examination.* Epidemic keratoconjunctivitis can spread easily to other patients by contact with areas touched by a previous infected patient. A 1% solution of bleach or isopropyl alcohol can be used.

Pearls and Pitfalls

1. Fluorescein staining will make corneal abrasions easier to visualize.
2. Topical anesthetic may be used to facilitate the examination in patients who have trouble keeping their eye open.

References

Müller O: Ocular examination with the slit lamp. Distributed with slit lamp manufactured by Carl Zeiss, Inc., One Zeiss Drive, Thornwood, New York 10594.

Schmidt TA: On slit lamp microscopy/theory and practice. Haag-Streit AG Ophthalmologic Instruments. W Junk, ed. The Hague, BV Publishers, 1975.

Vaughn D, Asbury T: General Ophthalmology. Palo Alto, CA, Lange Medical Publications, 1977.

22 Thoracentesis

KEVIN FERGUSON, MD

Thoracentesis is the percutaneous drainage of intrapleural fluid. For the most part, emergency thoracentesis is done to relieve acute respiratory distress. Although the procedure may be done for therapeutic reasons, the fluid obtained should routinely be sent for laboratory analysis.

Indications

Drainage of pleural effusion in a patient with respiratory compromise
Culture in patients with an infiltrate in the ipsilateral lung
Cytologic analysis if a patient has a mass in the mediastinum or ipsilateral lung
Relief of a small nontraumatic pneumothorax in a stable patient

Contraindications

Coagulopathy (relative)

Equipment

There are several brands of preassembled, disposable thoracentesis trays whose major advantage is convenience.

Betadine skin prep solution
Sterile drapes
Two 10-ml syringes
50-ml syringe
25-gauge, ⅝-inch needle
22 gauge, 2-inch needle
12-gauge, 4-inch introducer needle
16-gauge, 8-inch intravenous catheter
Local anesthetic
Three-way stopcock
Kelly clamp
1 foot of intravenous extension tubing

Laboratory specimen bottles and tubes

Plasma vacuum bottle (if cytologic specimen is to be sent, the larger the specimen, the better the yield)

Sterile gauze dressing

2-inch adhesive tape

Sterile gloves

Mask

Eye shield

Sterile gown

Universal Precautions

1. Wear sterile gown and gloves and a mask.
2. Use an eye shield.

Technique

1. Explain the procedure to the patient and obtain consent.
2. Position the patient based on whether the procedure is to remove air or liquid.
   a. The patient with a small pneumothorax should be supine with the head of the bed slightly elevated, 30 to 40 degrees.
   b. For the removal of an effusion, the patient should be as close to upright as can be securely maintained for the duration of the procedure. It may be easier to allow the patient to rest on his arms and lean over a table or Mayo stand.
   c. The effusion should be localized using posteroanterior and lateral chest x-ray films and by percussion of the chest wall. The change from tympany to dullness marks the border of the effusion. The site of the puncture is determined by the material to be removed and the location of the effusion. The preferred sites for effusions are the posterior axillary line at the sixth intercostal space and the angle of the rib posteriorly and just lateral to the paraspinous muscles. The midscapular line is also an

alternate site. For aspiration of air, entry should be on the anterior chest in the second intercostal space at the midclavicular line (Figure 22–1).

3. Put on mask, eye shield, and sterile gown and gloves.
4. Stand facing the patient.
5. Scrub the area widely with Betadine.
6. Drape area with sterile towels.

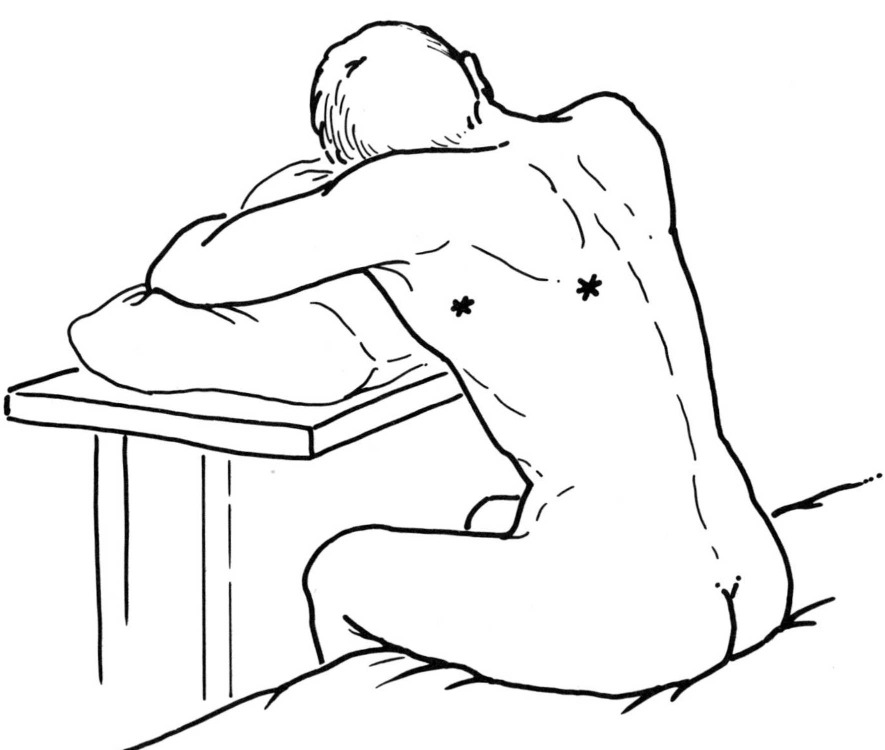

FIGURE 22–1. Asterisks indicate sites for thoracentesis.

7. Anesthetize the site with local infiltration of lidocaine. Use a 10-ml syringe and 25-gauge needle to raise a skin wheal, then switch to the 22-gauge needle for deeper infiltration. Infiltrate directly over the rib of the thoracentesis site and continue inward, aspirating back as the needle is advanced until the pleural fluid or air is aspirated. Clamp the needle at the skin with the Kelly clamp, and withdraw the needle. The distance from the tip of the needle to the hemostat is the chest wall thickness (Figure 22–2).

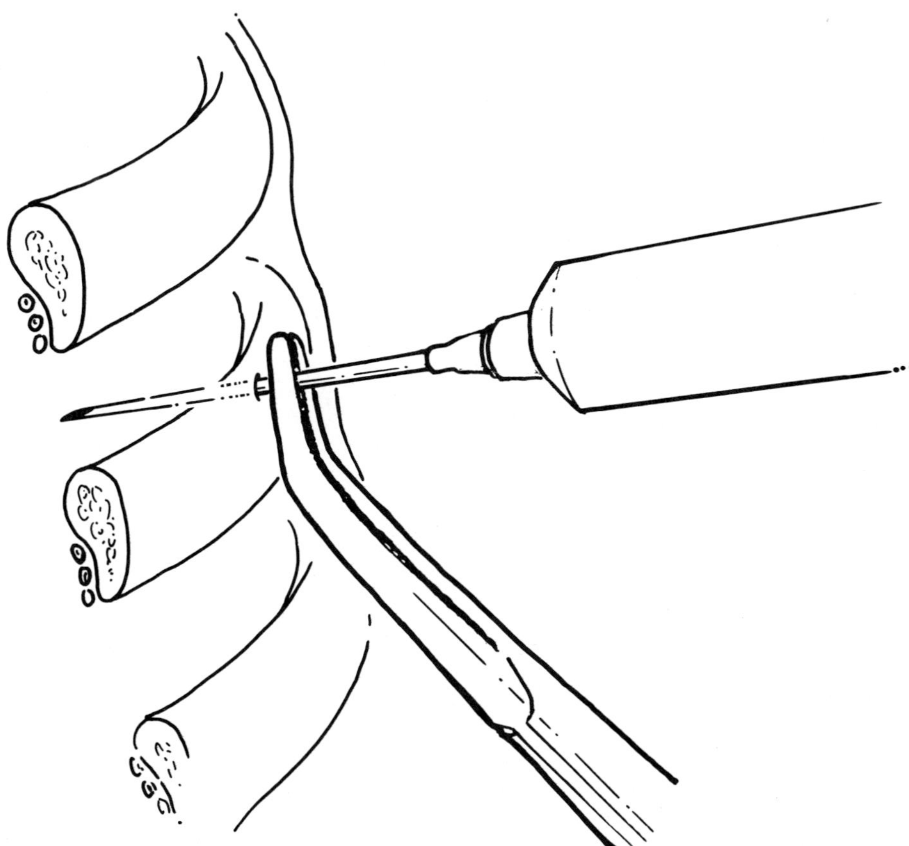

FIGURE 22–2. Determining chest wall depth.

8. Place a stopcock with a 10-ml syringe attached on the end of the introducer needle.
9. Using the distance marked by the Kelly clamp on the anesthetic needle that should correspond to the chest wall depth, grasp the introducer needle with the dominant hand at this point.
10. Using the other hand, stretch the skin around the site and puncture the skin directly over the rib. Then advance the introducer needle over the top of the rib to avoid the neurovascular bundle beneath the ribs. Advance the introducer to the distance measured by the anesthesia needle and open the stopcock and aspirate with the syringe. If no fluid is obtained, advance the needle while maintaining suction with the syringe.
11. Return of fluid indicates the introducer needle is in the pleural space. At this point, a soft catheter is introduced into the pleural space to complete the withdrawal of fluid with less risk of damage to the lung from a sharp needle. There are three catheter introduction methods:
    a. With the through-the-needle technique, the needle is advanced until the

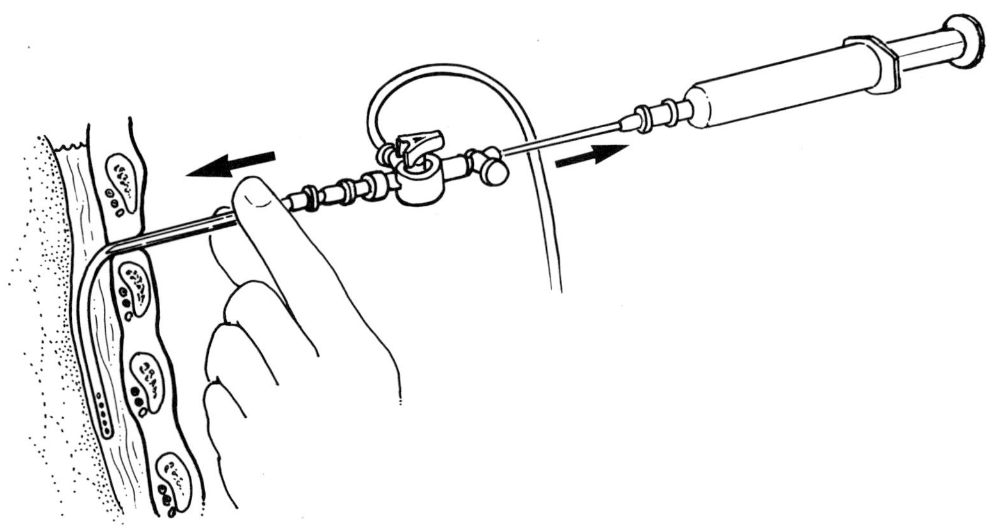

FIGURE 22–3. Introducing the catheter.

pleural space is entered and then the catheter is placed through the needle into the pleural space and the needle is removed.

b. With the over-the-needle method the catheter is over the needle as on an intravenous catheter, so that once the needle enters the pleural space the catheter is in place and is advanced over the needle, the needle is removed, and the stopcock assembly is attached (Figure 22–3).
c. In some prepared disposable kits there will be a guide wire that is placed through the needle into the pleural cavity, the needle is withdrawn, the catheter is then threaded over the guide wire, the wire is removed, and the collection is begun.

12. Attach the extension tubing apparatus to the catheter, the three-way stopcock to the extension tubing, and the 50-ml syringe to the three-way stopcock. Then the three-way stopcock is opened to the syringe and the syringe is filled. Then the stopcock is turned so the catheter going to the patient is closed to prevent air entry, and the syringe is removed. After enough fluid has been aspirated to fill the required specimen tubes (Table 22–1), the catheter is then attached to a vacuum bottle and the rest of the

TABLE 22–1. Pleural Fluid Specimens

Container	Volume	Studies
Sterile culture tube	10–20 ml	Gram stain Tuberculosis stain Bacterial cultures (aerobic and anaerobic) Tuberculosis culture Viral culture*
Heparinized syringe	3–5 ml	pH*
Lavender tube	5–10 ml	Cell count and differential
Red tube	5–10 ml	Glucose Lactate dehydrogenase Amylase* Rheumatoid factor* Protein*
Vacuum bottle	All remaining fluid	Cytology*

*If indicated by the clinical setting.

fluid is removed. The heparinized arterial blood gas syringe is filled directly from the stopcock (Figure 22–4).

13. Once the fluid is removed, the catheter and needle should be removed as a unit and a sterile occlusive dressing applied.
14. If the procedure is done for the removal of air, fill the syringe attached to the introducer needle with 3 ml of sterile saline to make it easier to perceive the air bubbles obtained when the pleural space is entered. Once the catheter is in place it can be placed on low suction and aspirated until the patient feels a pleuritic chest pain, indicating the irritation of the pleura by the suction. The stopcock is then turned off to the patient and a chest x-ray film obtained to document reduction. The catheter is left in place and the patient is observed for evidence of pneumothorax for 4 to 6 hours. If a 4- to 6-hour postprocedure, follow-up chest x-ray film demonstrates no pneumothorax and the patient's clinical condition is improved, the catheter may be removed.
15. Obtain and look at a chest x-ray film after the procedure.

Complications

Pneumothorax. Air is likely to be introduced when the patient breathes and the catheter is open to the environment or may also result from puncture of the lung parenchyma by the needle. A slow leak may result in a delayed pneumothorax and will not be appreciated on the initial postprocedure chest x-ray film. A 6-hour postprocedure chest x-ray film is advised if the patient is to be discharged.

Intercostal neurovascular bundle injury

Intra-abdominal visceral injury to liver, spleen, or bowel

Catheter-tip foreign body in the pleural space (never pull the catheter back through the needle)

Reexpansion hypoxia and unilateral pulmonary edema. This results from rapid reperfusion of atelectatic lung. This causes a rapid increase in pulmonary capillary pressure and transudation of fluid into the alveolar space and resulting ventilation–perfusion mismatch. This usually resolves with supplemental oxygen, and all patients undergoing thoracentesis should be on O_2 therapy. Patients who have had long-standing large effusions and those who had large volumes of fluid removed at one time seem to be most prone to severe post-thoracentesis pulmonary edema.

Infection

Pearls and Pitfalls

1. Determination of the span of the effusion is important to obtain the optimum placement of the catheter.
2. A stopcock should be placed on the introducer and catheters and turned off to the patient each time the system is opened to change to vacuum bottle or to change syringes. This prevents inspiration pneumothorax. Inspiration pneumothorax can also be avoided if the patient is instructed to do a forced expiratory maneuver each time the needle must be open (i.e., for passage of a catheter or guide wire).

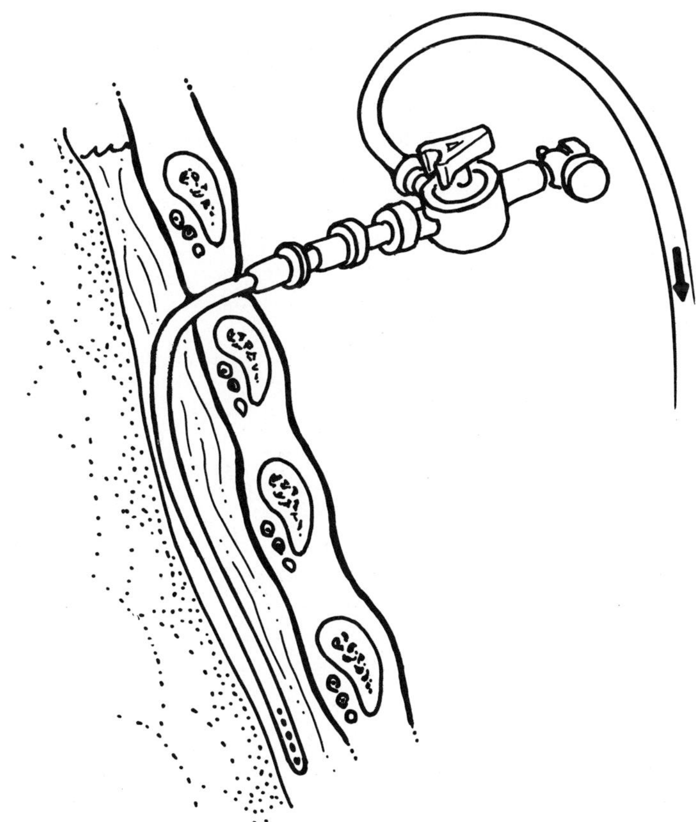

FIGURE 22–4. Arrow points to tubing connected to vacuum bottle.

3. Extreme caution is advised if the puncture is to be below the eighth rib owing to increased risk of intra-abdominal injury. Fluoroscopy or open technique is advised for procedures below this point.
4. If the thoracentesis is for purely diagnostic purposes, no more than 1 L of fluid should be removed. If the patient is in respiratory distress, the amount should be the least amount after the first liter necessary to relieve the symptoms, and in few cases should over 2 L be removed. If more is to be removed, it should be removed slowly and in small increments.
5. Pulling the catheter through the needle may shear off the catheter and create a foreign body in the pleural space.
6. Echocardiographic thoracentesis may be necessary for the successful and safe drainage of small loculated effusions.

References

Rosen P, Dailey R (eds): Emergency Medicine Concepts and Clinical Practice. St. Louis, CV Mosby, 1983.

Tintinalli J, Krome R (eds): Emergency Medicine: A Comprehensive Review Guide. New York, McGraw-Hill Book Company, 1988.

23

Tube Thoracostomy

JODY RIVA LEWINTER, MD

Indications

Drainage of air, blood, or fluid from the pleural space
Instillation of medications into the pleural space

Contraindications

Multiple adhesions
Giant blebs
Coagulopathy
Need for immediate open thoracotomy

Equipment

Antiseptic solution
Local anesthetic
Sterile gloves
Gown
Mask
Eye shield
Scalpel with No. 11 blade
Two large Kelly clamps
Thoracostomy tube (Nos. 32–40)
Underwater seal apparatus (e.g., Plurovac)
Needle holder
1-0 silk suture
Suture scissors
4 × 4-inch gauze pads
Wide adhesive tape for sterile dressing
Sterile petrolatum gauze
5-ml syringe
25-gauge, 1-inch needle
20-gauge, 1½-inch needle
Two hemostats
Sterile drapes

Universal Precautions

1. Wear gown, mask and sterile gloves.
2. Use an eye shield.

Technique

1. Explain procedure to patient and obtain informed consent if circumstances allow.
2. Prepare equipment:
   a. Ensure that all is present.
   b. Attach needle holder to suture.
   c. Clamp distal end of chest tube with a hemostat and apply large curved Kelly clamp to proximal end (Figure 23–1).
3. If patient's condition permits, position patient at a 45-degree angle with his arm on the side of insertion over the head (Figure 23–2).

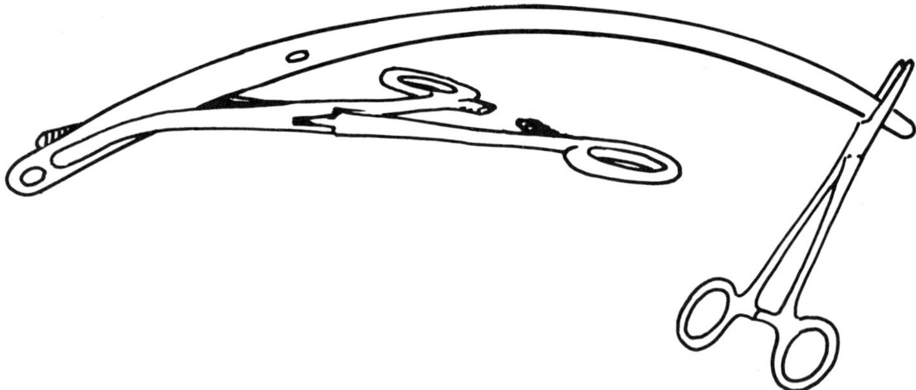

FIGURE 23–1. Preparation of the chest tube.

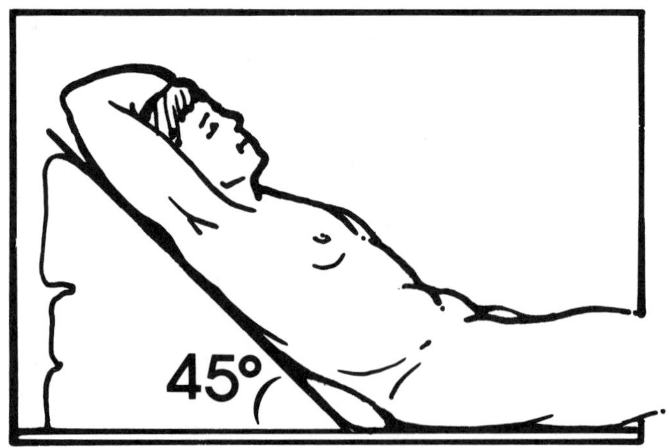

FIGURE 23–2. Position for tube thoracostomy.

4. Identify site of chest tube insertion: right or left fifth or sixth intercostal space in the anterior axillary line. Identify the incision site: one rib below the insertion site. For example, make an incision over the sixth rib for chest tube insertion in the fifth intercostal space. This creates a subcutaneous tunnel to ensure the tract seals (Figure 23–3).
5. Put on mask, eye shield, gown, and sterile gloves.
6. Surgically prepare area with Betadine and drape area surrounding the incision site.
7. Anesthetize the skin and subcutaneous tissue using a 5-ml syringe and a 25-gauge, 1-inch needle. Change to a 20-gauge, 1½-inch needle to anesthetize the periosteum of the rib underlying the interspace that the chest tube will enter.

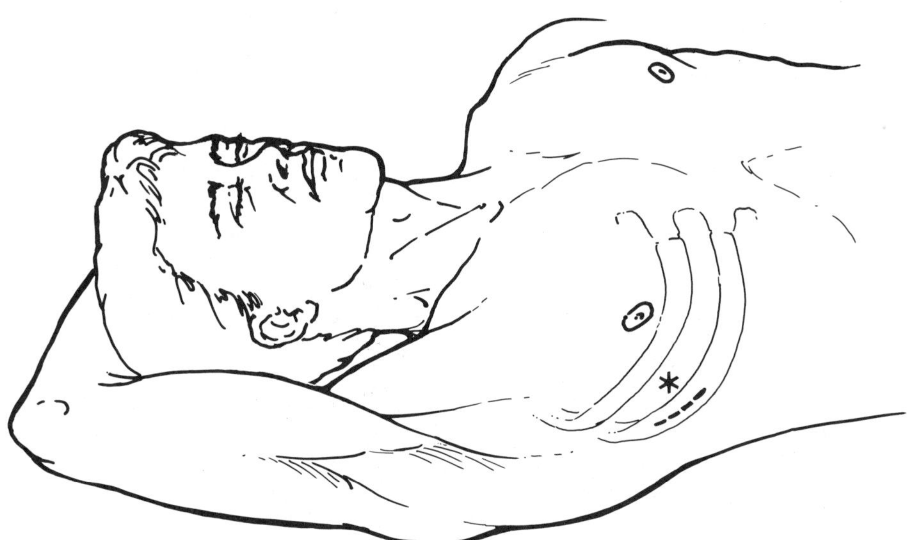

FIGURE 23–3. Asterisk indicates site for chest tube to enter the pleural space in the fifth intercostal space. Dotted line indicates the location of the incision.

8. Make a 3-cm transverse skin incision directly over the rib below the insertion site (Figure 23–4).
9. Use a large, curved Kelly clamp to bluntly dissect through the soft tissue passing over the superior aspect of the rib into the chosen intercostal space and puncturing the parietal pleura (see Figure 23–4, *arrows*).
10. Insert a finger through the incision and into the pleural space to verify position, widen the pleural opening, and ensure that there are no adhesions.

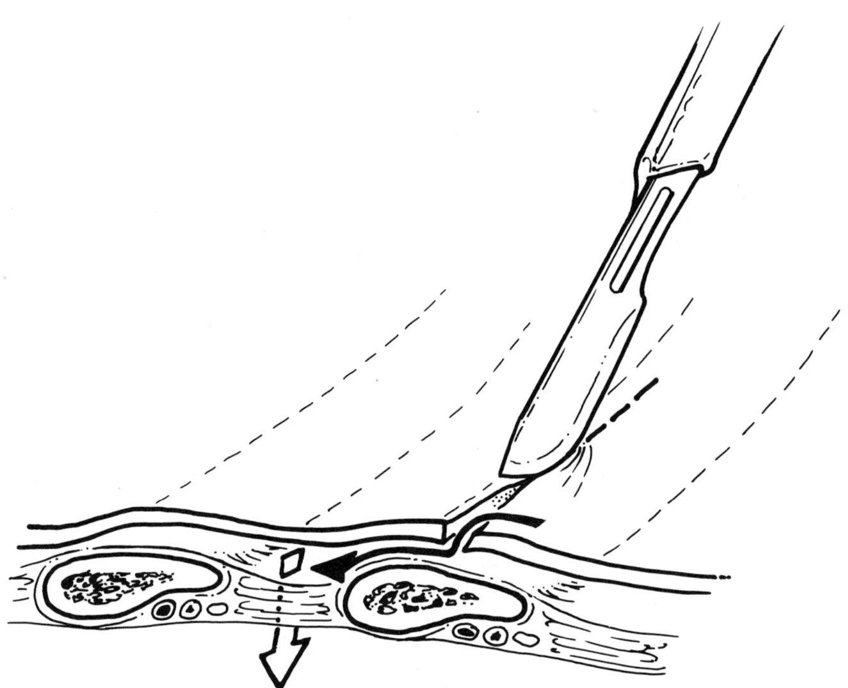

FIGURE 23–4. Tract through the chest wall.

11. Insert the thoracostomy tube through the incision into the chest cavity using the curved Kelly clamp, holding the proximal end to guide the tip into the pleural space (Figure 23–5). Remove the Kelly clamp and insert the rest of the chest tube into the pleural space, aiming posteriorly and superiorly toward the apex of the lung to drain air or inferiorly and posteriorly to drain fluid. Do not allow any of the side ports of the thoracostomy tube to remain outside the pleural space.

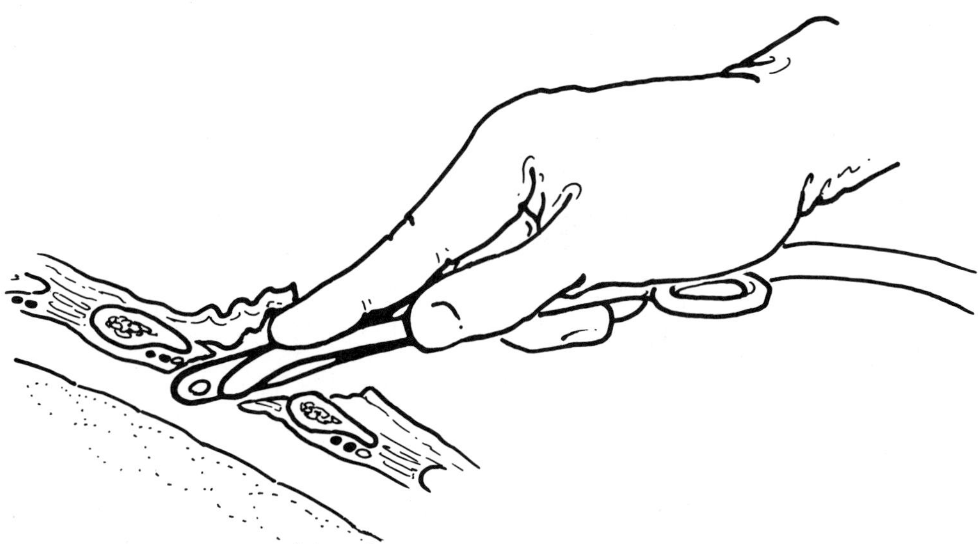

FIGURE 23–5. Insertion of the chest tube.

12. Remove the hemostat and connect the thoracostomy tube to the underwater seal apparatus.
13. Place a pursestring stitch around the thoracostomy tube and pass the free ends of the suture around it several times to secure the tube position (Figure 23–6).

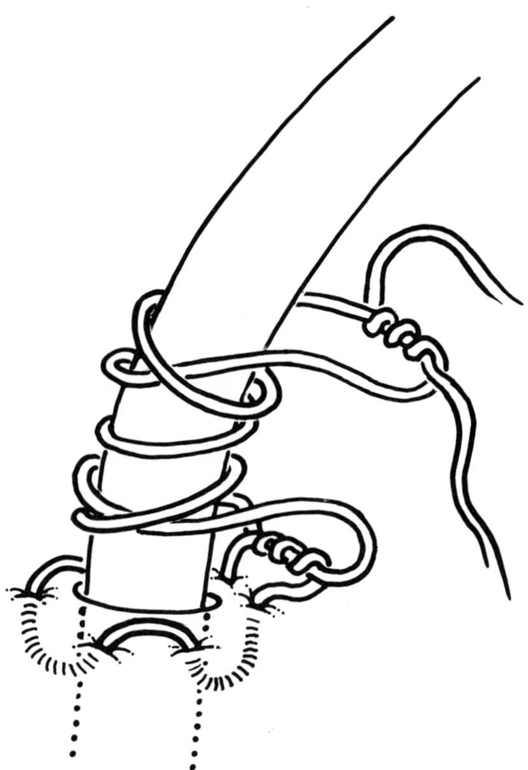

FIGURE 23–6. Suturing a chest tube.

14. Place sterile petrolatum gauze and then 4 × 4-inch gauze pads over the incision and around the base of the thoracostomy tube, and complete the dressing with adhesive tape (Figure 23–7).
15. Tape the connection between the chest tube and tubing to the underwater seal apparatus.
16. Tape the thoracostomy tube to the patient at a distal site to prevent dislodgement.
17. Obtain a chest x-ray film to confirm tube position and look at it.

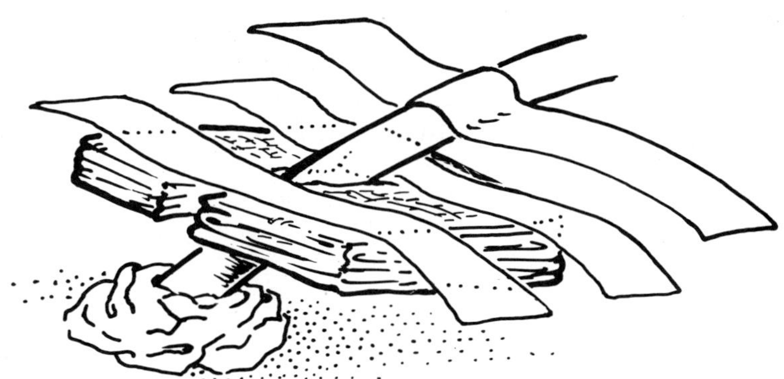

FIGURE 23–7. Chest tube dressing.

Complications

Thoracostomy tube becomes kinked or dislodged

Thoracostomy tube becomes separated from the underwater seal apparatus or underwater seal is not correctly assembled or attached to suction

Damage to the intercostal neurovascular bundle resulting in hemorrhage, neuropathy, or neuritis

Local or intrapleural infection

Subcutaneous or mediastinal emphysema

Laceration or puncture of intrathoracic structures

Laceration or puncture of intra-abdominal structures, including the liver or spleen

Chronic bronchopleural cutaneous fistula

Pearls and Pitfalls

1. Adequate local anesthesia and positioning will facilitate the procedure by opening the intercostal spaces.
2. Underwater seal apparatus must be kept below the level of the patient to prevent fluid flow into the thoracic cavity.
3. Never clamp a thoracostomy tube, since this may lead to lung collapse or a tension pneumothorax. If there is a problem with the system, leave the thoracostomy tube open to air while the problem is corrected.
4. When tube is being placed to drain fluid (as opposed to air), use a larger-sized tube and place the tube posteriorly and inferiorly to achieve dependent drainage.

References

American College of Surgeons Committee on Trauma: Advanced Trauma Life Support Program. Chicago, American College of Surgeons, 1989.

Simon R, Bailey T, Abraham E, Brenner B: A new technique for securing a chest tube. Ann Emerg Med 2:620, 1982.

Vascular Access 24

Arterial Blood Drawing

MICHAEL S. JASTREMSKI, MD

Indication

To obtain arterial blood sample for laboratory analysis, primarily for blood gas analysis

Contraindications (Relative)

Coagulopathy—for femoral route
Raynaud's phenomenon—for radial route
Local trauma

Equipment

Ice in a container
22-gauge needle: 1-inch for radial, 2-inch for femoral
3-ml syringe
Heparin
Betadine swab
Gauze pad
Sterile gloves
Eye shield
Mask
Stopper for syringe
Optional equipment if multiple samples needed:
Three-way stopcock
20-ml syringe
21-gauge butterfly catheter

Universal Precautions

1. Wear mask and sterile gloves.
2. Use an eye shield.

Technique

1. Explain the procedure to the patient and obtain consent if circumstances allow.
2. Choose the artery.
   a. Radial—preferred site since it is easily accessible and has minimal complications
   b. Femoral—alternate route if there are no radial pulses or both wrists are severely injured
3. Radial artery (Figure 24–1)
   a. Use the patient's nondominant arm. Fix the wrist on an armboard with the palmar surface up and a rolled-up pair of 4 × 4-inch gauze pads under the wrist to produce some extension.

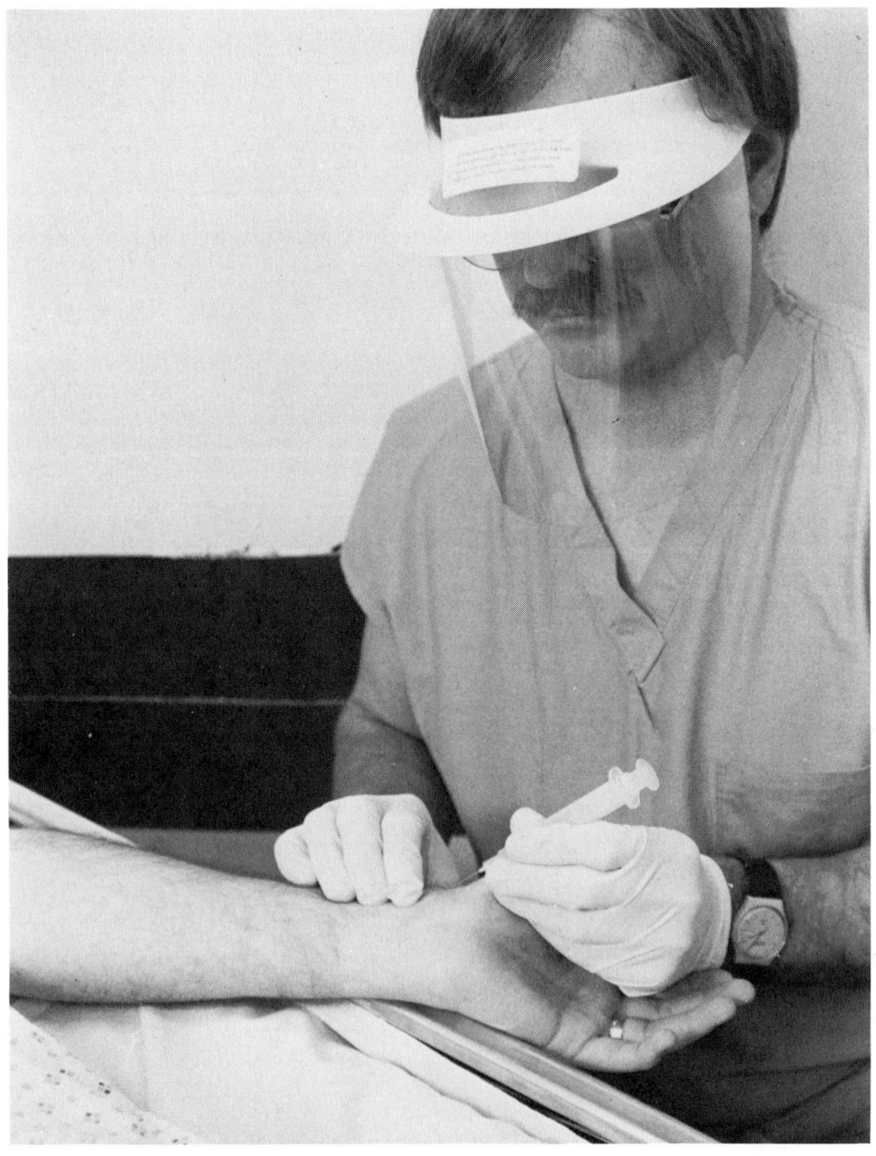

FIGURE 24–1. Radial artery puncture.

b. Stand on the same side as the chosen arm, facing the patient's head.
c. Put on mask, eye shield, and sterile gloves.
d. Swab the wrist over the radial artery with Betadine.
e. Attach the 22-gauge, 1-inch needle to the 3-ml syringe.
f. Draw up to 1 ml of heparin solution 1000 units/ml into the syringe. Pull the plunger all the way back to coat the entire barrel of the syringe and then discard the heparin, leaving only the needle filled with heparin.
g. Gently palpate the radial artery at a spot level with the radial styloid, using the first finger of your nondominant hand.
h. Hold the heparinized 3-ml syringe with the 22-gauge, 1-inch needle in your dominant hand as you would hold a pen or pencil.
i. Puncture the skin approximately 1 cm distal to the finger that is palpating the radial artery. The needle should be at a 20- to 30-degree angle to the skin with the bevel up.
j. Aim for the spot where the radial pulse is felt under the palpating finger of your nondominant hand, and slowly advance the needle toward this spot until blood flashes back into the hub of the syringe.
k. Allow the syringe to fill by the arterial pressure (i.e., do not aspirate by pulling back on the plunger of the syringe).
l. Withdraw the needle and maintain pressure on the puncture site for 5 minutes.
m. Immediately remove the needle, cap the hub of the syringe, place the syringe on ice, and send the specimen to the laboratory.
n. Assess the extremity for adequacy of perfusion.

4. Femoral artery (Figure 24–2)
   a. Position the patient supine with the chosen leg straight, externally rotated, and slightly abducted.
   b. Stand on the chosen side of the patient at the patient's hip, facing the patient's head.

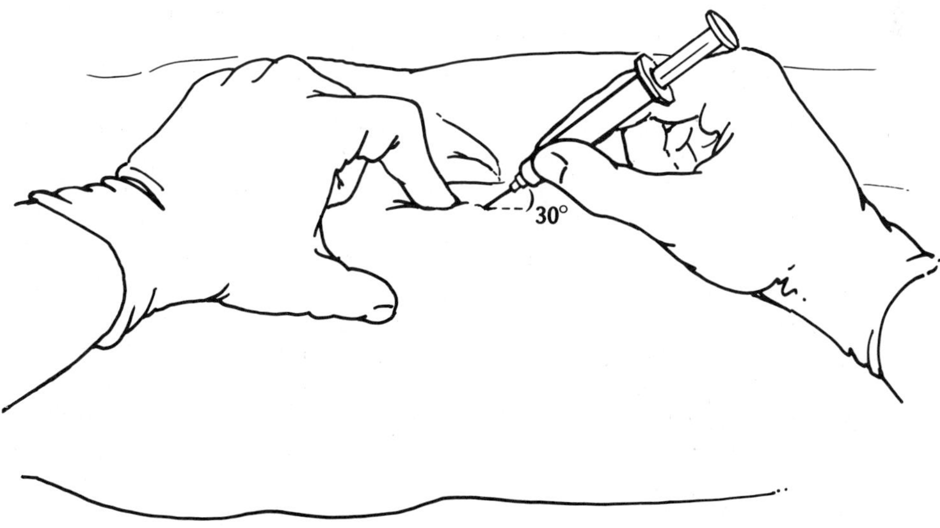

FIGURE 24–2. Femoral artery puncture.

c. Prep the chosen groin with Betadine.
d. Put on mask, eye shield, and sterile gloves.
e. Attach the 22-gauge, 2-inch needle to the 3-ml syringe.
f. Heparinize the syringe as described for the radial artery technique.
g. Palpate the femoral artery with the first finger of your nondominant hand 2 cm below the inguinal ligament.
h. Puncture the skin at a spot over the femoral artery 1 cm distal to the palpating finger, with the needle bevel up at a 30-degree angle to the skin.
i. Follow steps k through m as for the radial artery technique.

Complications

Bleeding—especially from the femoral artery
Distal ischemia
Infection
Arteriovenous fistula

Pearls and Pitfalls

1. The dorsalis pedis, superficial temporal, and axillary artery are alternative sites to consider if all radial and femoral arteries are not available. (I know a neurosurgeon who got his blood samples from the carotid artery because he was used to using this artery for angiograms, but I would not recommend this route).
2. Do not use the brachial artery. This is an end artery with no collaterals and, thus, at a much greater risk for distal ischemia.
3. Do not use the femoral artery if the patient has received thrombolytic therapy.
4. Do not use the femoral artery if the patient has a femoral bypass graft.
5. Multiple samples may be obtained from a single arterial puncture using one of the following techniques:
   a. Radial—use a 22-gauge butterfly catheter with attached tubing for the puncture. While you are carefully stabilizing the needle to keep it in the artery, have an assistant fill the heparinized 3-ml syringe with a blood sample for blood gas analysis and a second syringe of appropriate size to obtain blood to fill the required tubes for other laboratory tests.
   b. Femoral—interpose a three-way stopcock between the heparinized 3-ml syringe and the 22-gauge, 2-inch needle. While you carefully stabilize the needle, have an assistant fill the syringe with a blood sample for blood gas analysis and then turn the stopcock off. Attach a syringe of adequate volume to obtain the additional samples, open the stopcock, and fill the second syringe. Alternatively, the butterfly catheter technique may be used for the femoral artery, although the needle may not be long enough on obese patients.
6. Use a 25-gauge needle in infants and small children.

Reference

Extensive experience.

Arterial Cannulation

Indications

Continuous, real-time measurement of arterial pressure for monitoring and/or titration of vasoactive infusions

Provision of a more accurate blood pressure measurement than indirect techniques, especially in shock states

Facilitation of blood sampling for laboratory studies and elimination of patient discomfort from multiple venous or arterial punctures

Contraindications

Ischemia of the extremity

Raynaud's disease

Localized infection at the puncture site (use a different artery)

***Note:* The four techniques for arterial cannulation are presented in my order of preference: percutaneous radial, radial cutdown, femoral, and axillary.**

PERCUTANEOUS RADIAL ARTERY CANNULATION

MICHAEL S. JASTREMSKI, MD

Equipment

Short armboard
Cap, mask, eye shield, and gown
Sterile gloves
Betadine skin prep
Sterile drapes
1-foot pressure tubing
Three-way stopcock
Needle holder
Pressure monitor/flush system
3-0 nylon suture—curved needle
3-ml syringe with 25-gauge needle
Lidocaine 1% *without* epinephrine
20-gauge, 2-inch catheter over needle
4 × 4-inch gauze pads
Betadine ointment
Tape
Suture scissors

Universal Precautions

1. Wear mask and sterile gloves.
2. Use an eye shield.

Technique

1. If patient status and circumstances allow, explain the procedure to the patient and obtain consent.
2. Position patient's wrist on short armboard, palmar side up, in 60-degree extension (Figure 24-3).
3. Put on cap, mask, eye shield, gown, and sterile gloves.
4. Prep site with Betadine.
5. Drape site.
6. Attach needle to needle holder and three-way stopcock to 1-foot tubing (end opposite catheter).
7. Stand facing patient's arm and off to one side (so blood will not spurt on your clothes) such that your dominant hand is distal in relation to the patient's arm. Palpate radial artery at head of radius with index finger of your nondominant hand (Figure 24–3).
8. Infiltrate site of skin entry over radial artery approximately 1 cm distal to your index finger with a small amount of 1% lidocaine.
9. Remove cap from catheter-over-needle unit so blood flashback will be seen.
10. Holding catheter-over-needle unit in your dominant hand with it aligned at a 20-degree angle to the skin, enter skin over radial artery 1 cm distal to your index finger and advance catheter-over-needle unit aiming for radial pulse under your index finger (see Figure 24–3).

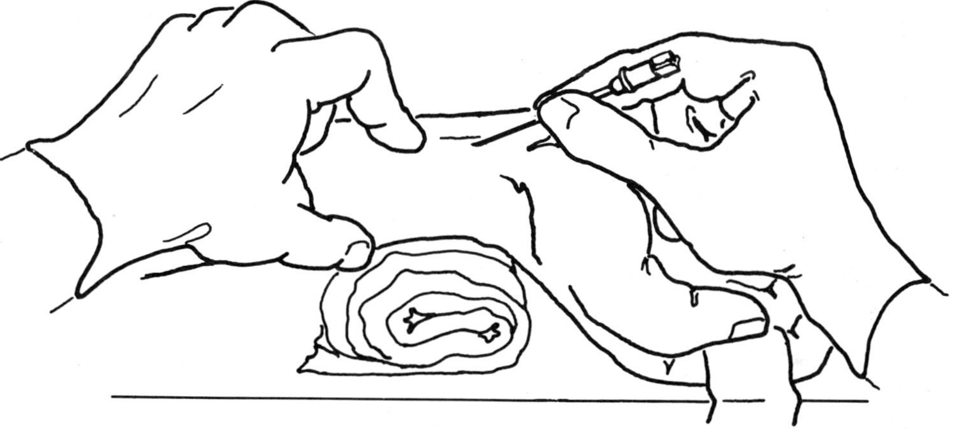

FIGURE 24–3. Percutaneous radial artery cannulation.

11. When blood flashes back, advance the catheter over the needle without moving the needle until the hub of the catheter is at the skin (Figure 24–4).
12. Remove needle.
13. Connect 1-foot tubing to catheter.
14. Secure catheter with one hand, open stopcock to allow back-bleeding to fill 1-foot tubing and stopcock, and attach tubing from monitor/flush system to stopcock.
15. Turn stopcock off to patient and flush the air bubble that was captured when tubing and stopcock were connected out of the sideport of the stopcock.
16. Turn stopcock on to patient and flush 1-foot tubing and catheter, watching for air bubbles. (If you see an air bubble, stop flushing and aspirate it back to the stopcock so the patient will not receive an arterial air embolism.)
17. Suture in place as illustrated in Figure 24–5.
18. Apply Betadine ointment to site.
19. Apply dressing. (Do not tape completely around the wrist since this can have a tourniquet effect.)

Complications

- Ischemia
  - Hand
  - Skin over distal forearm
  - Systemic with prolonged fast flush
- Bleeding
- Infection
- Inadvertent intra-arterial drug injection
- Aneurysm

Pearls and Pitfalls

1. Use nondominant arm so an ischemic injury would be less devastating than if it occurred in the dominant extremity.
2. The Arrow Radial Artery Catheterization Set, which combines needle, catheter, and guide wire, probably yields a higher success rate, especially for the beginner, than the catheter-over-needle alone.
3. The technique for cannulation of the dorsalis pedis or temporal artery is essentially the same as that described for percutaneous radial artery cannulation except for the obvious differences in positioning.
4. A simple device to give continuous monitoring of mean arterial pressure from an arterial catheter can be rapidly assembled from materials readily available in any emergency department. This device can be quite useful when electronic monitoring equipment is not immediately available or not convenient (helicopters, transport within the hospital, field conditions [I used this device to monitor a critically ill elephant at the local zoo]). Necessary equipment includes the pressure gauge from a blood pressure cuff, a length of oxygen tubing, and a three-way stopcock that can have all ports open

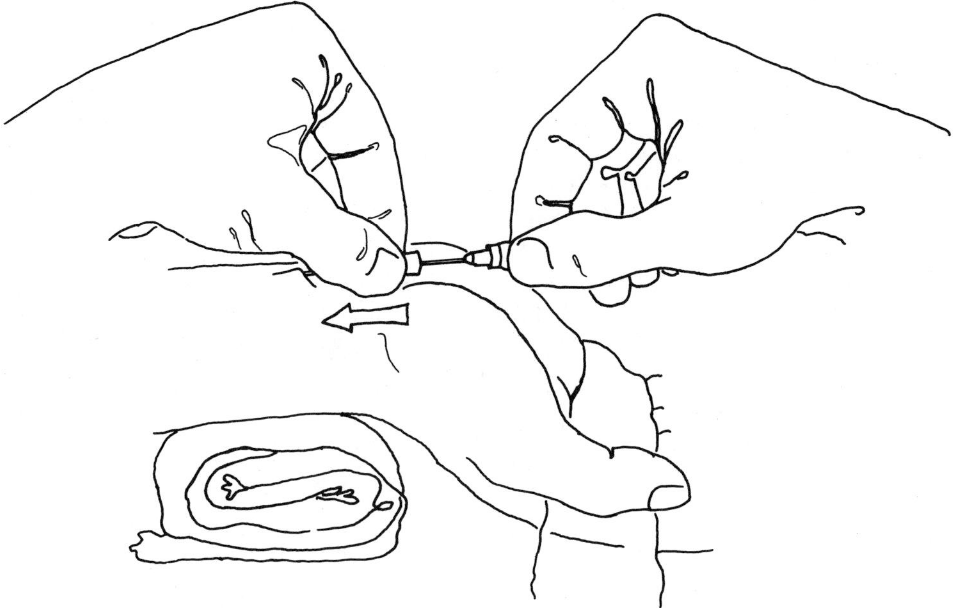

FIGURE 24–4. Percutaneous radial artery cannulation.

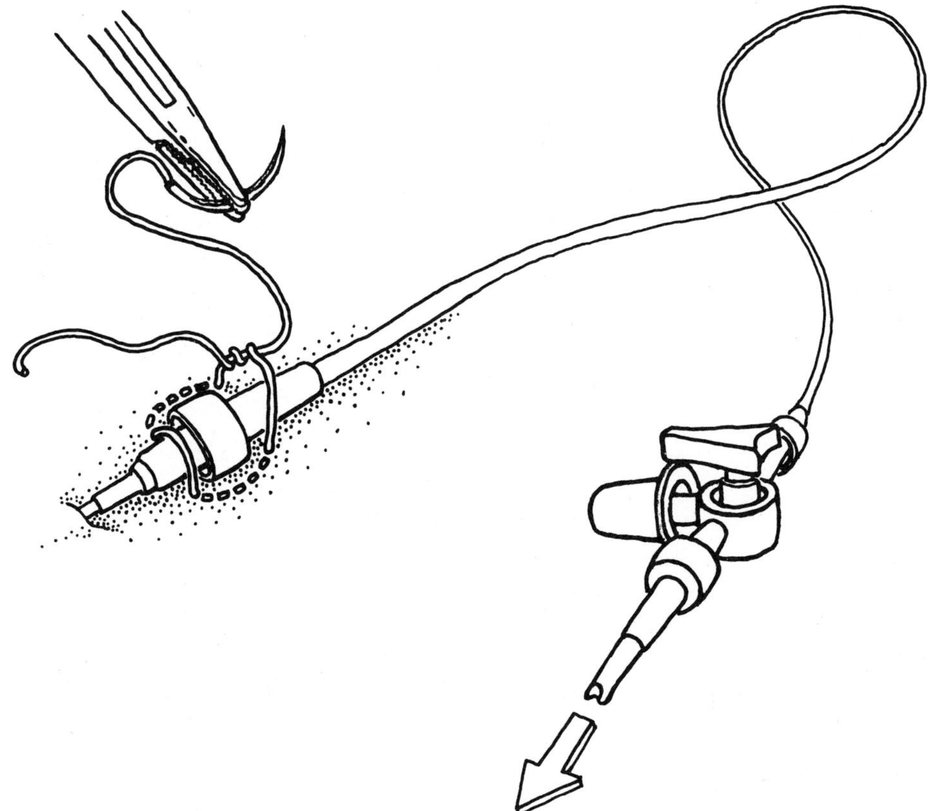

FIGURE 24–5. Securing an arterial catheter.

simultaneously. Figure 24–6 illustrates the configuration of this device. To construct this monitor:

a. Attach one end of the oxygen tubing to the pressure gauge and the other end to the top port of the three-way stopcock.
b. Turn the stopcock off to the patient and use the fast flush to fill two thirds of the tubing with saline.
c. Remove any air bubbles in the saline column by holding the tubing vertical with the pressure gauge up and tapping the tubing until the bubble rises to the top. Do not let any saline enter the pressure gauge.
d. Turn the stopcock so all ports are in the open position. The pressure gauge then displays mean arterial pressure, which can be used as a patient monitor or endpoint for vasoactive drug titration.

References

Extensive experience.

Slogoff S, Keats AS, Arlund C: On the safety of radial artery cannulation. Anesthesiology 59:42–47, 1983.

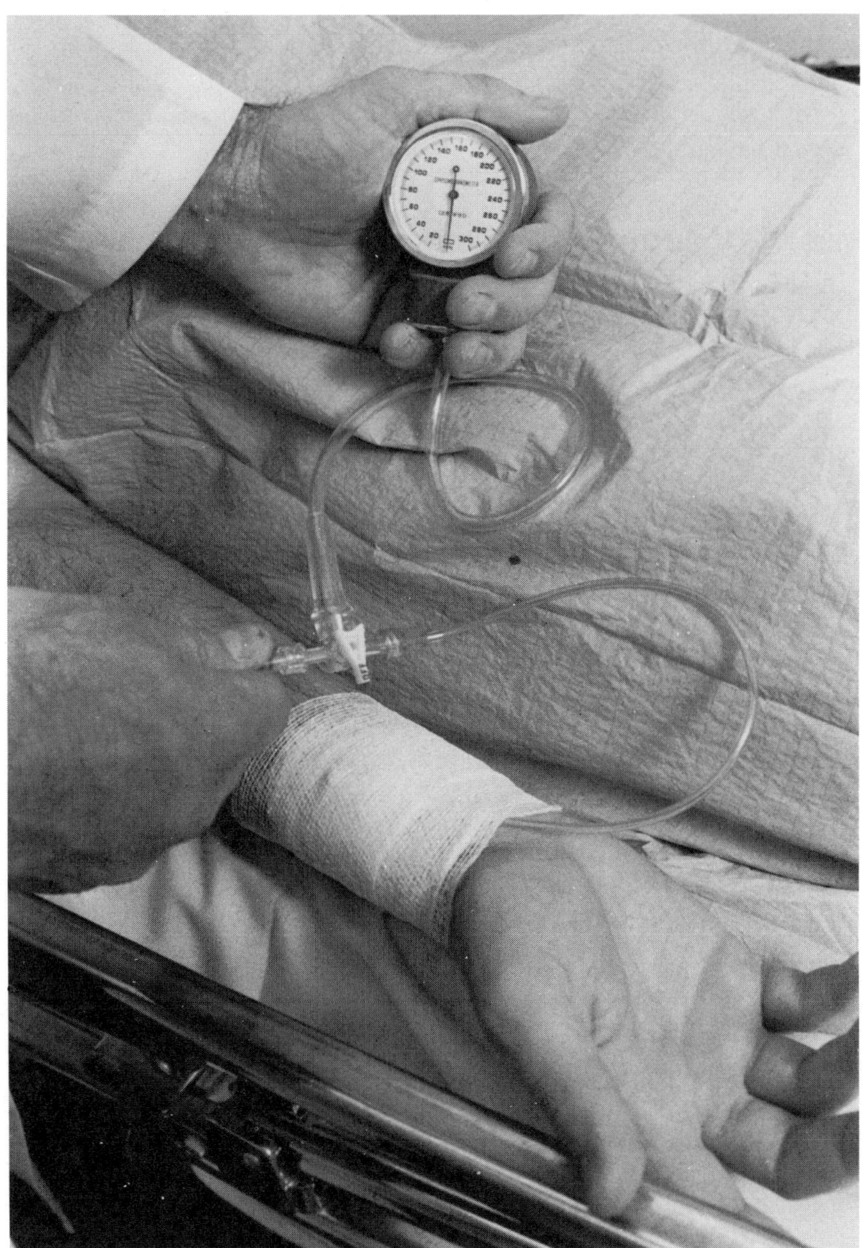

FIGURE 24–6. A simple mean arterial pressure monitor.

RADIAL ARTERY CUTDOWN

MICHAEL S. JASTREMSKI, MD

Equipment

Same as needed for percutaneous radial artery cannulation plus:

Scalpel with No. 15 blade	Two straight hemostats
Two curved mosquito clamps	4-0 silk ties

Universal Precautions

1. Wear mask, gown, and sterile gloves.
2. Use an eye shield.

Technique

1. If patient status and circumstances allow, explain the procedure to the patient and obtain consent.
2. Position patient's wrist on short armboard, palmar side up, in 60-degree extension (Figure 24–7).
3. Put on cap, mask, eye shield, gown, and sterile gloves.
4. Prep site with Betadine.
5. Drape the area.
6. Ready nylon sutures in needle holder, silk tie on hemostat (if you fold the tie in half and pass it around the artery at the bend, it can then be cut at the bend to produce the two ties needed, thus saving having to pass a second tie) and three-way stopcock on 1-foot tubing (stopcock on end opposite catheter, which is female end of tubing).
7. Stand facing the patient's arm and off to one side (so blood will not spurt on your clothes) such that your dominant hand is distal in relation to the patient's arm. Attempt to palpate the radial artery at the head of the radius; if you can feel a pulse, first attempt percutaneous cannulation.
8. The cutdown incision will be made perpendicular to the radial artery at the level of the radial styloid extending just to the radial side of the flexor carpi radialis tendon. Infiltrate the incision site and deeper tissues with 1% lidocaine (see Figure 24–7).
9. With the scalpel, make the initial incision through the *skin only,* avoiding any visible veins.
10. Spread the subcutaneous tissue in a plane parallel to the radial artery (perpendicular to the incision) with the curved mosquito forceps until the radial artery is exposed. Note the radial artery is approximately 0.5 cm in diameter, thick walled compared with the darker-colored vein usually found next to it, and *under* a fairly dense layer of fascia. There is often a much smaller branch artery found between the skin and fascia that can fool the unwary (Figure 24–8).
11. After the radial artery is located, gently use the mosquito clamp to dissect around a 1-cm length of the artery.

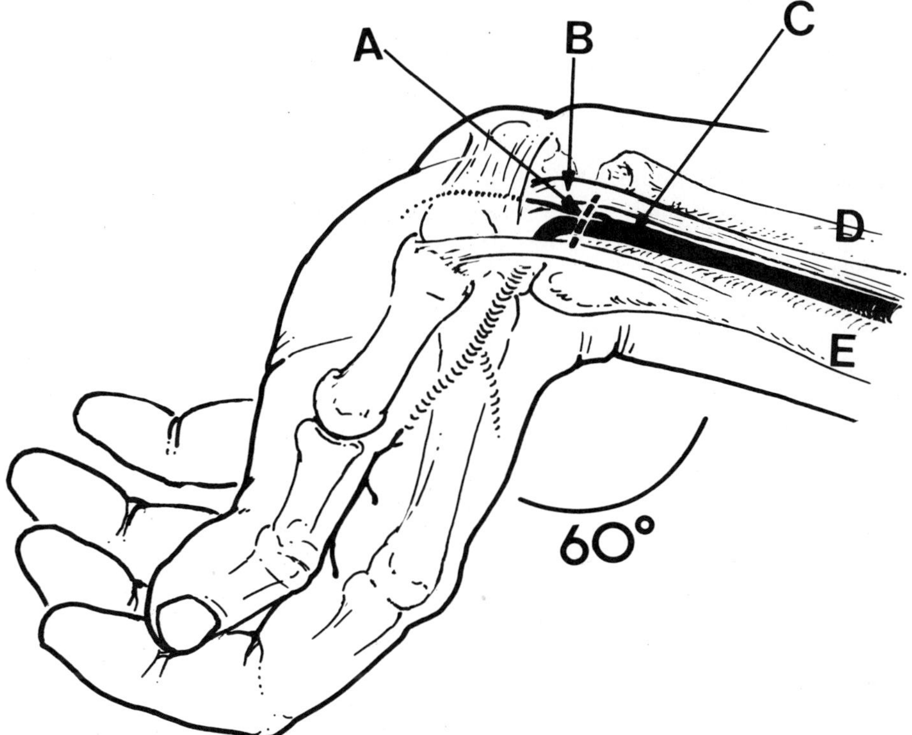

FIGURE 24–7. *A,* Incision; *B,* flexor carpi radialis tendon; *C,* radial artery; *D,* ulna; *E,* radius.

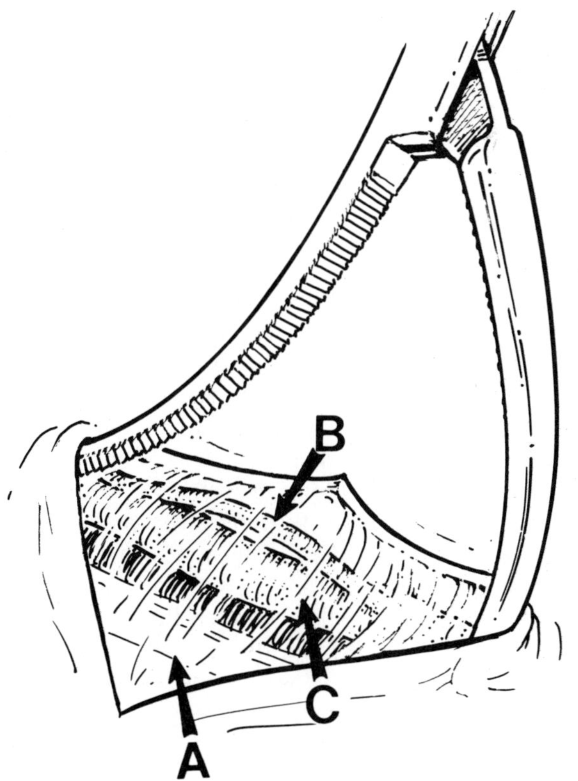

FIGURE 24–8. *A,* Fascia; *B,* superficial branch artery; *C,* radial artery.

12. Pass the doubled-over single tie around the artery and then cut it at the loop to produce two ties: one each for proximal and distal control. *Do not* tie the ties since they will not be left in place.
13. Use gentle traction on the distal tie to simultaneously lift the artery out of the incision and straighten it.
14. Holding the catheter-over-needle unit in your dominant hand, with it aligned at a 5-degree angle to the artery, cannulate the artery under direct vision at the point where it is being lifted and straightened by the distal tie (Figure 24–9).
15. As soon as blood flashes back, advance the catheter over the needle without moving the needle.
16. Remove the needle.
17. Secure the catheter with one hand, connect 1-foot tubing to the catheter, open stopcock to allow back-bleeding to fill 1-foot tubing and stopcock, and then attach tubing from monitor/flush system to stopcock.
18. Turn stopcock off to patient and flush the air bubble that was captured when tubing and stopcock were connected out of the sideport of the stopcock.
19. Turn stopcock on to patient and flush 1-foot tubing and catheter, watching for air bubbles. (If you see an air bubble, stop flushing and aspirate it back to the stopcock so the patient will not receive an arterial air embolism.)
20. Suture catheter in place as shown in Figure 24–5.
21. Remove ties and suture skin incision with 4-0 nylon suture.
22. Apply Betadine ointment to site.
23. Apply dressing.

Complications

The complications are the same as those for percutaneous cannulation, with hemorrhage more likely.

Pearls and Pitfalls

1. Do not be fooled by the small branch artery that supplies the dorsal surface of the forearm that may be encountered between the skin and fascia. The radial artery is *under* the fascia, deeper than the top of the radius.
2. It is not necessary to incise or tie off the artery. This technique is essentially percutaneous cannulation under direct vision.
3. If the field is obscured by bleeding (usually venous), temporary hemostasis can be achieved by inflating a blood pressure cuff on the arm to greater than arterial pressure. Just remember to deflate the cuff when you cannulate the artery or there will not be a blood return. Closure of the skin incision will provide permanent hemostasis.
4. As an alternative to inserting the catheter through the incision, it may be inserted through intact skin 0.5 cm distal to the incision and then inserted into the radial artery under direct vision, as described above. This approach allows better approximation of the skin edges and thus better hemostasis and may reduce the incidence of localized wound infections.

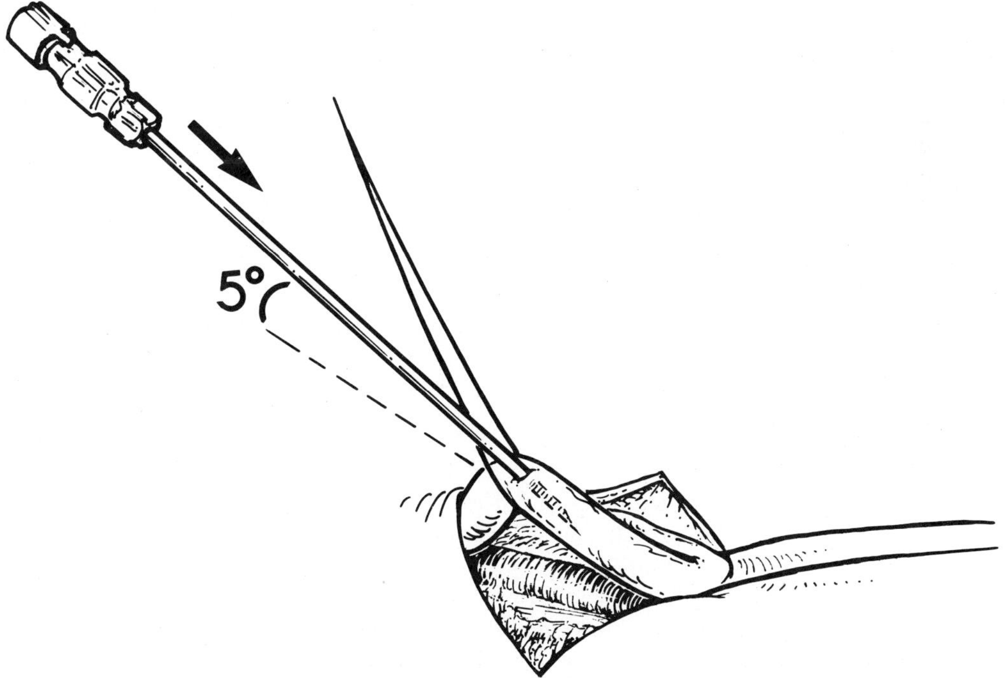

FIGURE 24–9. Cannulating the radial artery.

PERCUTANEOUS FEMORAL ARTERY CANNULATION

JONATHAN WARREN, MD

Equipment

Cap, mask, gown, and eye shield
Sterile gloves
Sterile drapes
Betadine skin prep
1-foot pressure tubing
Three-way stopcock
Needle holder
Suture scissors
3-0 nylon suture on curved needle
3-ml syringe with 25-gauge, 1½-inch needle
1% lidocaine *without* epinephrine
20-gauge, 2½-inch thin-walled needle
0.025-inch diameter (40 cm) guide wire
20-gauge internal diameter (12 cm) polyethylene catheter
Betadine ointment
Pressure monitor/flush system
Sterile 4 × 4-inch gauze pads
Tape

Universal Precautions

1. Wear mask, gown, and sterile gloves.
2. Use an eye shield.

Technique

1. If patient status and circumstances allow, explain the procedure to the patient and obtain informed consent.
2. Position the patient supine and flat in bed, with knees slightly apart. Stand on the side of the patient you will cannulate.
3. Shave patient's groin area.
4. Put on cap, mask, eye shield, gown, and sterile gloves.
5. Prep the patient's groin and immediate surrounding area with Betadine.
6. Drape the area.
7. Attach the three-way stopcock to the 1-foot pressure tubing on the end opposite the attachment to the catheter. Close the stopcock to its sideport. Attach the suture to the needle holder. Check to ensure that the guide wire fits through the needle and the catheter fits over the guide wire. Ensure that all these items are within reach on a sterile surface.
8. Draw up the 1% lidocaine into the 3-ml syringe with the 25-gauge needle.
9. Palpate the femoral artery just inferior to the inguinal ligament.
10. Infiltrate the skin over this area with 1% lidocaine.
11. Hold the 20-gauge needle with your dominant hand at a 15-degree angle from the midline and at a 45-degree elevation. Palpate the femoral artery with your other hand. Position the needle tip over the artery just inferior to the inguinal ligament (Figure 24–10). Enter the skin over the artery and advance the needle toward the pulse.

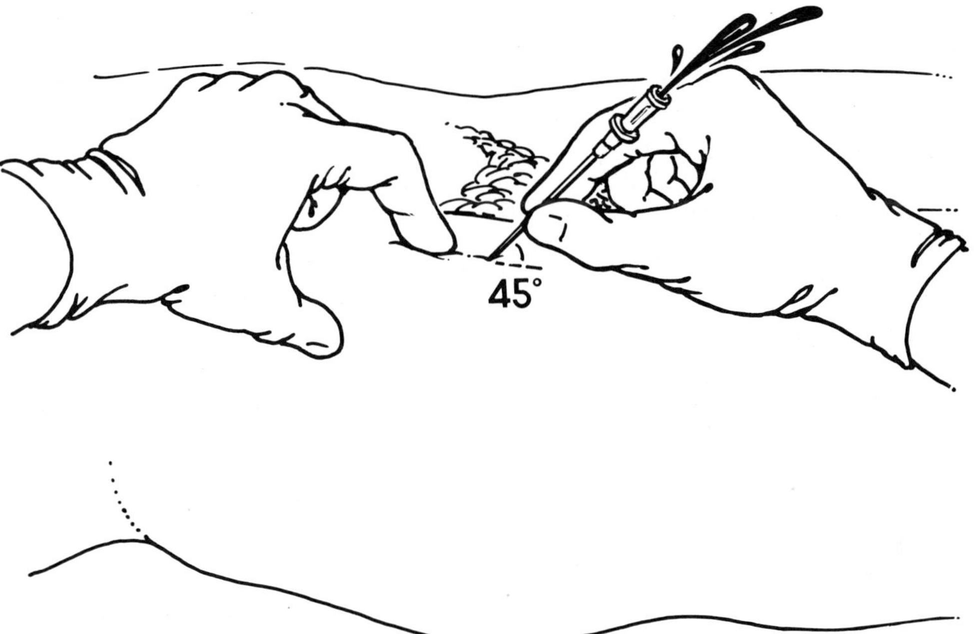

FIGURE 24–10. Femoral artery cannulation.

12. When blood pulses from the hub of the needle, pick up the guide wire with your palpating hand and pass the guide wire through the needle into the femoral artery. Continue to pass the guide wire until one half of its length is within the artery.
13. Remove the needle over the guide wire.
14. Pass the polyethylene catheter over the guide wire and through the skin into the femoral artery. The catheter should be advanced as far as possible.
15. Remove the guide wire while firmly stabilizing the catheter. Blood should flow freely from the catheter.
16. Attach the 1-foot tubing to the catheter at the end opposite the stopcock, and allow back-bleeding to fill both tubing and stopcock. Then attach the stopcock to a monitor/flush system.
17. Close the stopcock to the patient and flush to remove any air bubbles from the flush tubing and stopcock.
18. Turn the stopcock to connect patient to flush, and flush to clear blood from the 1-foot tubing, watching for air bubbles. (If you see any air bubbles, stop flushing and aspirate the system with syringe until all air is removed.)
19. Suture the catheter to the skin of the upper thigh (see Figure 24–5).
20. Apply Betadine ointment to puncture and suture sites.
21. Apply a sterile dressing.

Complications

Ischemia of leg
Thrombosis (arterial or venous)
Embolism of thrombus
Bleeding
Peripheral neuropathy (accidental puncture of femoral nerve)
Air embolism
Infection
Puncture of an abdominal organ

Pearls and Pitfalls

1. The femoral insertion site has the same number of infectious complications as other insertion sites, provided adequate site care can be provided. Patients with frequent diarrhea, with urinary incontinence, or who have central obesity with a large abdominal panniculus may not be suitable candidates for the use of this insertion site.
2. The appearance of small cutaneous infarctions of the distal lower extremity on the side of the arterial catheter suggests a thromboembolic source, which could be the arterial catheter. One should consider removing the catheter under these circumstances.
3. The Cook 4 F single-lumen central venous catheter set is ideally suited for femoral arterial access. It contains the proper size and type of needle, guide wire, and catheter in one sterile container.

References

Kaye W: Venous and arterial catheterization. In Sprung CL, Grenvik A (eds): Invasive Procedures in Critical Care, pp 1–48. New York, Churchill Livingstone, 1985.
Norwood SH, et al: Prospective study of catheter-related infection during prolonged arterial catheterization. Crit Care Med 16:836–839, 1988.
Puri VK, et al: Complications of vascular catheterization in the critically ill. Crit Care Med 8:495–499, 1980.
Thomas F, et al: The risk of infection related to radial vs. femoral sites for arterial catheterization. Crit Care Med 11:807–812, 1983.

PERCUTANEOUS AXILLARY ARTERY CANNULATION

JONATHAN WARREN, MD

Equipment

Cap, mask, gown, and eye shield
Sterile gloves
Sterile drapes
Betadine skin prep
1-foot pressure tubing
Three-way stopcock
Needle holder
3-0 nylon suture on curved needle
3-ml syringe
25-gauge, 1½-inch needle
1% lidocaine *without* epinephrine
20-gauge, 2½-inch thin-walled needle
0.025-inch diameter (40 cm) guide wire
20-gauge internal diameter (12 cm) polyethylene catheter
Betadine ointment
Suture scissors
Pressure monitor/flush system
Sterile 4 × 4-inch gauze pads
Tape

Universal Precautions

1. Wear cap, mask, gown, and sterile gloves.
2. Use an eye shield.

Technique

1. If patient status and circumstances allow, explain the procedure to the patient and obtain informed consent.
2. Position the patient supine with the arm to be catheterized in 120-degree abduction at the shoulder, with the elbow flexed (Figure 24–11).
3. Shave the patient's axilla.
4. Put on cap, mask, eye shield, gown, and sterile gloves.
5. Prep the patient's axilla and immediate surrounding area with Betadine.
6. Drape the area.
7. Attach the three-way stopcock to the 1-foot tubing at the end opposite the attachment to the catheter and close the stopcock to its sideport. Attach the suture to the needle holder and check to ensure that the guide wire fits through the needle and the catheter fits over the guide wire. Ensure that all these items are within reach on a sterile surface.
8. Draw up the 1% lidocaine into the 3-ml syringe with the 25-gauge needle.
9. Stand in between the patient and the abducted arm, facing the axilla.
10. Palpate the axillary artery against the humerus as high into the axilla as possible.
11. Infiltrate the skin over this area with 1% lidocaine.
12. Hold the 20-gauge needle in your dominant hand at a 45-degree angle to the skin of the upper arm. Palpate the artery using your opposite hand. Position the needle tip such that the artery is directly between the needle tip and the humerus. Enter the skin over the artery and advance the needle toward the pulse (Figure 24–12).
13. When blood pulses from the hub of the needle, pick up the guide wire with the palpating hand and pass the guide wire through the needle into the

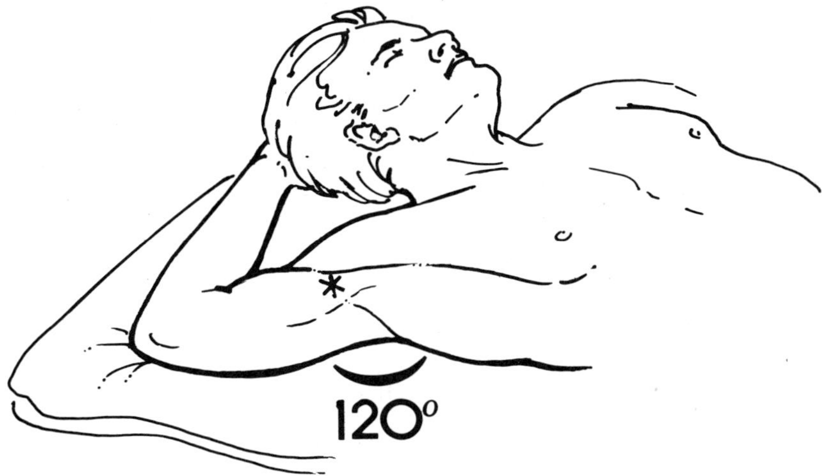

FIGURE 24–11. Position for axillary artery cannulation.

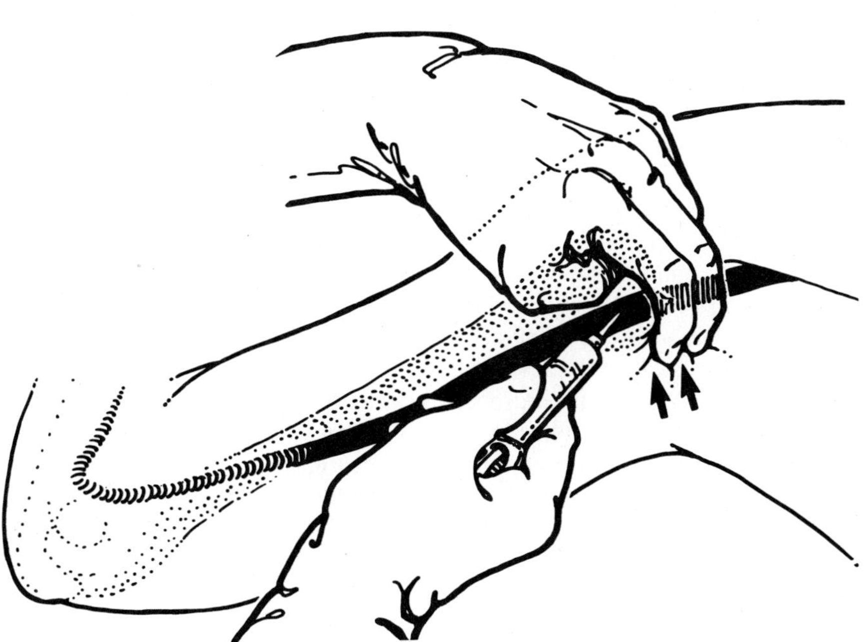

FIGURE 24–12. Axillary artery cannulation.

axillary artery. If passage of the guide wire is difficult, angle the needle slightly closer to the arm. Continue to pass the guide wire until one half of its length is within the artery.

14. Remove the needle over the guide wire.
15. Pass the polyethylene catheter over the guide wire and through the skin into the artery. The catheter should be advanced as far as possible.
16. Remove the guide wire. Blood should flow freely from the catheter.
17. Attach the 1-foot tubing to the catheter at the end opposite the stopcock, and allow back-bleeding to fill both tubing and stopcock. Then attach the stopcock to a monitor/flush system.
18. Close the stopcock to the patient and flush to remove any air bubbles.
19. Turn the stopcock to connect patient to flush, and flush to clear blood from the stopcock and 1-foot tubing, watching for air bubbles. (If you see any air bubbles, stop flushing and aspirate the system with a syringe until all air is removed.)
20. Suture the catheter to the skin of the upper arm, not the chest wall (see Figure 24–5).
21. Apply Betadine ointment to puncture and suture sites.
22. Apply a sterile dressing.

Complications

Ischemia of arm
Thrombosis
Bleeding
Peripheral neuropathy (bleeding into axillary sheath)
Cerebral embolism (air or thrombotic)
Infection

Pearls and Pitfalls

1. The catheter should be placed as high in the axilla as possible, to ensure placement in the axillary artery rather than the brachial artery. Since the latter is an end-artery, thrombosis carries a greater morbidity. Collateral circulation provides adequate blood flow to the distal circulation in the event of thrombosis of the axillary artery.
2. Use the left axilla whenever possible. Air accidentally injected into the catheter is less likely to cause cerebral air embolism, since the left axillary artery is downstream from the carotid arteries.
3. The Cook 4 F single-lumen central venous catheter set is ideally suited for axillary arterial access. It contains the proper size and type of needle, guide wire, and catheter in one sterile container.

References

Bryan-Brown, CW, Kwun KB, Lumb PD, et al: The axillary artery catheter. Heart Lung 12:492, 1983.
De Angelis J: Axillary arterial monitoring. Crit Care Med 4:205, 1976.
Sladen A: Complications of invasive hemodynamic monitoring in the intensive care unit. Curr Probl Surg 25(2):69–145, 1988.

Femoral Vein Catheterization

THOMAS TERNDRUP, MD

Indications

Central intravenous access

The femoral vein is a safe and rapidly accessible, but often underused, vessel for intravenous access. It is the preferred intravenous access method in unstable infants. The femoral vein may be the only possible route for large-bore venous cannulation in patients without available veins, such as intravenous drug abusers, those with a history of previous peripheral vein cutdowns, or patients without available veins with no apparent peripheral venous access sites. The femoral vein allows direct access to the central circulation and is one possible route for passage of pressure monitoring catheters and temporary transvenous pacers.

Contraindications

Coagulopathy (relative—must balance risk against need for central intravenous access)
Venous thrombosis of leg
Ischemia of leg
Localized infection at site

Equipment

Betadine
Sterile towels
4 × 4-inch gauze pads
1% lidocaine
10- and 20-ml syringes
25-gauge, 1-inch needle
20-gauge, 1½-inch needle
18-gauge, 2½-inch thin wall catheter over needle
Three-way stopcock
Suture scissors
Intravenous tubing and solution
Guide wire—0.035-inch diameter × 25–30-inch length
Single- or triple-lumen catheter
Heparin flush
3-0 nylon suture on curved needle
No. 11 blade
Vein dilator
Mask
1-foot extension tubing
Sterile gown and gloves
Cap, mask, and eye shield

Universal Precautions

1. Wear mask and sterile gown and gloves.
2. Use an eye shield.

Technique

1. If patient status and circumstances allow, explain the procedure to the patient and obtain consent.
2. Place the patient's leg on the chosen side in slight external rotation at the hip.
3. Put on cap, mask, eye shield, gown, and sterile gloves.
4. Prep the patient's groin with Betadine and drape.
5. Stand on the chosen side of the patient between the hip and knee of the patient's leg. In patients with a pulse, locate the femoral arterial pulsation about 2 cm below the inguinal ligament. The femoral vein is located approximately 1 cm medial to the femoral arterial pulsation. In patients who are pulseless, the femoral vein can be located by placing the fifth finger on the pubic symphysis and the thumb on the anterior-superior iliac spine and flexing the middle finger toward the patient's foot. The femoral vein runs under the middle finger. The skin puncture should occur 2 cm inferior to the inguinal ligament (Figure 24–13).
6. Anesthetize the skin and subcutaneous tissues with 1% lidocaine administered through a 25-gauge needle.
7. After the vein is located, a short, small-diameter catheter-over-needle device, attached to a syringe, is inserted with the needle oriented cephalad, at 45 degrees to the skin and with constant suction (Figure 24–13). As the vein is entered and blood returns, reduce the angle to the skin to about 15 degrees, and advance the needle and catheter 1 to 2 mm. The catheter is then advanced over the needle, the needle removed, and the catheter aspirated to confirm intravenous placement.
8. If a longer central-line or large-bore catheter introducer is to be placed, do the following:
   a. Pass the guide wire through the initial short catheter (Figure 24–14).
   b. Remove the short catheter, being careful not to remove the guide wire.
   c. Pass the vein dilator over the guide wire to create a tract.
   d. Remove the vein dilator, being careful not to remove the guide wire.

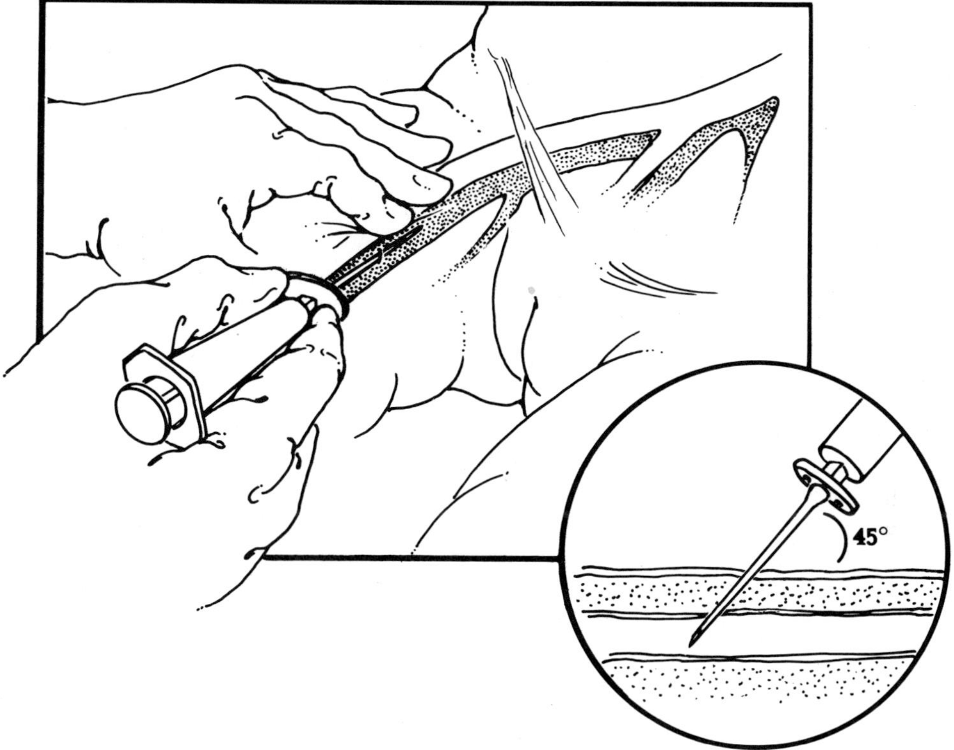

FIGURE 24–13. Femoral vein cannulation: Step 1.

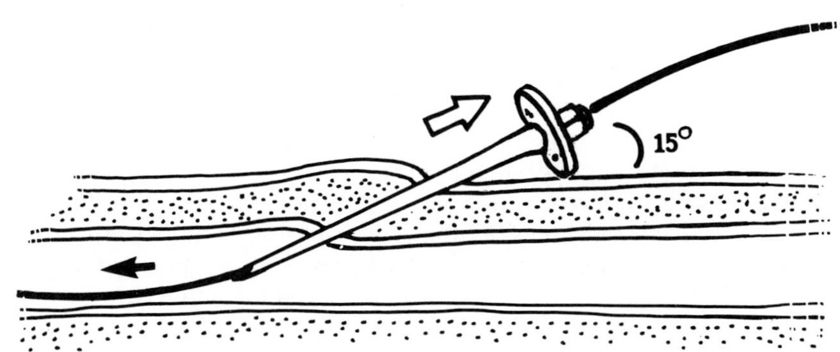

FIGURE 24–14. Femoral vein cannulation: Step 2.

e. Insert the long catheter or introducer over the guide wire (*Note:* the dilator needs to be inside an introducer during this step) (Figure 24–15).
f. Remove the guide wire (Figure 24–16).
g. Aspirate blood to ensure proper position.

If using a triple-lumen catheter, the two proximal ports should be flushed with heparin solution (1 unit/ml) and capped before the catheter is inserted.

---

9. Attach the 1-foot extension tubing to the catheter, the three-way stopcock to the extension tubing, and the intravenous tubing to the stopcock.
10. Stabilization of the catheter is best performed by suturing the hub of the catheter to the skin (Figure 24–5).
11. Apply a dab of Betadine ointment over the skin puncture site.
12. Cover the site with a sterile dressing (I use Tegoderm).

Complications

Femoral arterial puncture and bleeding
Injury to the femoral nerve
Retroperitoneal bleeding (if the external iliac is punctured)
Potential for bladder or bowel injury (with an inappropriately placed needle)
Thrombophlebitis and thromboembolic disease (high incidence with large catheters)
Infection

Pearls and Pitfalls

1. The femoral vein is one of the largest and most accessible sites for quick, large-bore intravenous access in all age groups.
2. Previous concerns over septic hip complications in infants are distinctly unusual.
3. Placement of the catheter is facilitated by having a cooperative patient.
4. As always, careful asepsis is required, and when any violation occurs, sites of alternative intravenous access should be pursued and the femoral line removed as soon thereafter as possible.
5. Transvenous pacers usually pass readily to the apex of the right ventricle when inserted through the femoral vein. Unfortunately, so do Swan-Ganz catheters, so it is often very difficult to pass a Swan-Ganz catheter out of the right ventricle into the pulmonary artery when coming from the femoral vein.

Reference

Swanson RS, Uhlig PN, Gross PL, et al: Emergency intravenous access through the femoral vein. Ann Emerg Med 244:51, 1984.

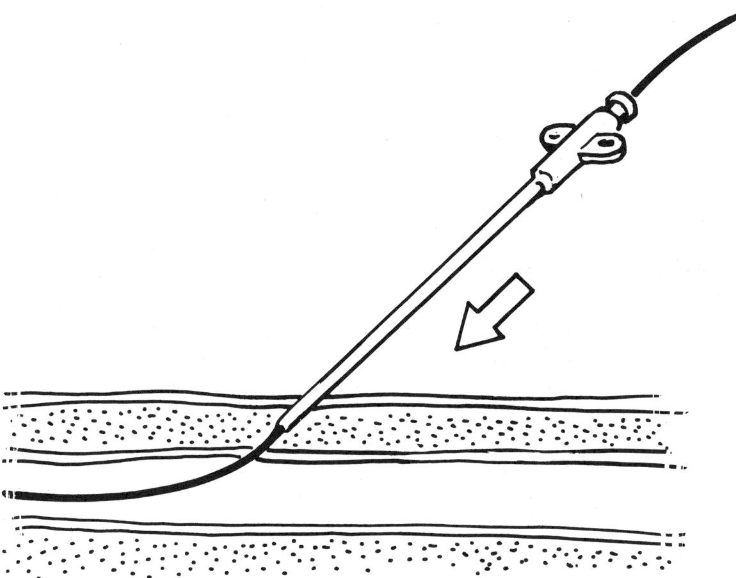

FIGURE 24–15. Femoral vein cannulation: Step 3.

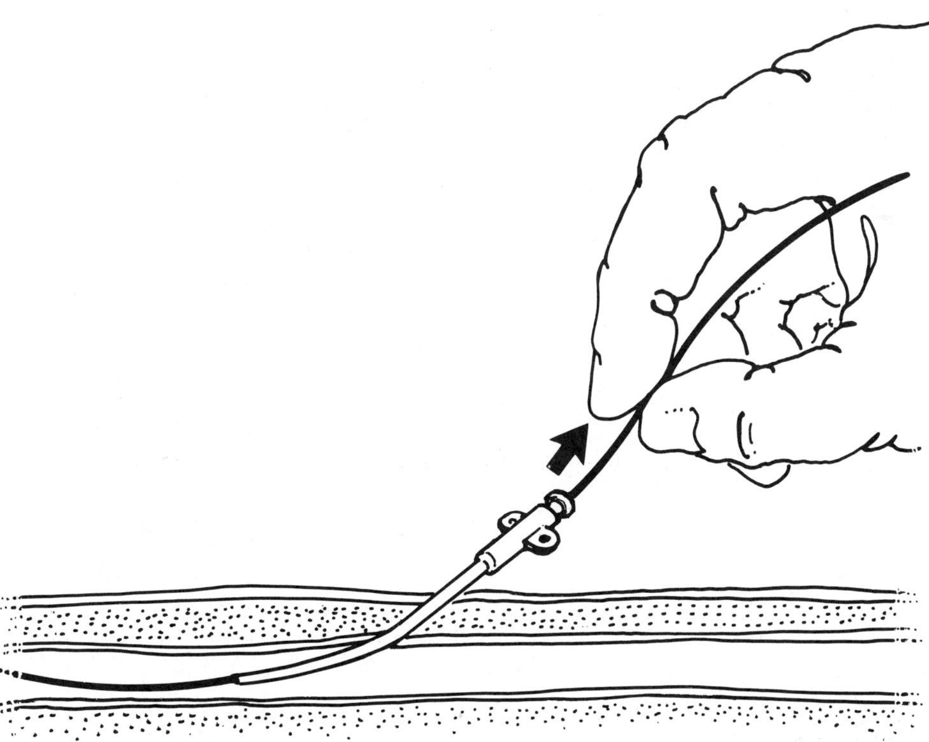

FIGURE 24–16. Femoral vein cannulation: Step 4.

Internal Jugular Vein Catheterization

PETER MARIANI, MD

Indications

Central delivery of cardiac arrest medications

Central venous pressure monitoring

Introduction of Swan-Ganz catheter or transvenous pacer

Introduction of multiple-lumen catheter for delivery of incompatible medication drips, medications whose peripheral administration is contraindicated, or hyperalimentation

Large-bore intravenous volume resuscitation in absence of peripheral access

Need for rapid vascular access (for any reason) where peripheral access is lacking and/or other central routes are unavailable or contraindicated

Contraindications

Absolute

Massive soft tissue neck trauma

Significant anatomic distortion of any etiology

Overlying cellulitis

Patients with cervical collar that cannot be temporarily removed

Relative

Overlying burn

Carotid atherosclerosis (plaque embolization may result with inadvertent arterial puncture)

Patient taking anticoagulants or with coagulopathy

Patient may be candidate for thrombolytic therapy (beware the contraindications contained in your own institutional policy!)

Equipment

Self-contained kits are ideal. In the absence of a kit the following equipment is needed:

- Drapes
- Mask, gown, eye shield, and sterile gloves
- Betadine antiseptic solution
- 1% lidocaine
- Syringes
- 25- to 27-gauge, 1¼-inch anesthetic needle
- Venipuncture needle accepting guide wire
- J-shaped guide wire and wire introducer
- Catheter/introducer unit
- No. 11 scalpel
- Hemostat
- Suture scissors
- 3-0 nylon suture on straight needle
- Antibiotic ointment
- Clear plastic dressing

Universal Precautions

1. Wear gown, mask, and sterile gloves.
2. Use an eye shield.

Technique

Posterior Approach

1. Prior to its undertaking, briefly explain the procedure to the alert patient and, if time permits, obtain formal written consent.
2. Be sure that nurses will have an intravenous line ready for you to connect at the procedure's end.
3. Assume a position at the head of the bed on the side of the patient you wish to cannulate. Place the patient in the Trendelenburg position with the head rotated approximately 45 degrees away from the planned side of venipuncture.
4. If time permits, prep and drape the venipuncture area in a sterile manner. Include the sternal notch, since this needs to be palpated during the procedure.

5. In the conscious patient, infiltrate the skin with anesthetic at a site just posterior to the posterior belly of the sternocleidomastoid muscle, between one third and one half of the way up from the clavicle to the mastoid (Figure 24–17). Deposit 1 to 2 ml of anesthetic subcutaneously toward the sternal notch, along the subsequent path of the venipuncture needle. Aspirate the needle on advancement to avoid intravenous injection.
6. After repalpating the location of the sternal notch, grasp the sternocleidomastoid muscle between the thumb and index finger of your nondominant hand, lightly retracting the muscle upward (Figure 24–18). (Simultaneous middle finger palpation of the sternal notch may be maintained by operators with sufficiently large hands.)
7. Introduce and advance the venipuncture needle under the belly of the sternocleidomastoid muscle toward the sternal notch, aspirating the needle on the way (Figure 24–18).
8. On vessel entry, stabilize the needle, disconnect the syringe, and introduce and advance the guide wire 10 to 15 cm.

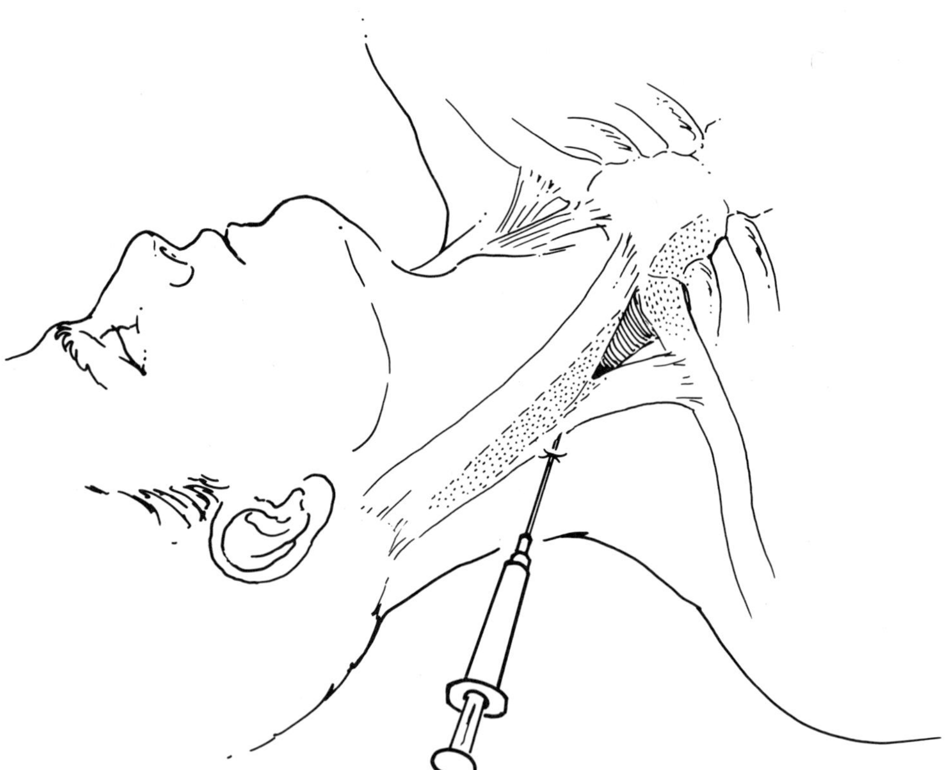

FIGURE 24–17. Internal jugular catheterization: Posterior approach.

9. Slide the needle off the wire and incise the skin around the wire to accommodate the diameter of the catheter.
10. Thread the catheter-introducer unit over the wire to the skin surface. Retract the wire as needed until a graspable length of wire protrudes through the hub of the unit.
11. Advance the unit over the wire into the central circulation with a twisting motion about its long axis, making sure that the end of the wire is well within grasp.
12. Remove the wire and introducer in toto, immediately covering the exposed catheter hub with the gloved thumb. Intraluminal location is confirmed by a nonpulsatile backflow of dark blood.
13. Obtain blood specimens and/or connect the intravenous tubing to the catheter.
14. Anesthetize as needed an area of skin adjacent to the catheter hub.
15. Place a suture through this area, knot it, and then secure it to the hub.

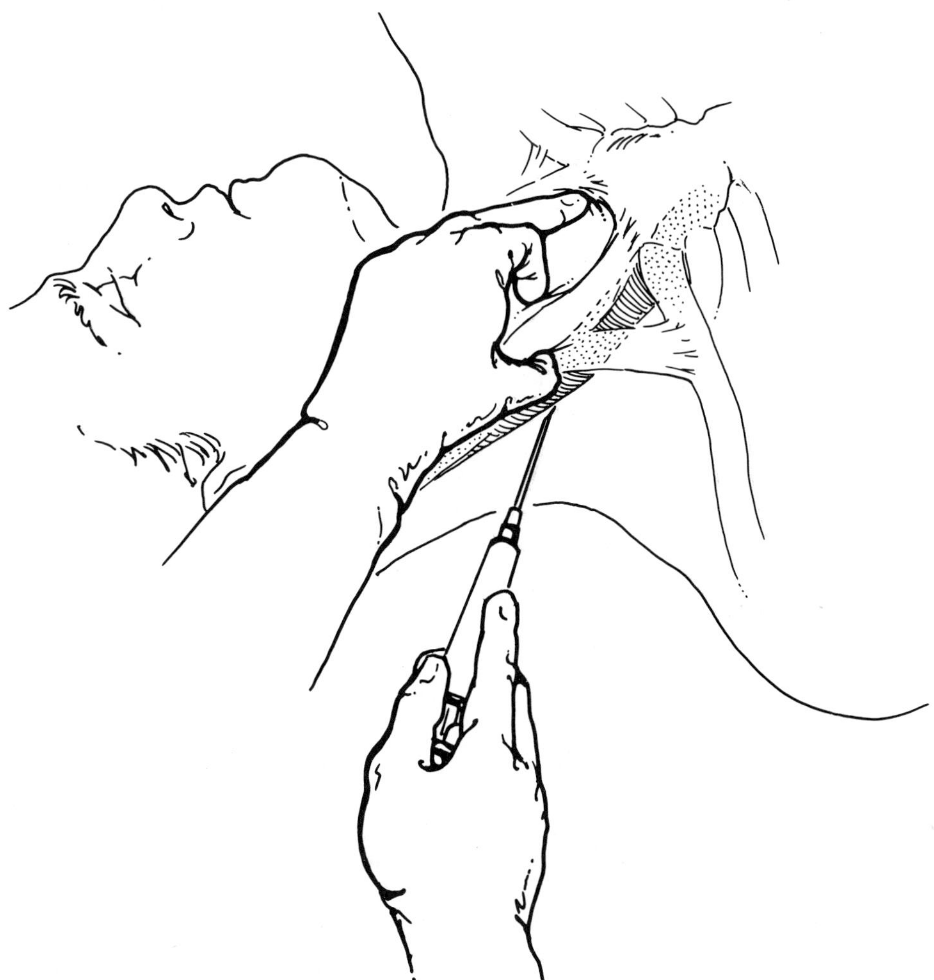

FIGURE 24–18. Internal jugular catheterization: Posterior approach.

16. After application of antibiotic ointment to the puncture site, apply a clear plastic dressing over the area, arranging for the intravenous tubing to loop around the patient's ear (Figure 24–19).
17. Obtain and examine a chest x-ray film to rule out pneumothorax and, if it is radiopaque, to confirm catheter position.

Supraclavicular Approach

1. Prior to its undertaking, briefly explain the procedure to the alert patient and, if time permits, obtain formal written consent.
2. Be sure that nurses will have an intravenous line ready for you to connect at the procedure's end.
3. Assume a position at the head of the bed on the side of the patient you wish to cannulate. Place the patient in the Trendelenburg position with the head rotated approximately 45 degrees away from the planned side of venipuncture.
4. If time permits, prep and drape the venipuncture area in a sterile manner.
5. Locate the triangle formed by the clavicle and the clavicular and sternal heads of the sternocleidomastoid muscle (Figure 24–20).
6. Infiltrate skin and subcutaneous tissue with a local anesthetic using a 5-ml syringe and 25-gauge, 1-inch needle, inserting the needle at the apex of the triangle and advancing it toward the patient's sternum.
7. Introduce the venipuncture needle on a 10-ml syringe at the apex of the triangle and advance it caudally at a 30-degree angle in the sagittal plane. Maintain negative pressure in the syringe constantly while advancing the needle. Blood return indicates vessel entry (Figure 24–20).
8. On vessel entry, stabilize the needle, disconnect the syringe, and introduce and advance the guide wire 10 to 15 cm.
9. Slide the needle off the wire, and incise the skin around the wire to accommodate the diameter of the catheter.
10. Thread the catheter-introducer unit over the wire to the skin surface. Retract the wire as needed until a graspable length of wire protrudes through the hub of the unit.
11. Advance the unit over the wire into the central circulation with a twisting motion about its long axis, making sure that the end of the wire is well within grasp.
12. Remove the wire and introducer in toto, immediately covering the exposed catheter hub with the gloved thumb. Intraluminal location is confirmed by a nonpulsatile backflow of dark blood.
13. Obtain blood specimens and/or connect the intravenous tubing to the catheter.
14. Anesthetize as needed an area of skin adjacent to the catheter hub.
15. Place a suture through this area, knot it, and then secure it to the catheter hub.
16. After application of antibiotic ointment to the puncture site, apply a clear plastic dressing over the area, arranging for the intravenous tubing to loop around the patient's ear (Figure 24–19).
17. Obtain and examine a chest x-ray film to rule out pneumothorax and, if it is radiopaque, to confirm catheter position.

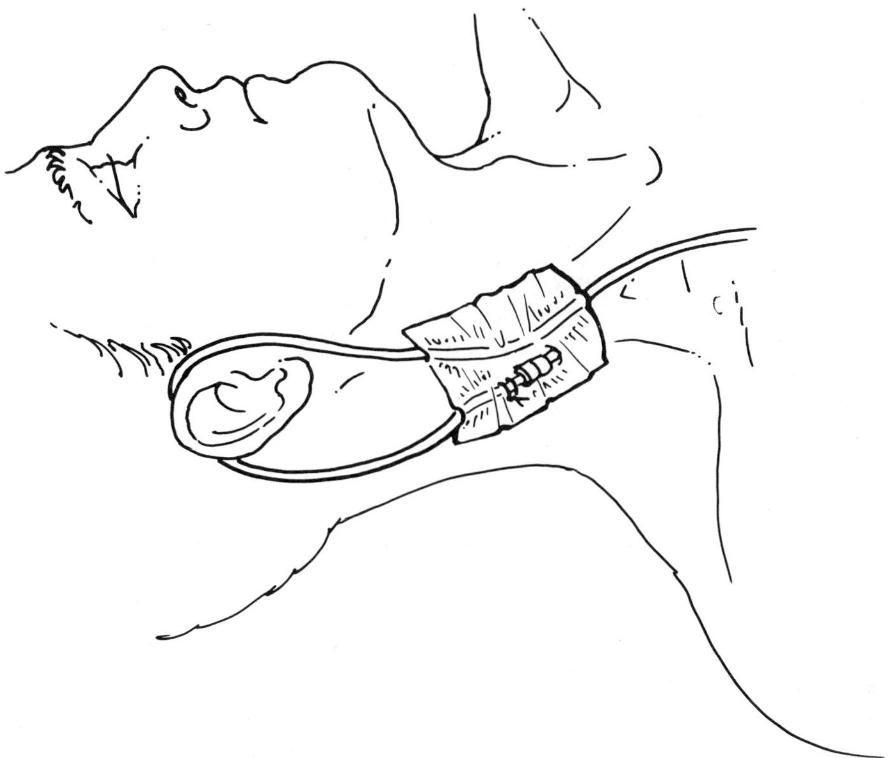

FIGURE 24–19. Securing an internal jugular catheter.

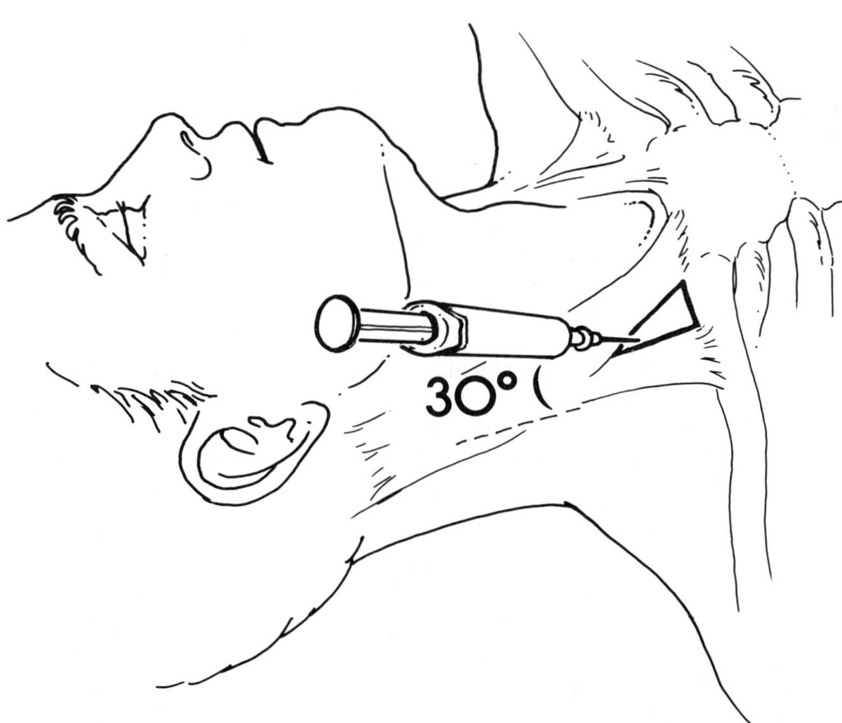

FIGURE 24–20. Internal jugular catheterization: Supraclavicular approach.

Complications

1. Pneumothorax. A finite number will occur despite the best of technique. Risk is, however, less with the internal jugular approach than with the subclavian approach. Always check with a postprocedure chest x-ray film.
2. Air embolism. Always quickly cover an exposed needle or catheter hub with the thumb. The Trendelenberg position will maximize the patient's central venous pressure and minimize the risk.
3. Vascular perforation. The infusion may be delivered into the pleural space, mediastinum, or pericardium. Results range from development of "pleural effusion" on chest x-ray film, to rapid clinical development of cardiac tamponade. To minimize risk:
   a. Favor catheter introducers that are not excessively stiff.
   b. Never thread an introducer over a guide wire that is insufficiently advanced into the central circulation.
   c. Never begin intravenous infusion unless good backflow of blood is obtained after catheter advancement and/or catheter position is confirmed on chest x-ray film.
4. Arterial puncture. Actually, the consequences are less risky than with the subclavian route since the internal jugular site is compressible. Should arterial puncture occur, compress the site for a minimum of 5 minutes.
5. Phrenic nerve injury. This can result from direct needle trauma or from compression by adjacent hematoma. Hypocoagulable patients are at increased theoretical risk of injury from a hematoma.
6. Guide wire embolization. Do not lose control of the protruding wire!
7. Dysrhythmias. These usually occur from guide wire irritation of the right atrium or ventricle and resolve when the guide wire is withdrawn.
8. Venous thrombosis, septic phlebitis, and thoracic duct injury. Should these problems manifest, they will do so long after the patient leaves the emergency department.

Pearls and Pitfalls

1. Always use the described guide wire (i.e., "Seldinger") technique in preference to those using large-bore needles and "through-the-needle" cannulas. Morbidity will be reduced when venipuncture is achieved with the narrowest needle possible.
2. Favor right-side access over left-side access since the course to the superior vena cava is more direct. It is also the more "natural" approach for right-handed operators.
3. When not using prefabricated kits, be sure prior to undertaking the procedure that all your equipment is compatible. (It is embarrassing to find out during the procedure that your venipuncture needle is too narrow to accommodate your guide wire.)
4. When prepping the area with antiseptic solution, be sure to include alternate central line sites (e.g., supraclavicular and infraclavicular subclavian) in case the internal jugular route is unsuccessful. You can thereby avoid reprepping and redraping.
5. In the event of failure, initially favor these alternate ipsilateral routes over "crossing over" and attempting the contralateral internal jugular catheterization. Bilateral pneumothoraces are a "worst case" scenario and must be avoided.

6. Do not couple your venipuncture syringe and needle with excessive tightness—they may be difficult to disconnect when you are ready to thread the wire. (Have a small sterile clamp ready just in case you cannot get them apart by hand.)
7. The most common technical error responsible for the inability to find the vein during the posterior approach is directing the syringe/needle too posteriorly (i.e., plunger end too high). In truly aiming for the sternal notch, the syringe should either parallel the surface of the stretcher or, in fact, be angled upward in relation to it.
8. If guide wire threading is met with resistance, retract it back into the needle, rotate it about a quarter turn, and then readvance it. Subtle rotation and angulation adjustments to the needle, itself, may also prove helpful. Inability to thread the guide wire probably occurs more often with straight wires than with J-wires, so favor using the latter. *Never* try to overcome threading problems by introducing the nonfloppy end of the wire. The risk of perforation is too great.
9. Unless high flow/volume is needed, attach a diaphragmed port to all catheter hubs after insertion while the site is freshly sterile. This will maximize future options for pacing, Swan-Ganz, and multiple-lumen catheter introduction should the need later arise.
10. For pediatric patients in need of rapid central venous access for whom femoral vein catheterization is unsuccessful, the internal jugular route is preferred over subclavian routes.
11. The sternocleidomastoid muscle of obese, stocky, or "thick-necked" patients may be more easily palpated when wet with antiseptic solution. If you loose your landmarks, try reapplying Betadine.
12. When the procedure is undertaken emergently with suboptimal sterile technique, consider a dose of intravenous antibiotics in the emergency department.

References

Parsa MH, Tabora F: Central venous access in critically ill patients in the emergency department. Emerg Med Clin North Am 4:709–744, 1986.

Sanford TJ: Internal jugular vein cannulation versus subclavian vein cannulation: An anesthesiologist's view: The right internal jugular vein. J Clin Monit 1:58–61, 1985.

Sessler CN, Glausser FL: Central venous cannulation done by house officers in the intensive care unit: A prospective study. South Med J 80:1239–1243, 1987.

Sterner ST, Plummer D, Clinton J, Ruiz E: A comparison of the supraclavicular approach and the infraclavicular approach for subclavian vein catheterization. Ann Emerg Med 15:421–424, 1986.

Implantable Venous Access Devices

JUDY KILPATRICK, RN, MSN

ACCESSING PORT DEVICES

Indications

For use in administering long-term intravenous fluids, blood products, medication, and parenteral nutrition when other forms of venous access are not indicated

For use in obtaining blood specimens

Contraindications

1. Do not draw coagulation studies since it is a heparinized catheter.
2. Large volume fluid replacement in emergencies is usually not possible owing to small size of catheter.

Equipment

Venous access device (Figure 24–21)
Sterile drape
Sterile towel
Hemostat (booted)
Two 2×2-inch gauze pads
Two 4×4-inch gauze pads
20- or 22-gauge right-angled Huber needle
Sterile gloves
Three Betadine swabs
10-ml syringe of normal saline
Syringe of heparin solution 100 units/ml for instillation
  Pediatric: 4 ml
  Adult: 6 ml
Extension set with T—as needed
Three-way stopcock with Luer-Lok—as needed
22-gauge needle—as needed
Bio-occlusive dressing

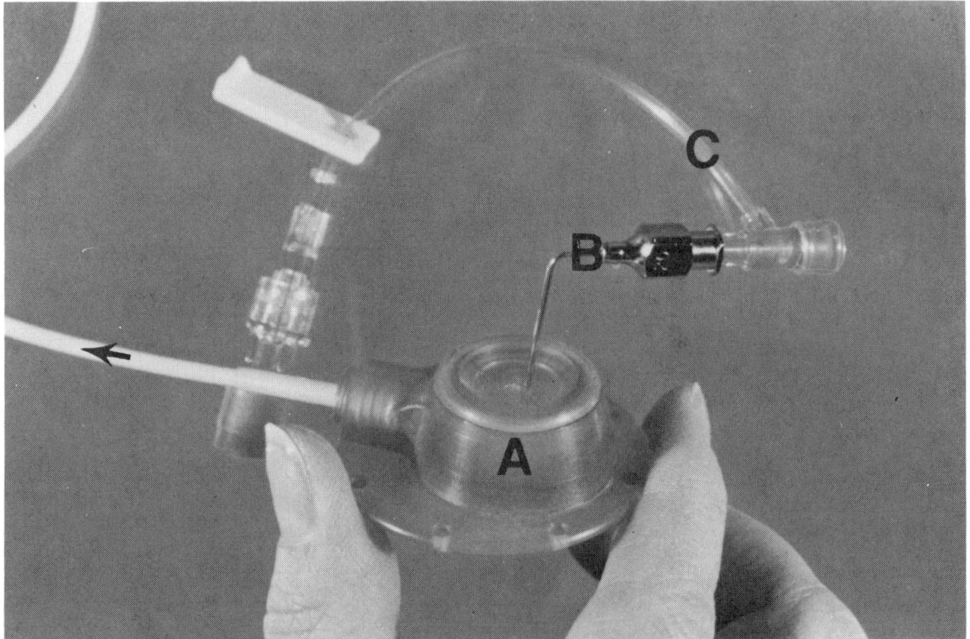

FIGURE 24–21. Implantable venous access device in vitro. *A,* Subcutaneous port; *B,* right-angle Huber needle; *C,* IV tubing or heparin lock; arrow points in direction to vein.

Universal Precautions

1. Wear mask and sterile gloves.

Technique

1. Observe the site for signs of infection, hematomas, distended veins across the top of the injection site, and serous fluid accumulation in the pocket.
2. Palpate for device rotation and location of access port septum and outflow track.
3. Cleanse a 4-inch area around device with Betadine. Allow to air dry.
4. Connect extension T-set to right-angle needle. Flush setup with normal saline solution, leaving syringe and needle inserted in extension tubing.
5. Apply drape.
6. Palpate the access port septum.
7. Insert the right-angled needle into the septum until the solid posterior surface of port is felt.
8. Aspirate slightly to ascertain blood return and then flush with remaining saline. Switch to heparin solution (100 units/ml) and flush. While flushing last milliliter, withdraw needle from extension tubing. If unable to obtain blood return:
   a. Connect 1-ml syringe of normal saline directly to extension T-set and aspirate slowly.
   b. Have patient deep breathe and cough.

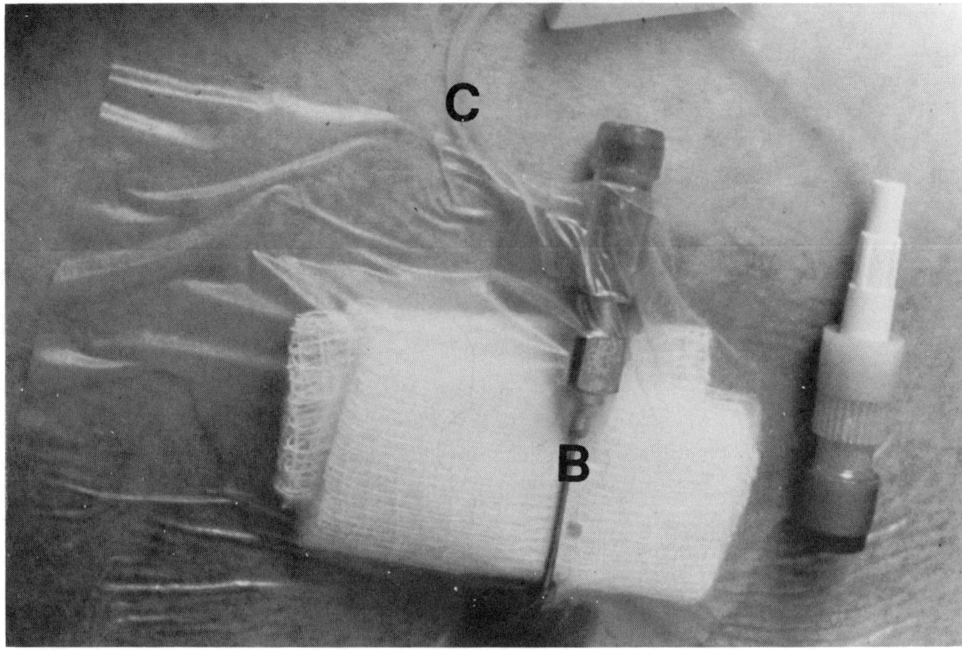

FIGURE 24–22. Implantable venous access device in vivo. *B,* Right-angle Huber needle; *C,* IV tubing or heparin lock.

c. Change patient's position by:
 1) Lowering head of bed
 2) Elevating shoulders by placing hands over head
 3) Turning patient to either side

If still unable to aspirate from port, it may be necessary to verify position of catheter by radiographic injection under fluoroscopy.

9. Apply dressing (change every 72 hours) (Figure 24–22).
10. To start intravenous infusion:
 a. Cleanse PRN adapter with alcohol wipe.
 b. Insert 22-gauge needle attached to syringe with normal saline into PRN adapter and aspirate to ensure blood return. Remove needle and syringe.
 c. Insert 22-gauge needle attached to primed intravenous tubing and solution into PRN adapter.
 d. Tape connections securely.
 e. When disconnecting intravenous line, flush PRN adapter with normal saline followed by appropriate heparin flush solution.
11. To obtain blood specimens:
 a. If device is connected to heparin lock:
  1) Clamp T-connector.
  2) Remove Luer-Lok heparin cap and place 5-ml syringe on extension set. Withdraw 5 ml of heparin and blood for discard.
  3) Place syringe for aspirating specimen onto extension T-set and withdraw required amount and place in required tubes.
  4) Flush with 10 ml of normal saline.
  5) Replace *new* heparin lock cap and flush with required amount of heparin solution (100 units/ml). While flushing last milliliter, withdraw needle from PRN adapter.

b. If device is connected to continuous infusion:
   1) Clamp connector on extension T-set and solution administration set. Remove needle from PRN adapter and replace with new needle.
   2) Remove Luer-Lok heparin cap and place 5-ml syringe on extension set. Withdraw 5 ml of solution and blood for discard.
   3) Place syringe for aspirating specimen onto extension T-set and withdraw required amount. Place in required tubes.
   4) Flush with 10 ml of normal saline.
   5) Replace *new* heparin lock cap. Insert 22-gauge needle attached to primed intravenous tubing and solution into PRN adapter. Restart continuous infusion.
   6) Tape connections securely.

Complications

Air embolism if system is broken or open to air

Hematoma at puncture site

Infection noted at tunnel or reservoir pocket

Partial withdrawal of needle from septum and infusion of drug, blood, or intravenous fluid into subcutaneous tissue or reservoir pocket

Pearls and Pitfalls

1. Sterile technique is used in all manipulations of the catheter.
2. The port is flushed with normal saline before and after intravenous administration of medication and blood products to ascertain patency and to clear the line of blood products and medications incompatible with heparin.
3. Catheter and port area should be avoided with defibrillation. If patient is defibrillated, port should be checked for function.
4. A 20-gauge (rather than 22-gauge) right-angled needle is recommended for infusion of blood products.
5. Attempting to bend a straight needle to form a right angle will change the size of the lumen at the point in the bend and getting fluid or blood to run is impossible.
6. Right-angled Huber butterfly sets with extensions may be substituted for the plain needle and extension T-set.
7. If device appears to be filled with debris or clots, cleanse with 1 to 2 ml of urokinase solution (5000 IU/ml). Instill solution and clamp device for 15 to 45 minutes, followed by normal saline instillation.

Hickman Catheter

CONNIE WALLECK, RN

FOR DRAWING BLOOD (Figure 24–23)

Indication

Need for blood sample in patient with poor venous access

Contraindication

Do not draw coagulation studies from a Hickman catheter since it is heparinized.

Equipment

Sterile barrier
Two 6-ml syringes (one with 22-gauge needle, one without)
3-ml syringe (with 22-gauge needle)
Bacteriostatic saline
Heparin flush, 10 units/ml
Alcohol swabs
Tubes for blood samples
Syringe large enough for blood sample needed
New heparin lock cap
Sterile gloves
Sterile 4 × 4-inch gauze pads

Universal Precautions

1. Wear sterile gloves.

Technique

1. Clamp catheter and remove heparin lock cap or disconnect intravenous drip if one is infusing.
2. Don gloves.
3. Thoroughly clean junction with alcohol swab.
4. Attach empty 6-ml syringe to catheter.
5. Open clamp and draw back 5 ml of blood. Reclamp catheter and discard blood.
6. Apply a new syringe of the size appropriate for the sample needed.

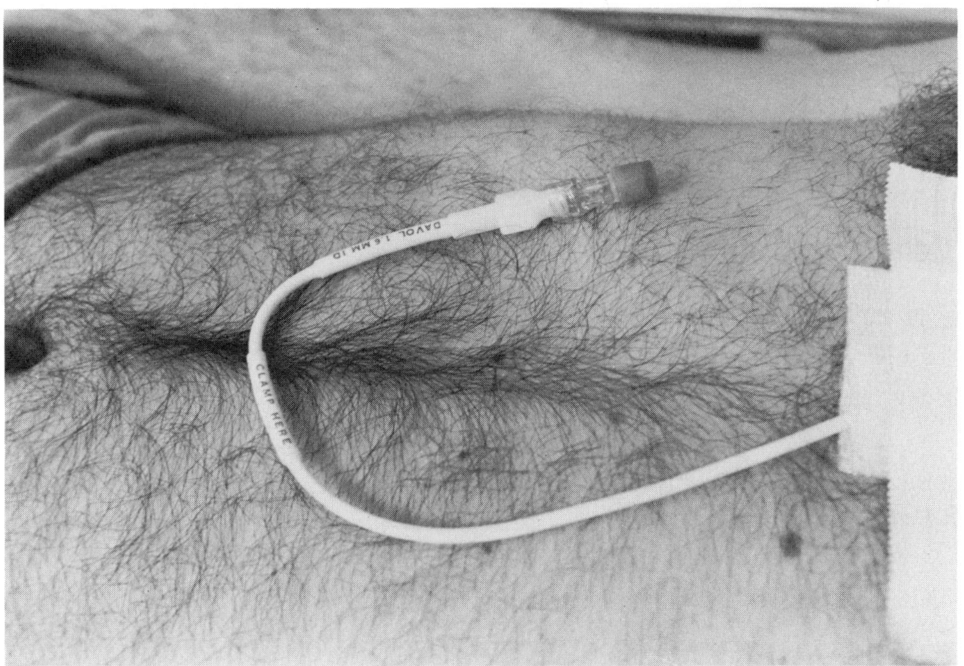

FIGURE 24–23. Hickman catheter.

7. Unclamp catheter and draw back appropriate amount of blood. Reclamp catheter.
8. Apply new heparin lock cap if needed.
9. Flush per Hickman flush protocol (see below) or restart intravenous infusion.

Complications

Air embolization if clamp left open
Bleeding through catheter
Infection
Dislodgement of Hickman catheter

Pearls and Pitfalls

1. Stop the injection before syringe is totally empty to prevent air from entering the catheter.
2. Make sure system is tightly clamped when not being used.
3. Clamp catheter only on soft portion to avoid severing of the catheter.

INTERMITTENT INFUSION

Indication

Intermittent intravenous infusions with a Hickman catheter in place

Contraindications

None

Equipment

Bacteriostatic normal saline
Heparin, 10 units/ml
3-ml syringe with 22-gauge needle
Two 6-ml syringes with 22-gauge needles
Alcohol swabs
Tape
Clamps (latex covered if permanent clamp not on Hickman)
Medication to be administered, intravenous tubing, and 22-gauge needle
Sterile gloves

Universal Precautions

1. Wear sterile gloves.

Technique

1. Swab tops of normal saline and heparin vials with alcohol swab.
2. Fill two 6-ml syringes with saline and one 3-ml syringe with heparin solution.
3. Don gloves.
4. Swab the heparin lock cap with alcohol swab.
5. Insert 6-ml normal saline–filled syringe with 22-gauge needle into cap. Unclamp the Hickman catheter while slowly injecting the saline until 0.5 ml of saline remains. Remove needle and syringe.
6. Attach a 22-gauge needle to the intravenous tubing, insert it into cap, and begin infusion.
7. Prior to end of infusion (before tubing is empty) clamp Hickman catheter and turn off infusion.
8. Remove infusion, insert 6-ml normal saline–filled syringe via 22-gauge needle into cap. Unclamp Hickman catheter and inject saline slowly until 0.5 ml of saline remains and clamp the catheter.
9. Attach 3-ml heparin-filled syringe to cap via 22-gauge needle and follow procedures in step 8.
10. Inspect catheter for leaking after removing the 3-ml syringe.

Complications

Air embolization if clamp is left open
Bleeding through catheter
Infection
Dislodgement of Hickman catheter

Pearls and Pitfalls

1. Stop the injection before the syringe is totally empty to prevent air from entering the catheter.
2. Make sure the system is tightly clamped when not being used.
3. Clamp the catheter only on the soft portion to avoid severing.

FLUSHING THE CATHETER (Figure 24–24)

Indications

Ensure continued patency of Hickman catheter

Contraindication

Abnormally elevated prothrombin and partial thromboplastin times

Equipment

Sterile barriers (2)
Clamp (should be permanently on Hickman or latex-covered catheter)
Alcohol swabs
3-ml syringe with 22-gauge needle (two for double lumen)
6-ml syringe with 22-gauge needle (two for double lumen)
Bacteriostatic saline solution
Heparin, 10 units/ml
Disposable heparin lock cap (two for double lumen)
Sterile gloves

Universal Precautions

1. Wear sterile gloves.

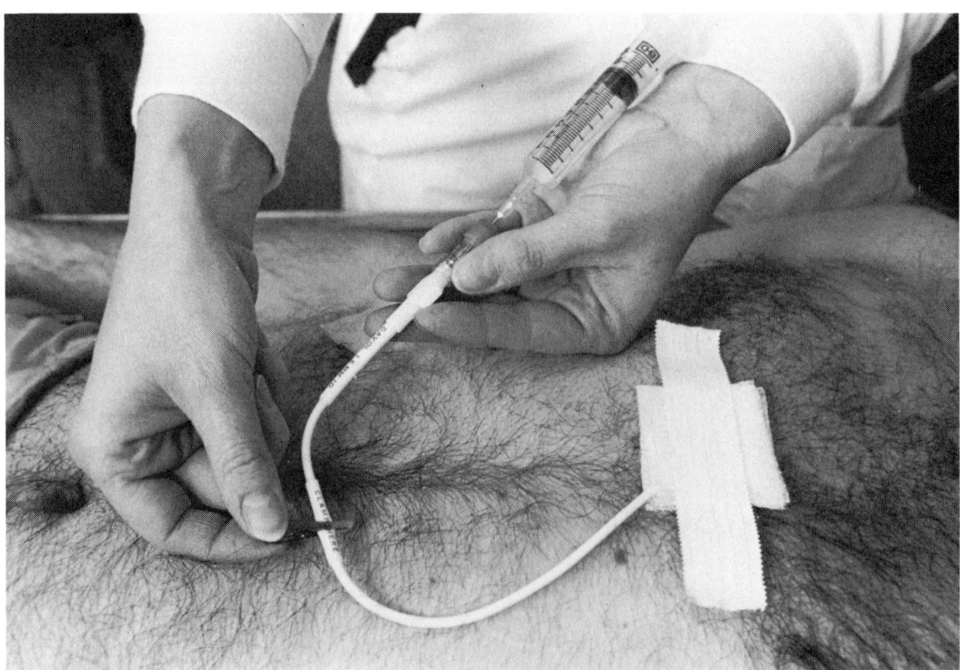

FIGURE 24–24. Flushing a heparin-locked Hickman catheter.

Technique

1. Open sterile barrier and place supplies on it.
2. Swab top of saline and heparin vials with alcohol pad.
3. Fill 6-ml syringe(s) with normal saline and fill 3-ml syringe(s) with 10 units/ml of heparin flush solution.
4. Don gloves.
5. Place a sterile barrier under the connection site.
6. If converting a continuous infusion to heparin lock, thoroughly cleanse site where intravenous tubing is attached to catheter hub with alcohol. Clamp catheter and then disconnect intravenous tubing.
7. Attach 6-ml syringe filled with normal saline to catheter hub after removing the needle. If catheter has previously been used as a heparin lock, cleanse cap(s) with alcohol swab and puncture heparin lock cap with the needle.
8. With one hand on catheter clamp and other thumb on plunger of syringe, begin injecting normal saline slowly as you release the clamp.
9. With 0.5 ml of normal saline left in the syringe, clamp the catheter. Remove the syringe from the catheter.
10. Repeat steps 7 through 9 with 3-ml heparin-filled syringe.
11. If converting continuous IV to heparin lock, place sterile heparin lock cap on catheter.
12. Repeat for additional lumens.

Complications

Air embolization if clamp left open
Bleeding through catheter
Infection
Dislodgement of Hickman catheter

Pearls and Pitfalls

1. Stop the injection before the syringe is totally empty to prevent air from entering the catheter.
2. Make sure system is tightly clamped when not being used.
3. Clamp catheter only on soft portion to avoid severing.
4. Infusaport system uses 100 units/ml heparin.

Peripheral Venous Cannulation

MICHAEL S. JASTREMSKI, MD

Indication

Interface with the vasculature for the administration of fluids and medications or the withdrawal of large amounts of blood (blood donation, dialysis, plasmapheresis)

Contraindications

None

Equipment

Intravenous solution and administration tubing selected based on clinical situation
Tourniquet
Gloves
Catheter over needle—size and type based on clinical situation (Figure 24–25)
Alcohol or Betadine swabs
Transparent, self-adhesive plastic dressing
4 × 4-inch gauze pads
1-inch tape

For heparin lock you also need:

Intermittent infusion cap
3-ml syringe
22-gauge, 1-inch needle
Heparin flush solution

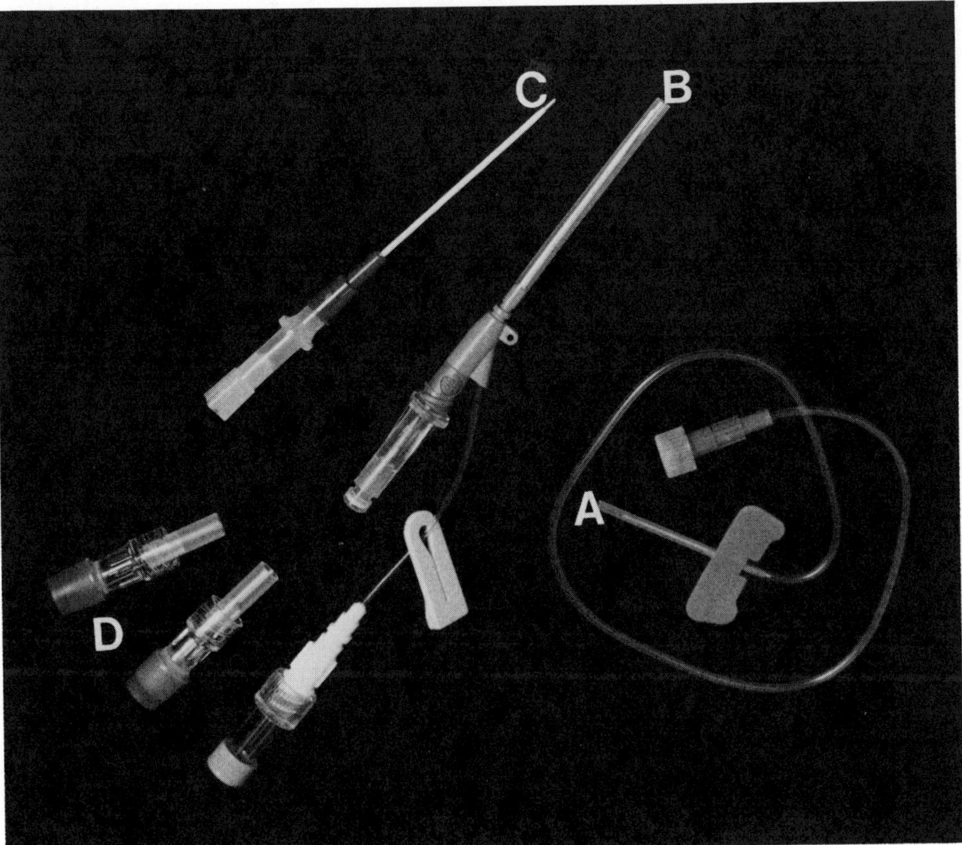

FIGURE 24–25. Venous cannulation devices. *A,* Butterfly needle; *B,* double-lumen catheter; *C,* catheter over needle; *D,* intermittent infusion caps.

Universal Precautions

1. Wear gloves.
2. Dispose of needles properly.

Technique

1. Explain the procedure to the patient and obtain consent.
2. Position the patient supine on a bed or stretcher.
3. Stand next to the arm you will use.
4. Apply a tourniquet to the mid upper arm.
5. Prepare your equipment and have it within reach:
   a. Intravenous tubing hooked to container of intravenous solution and flushed with the solution or heparin flush solution drawn up into the 3-ml syringe with 22-gauge needle
   b. 4 × 4-inch gauze pad opened
   c. Transparent dressing opened
   d. Several 3- to 4-inch pieces of tape
   e. Appropriate catheter
6. Put on gloves.

7. Using sight and palpation, identify a suitable vein—one that is visible, straight, larger than the chosen catheter, and not over a joint. Realistically, many persons do not have such ideal veins so you will have to find the best they have. As you develop skill and experience in this technique, you will become better and better at finding and cannulating small, invisible veins.
8. Cleanse the skin surrounding the puncture site with alcohol or Betadine. Allow to dry or wipe off with the 4 × 4-inch pad.
9. Remove the cap from the needle hub (so blood return will be more obvious) and ensure that the catheter slides easily off the needle.
10. Firmly palpate the chosen vein with the index finger of your nondominant hand 2 to 3 cm distal to the puncture site. This helps to fix the vein (Figure 24–26).
11. Hold the catheter-over-needle unit with your dominant hand so that the hub of the catheter is between the thumb and index finger and the hub of the needle is braced against the third and fourth fingers (see Figure 24–26).
12. Enter the skin directly over the vein with the needle bevel up, parallel to the vein, and at a 10- to 15-degree angle with the skin.
13. Slowly advance the needle into the vein until blood returns from the needle.
14. Fully advance the catheter over the needle into the vein using the thumb and index finger of your nondominant hand to advance the catheter as the needle is held in a fixed position by the thumb and middle finger of your dominant hand. If the catheter does not advance easily, try flattening the angle with the skin and/or moving the needle in or out a millimeter or so.
15. Place the 4 × 4-inch gauze pad under the catheter hub, and then remove the needle from the catheter.
16. Release the tourniquet.

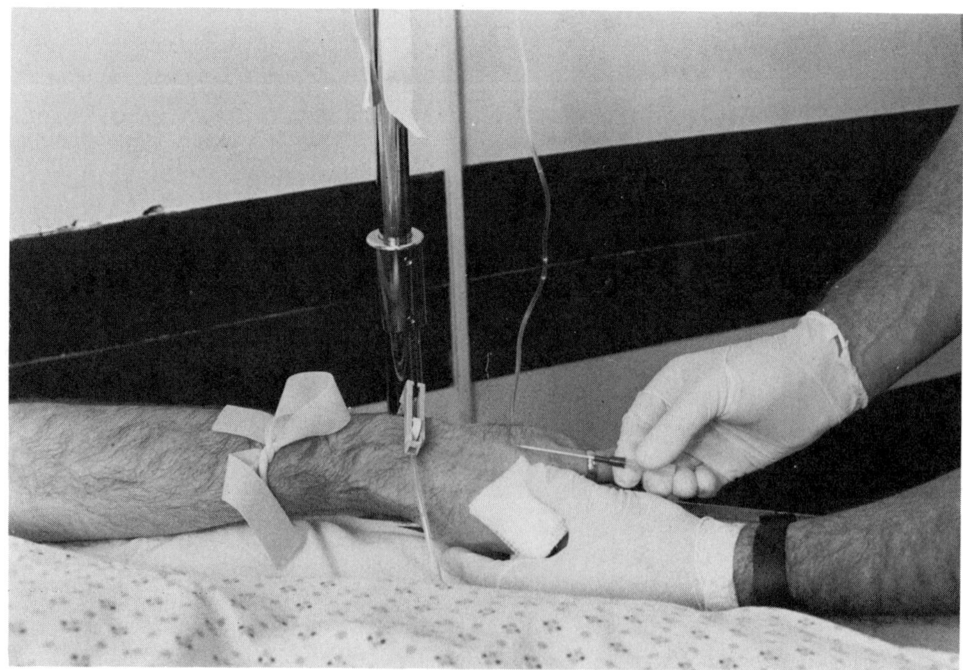

FIGURE 24–26. Peripheral venous cannulation.

17. Attach the intravenous tubing to the catheter and ensure that the intravenous solution flows freely. If there is not a free flow of intravenous fluid, pull the catheter back several millimeters. If you wish to have a heparin lock, attach the intermittent infusion cap to the catheter and flush it with 3 ml of heparin flush solution using the 3-ml syringe and 22-gauge needle.
18. Clean up any blood with the 4 × 4-inch gauze pad.
19. Apply a transparent, self-adhesive dressing over the site.
20. Tape the intravenous tubing to the arm in several places.
21. Recheck to ensure that the intravenous solution is still flowing.
22. Carefully dispose of the needle in an appropriate safety container.

Complications

Thrombosis

Phlebitis

Unsuccessful cannulation

Extravasation of intravenous solution or medications

Hematoma

Catheter shearing

Needle puncture of operator or assistant (Have you had your hepatitis B vaccine?)

Pearls and Pitfalls

1. Warming the arm with a heating pad or moist towels helps find veins in some patients.
2. Alternative peripheral veins to consider if you cannot find an arm vein are the lower extremities or the external jugular vein or, in infants, the scalp. Phlebitis seems to be more common with lower-extremity intravenous cannulation and has the potential for progressing to deep venous thrombosis.
3. The external jugular vein is often large and easily cannulated, especially during cardiac arrest. The technique for external jugular vein cannulation is essentially the same as for an arm vein except you do not use a tourniquet.
4. The incidence of phlebitis is lessened by changing the IV to a new site every 48 hours.
5. Rapid fluid resuscitation requires big (14- or 16-gauge), short catheters.
6. If the patient does not require a continuous intravenous infusion, use a heparin lock. This gives the patient much more mobility since he is only hooked to an intravenous setup pole during the periods when medications are being given.
7. Double-lumen peripheral intravenous catheters are available for use in patients who need multiple intravenous medications (e.g., the patient receiving thrombolytic therapy for an acute myocardial infarction).

Subclavian Vein Catheterization

MARCY LAYTON, MD

Indications

Intravenous access
Need for multiple intravenous solutions
Hyperalimentation
Vasoactive drug infusion
Vascular access for pulmonary artery catheter, transvenous pacer, or hemodialysis

Contraindication

Coagulopathy (relative—must balance risks against need for central intravenous access)

Equipment

A prepackaged kit is most useful.

Betadine
Sterile towels
4 × 4-inch gauze pads
1% lidocaine
10- and 20-ml syringes
25-gauge, 1-inch needle
20-gauge, 1½-inch needle
18-gauge, 2½-inch thin-wall needle
Three-way stopcock
Guide wire—0.035-inch diameter, 25- to 30-inch length
Single- or triple-lumen catheter
Heparin flush
3-0 nylon suture on needle
No. 11 blade
Vein dilator
Mask, cap, and eye shield
1-foot extension tubing
Sterile gown and gloves
Suture scissors
Needle holder

Universal Precautions

1. Wear mask and sterile gown and gloves.
2. Use an eye shield.

Technique

1. If patient status and circumstances allow, explain the procedure to the patient and obtain consent.
2. Position patient in the supine, Trendelenburg position with a towel between the scapulae.
3. Put on cap, mask, eye shield, and sterile gown and gloves.
4. Prep area with Betadine and widely drape.
5. Determine needle entry site by locating the angle made by the first rib and clavicle. Needle entry site will be 1 fingerbreadth lateral to this angle below the clavicle (Figure 24–27).
6. Anesthetize entry site with 1% lidocaine first using the 25-gauge, 1-inch needle for the skin, then using the 20-gauge, 1½-inch needle for the deeper tissues around the inferior surface of the clavicle.
7. Attach a 10-ml syringe to the 18-gauge thin-wall needle. The needle should be directed toward the angle formed by the clavicle and first rib so it initially hits the underside of the clavicle.
8. Apply negative pressure to the syringe as the needle is advanced under the clavicle aiming toward the thyroid.
9. Once adequate venous blood flow is obtained, the syringe is removed and a finger quickly placed over the open needle to prevent air embolism.

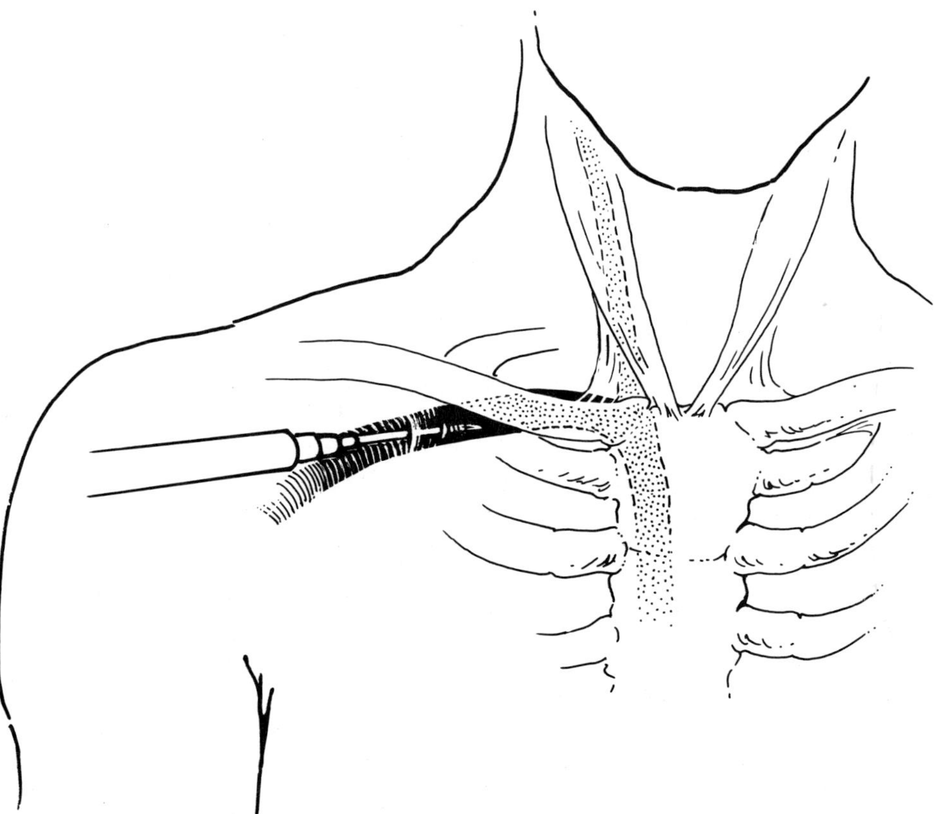

FIGURE 24–27. Subclavian catheterization.

10. A guide wire is then advanced through the needle as long as no resistance is met.
11. The needle is removed back over the guide wire. (Have your hand on the guide wire at all times.)
12. A small incision may be made at the entry site with a blade to allow easier catheter insertion.
13. A venous dilator is then introduced over the guide wire and inserted 10 cm beyond the entry site, if it passes easily.
14. After the dilator is removed, with the guide wire still in place, the chosen catheter is placed over the guide wire to 12 to 15 cm.
15. Remove the guide wire and aspirate through the catheter so that good venous flow is demonstrated.
16. Each lumen of the catheter should be flushed with heparin solution or hooked up to a running intravenous line.
17. If this is an introducer for another catheter (i.e., Swan, pacer), proceed with inserting that line. If this is a simple single-lumen central venous pressure catheter, attach 1-foot tubing and three-way stopcock and suture as shown in Figure 24–28. If this is a triple-lumen catheter, suture tab to skin.
18. Apply dressing (I use Tegoderm).
19. Obtain and review a chest x-ray film to confirm catheter position and rule out pneumothorax.

Complications

Arterial catheterization/laceration
Pneumothorax
Hematoma
Catheter embolus
Internal jugular catheterization
Hydrothorax
Thoracic duct laceration
Air embolus
Nerve laceration (brachial plexus, phrenic, recurrent laryngeal)
Perforation of superior vena cava
Cardiac tamponade (from right atrial perforation)
Dysrhythmias (usually from guide wire)

Pearls and Pitfalls

1. Traction on the ipsilateral arm may facilitate venous access.
2. If guide wire is difficult to advance, never force it. If the bevel of the needle is turned face down during insertion of the guide wire, internal jugular catheterization may be avoided.
3. Sometimes it may be difficult to rule out arterial cannulation (hypoxic, hypotensive patient), a pressure monitor may help in the differentiation.
4. When the subclavian vein is not entered on the initial pass of the needle, pull it back to the skin and then readvance, aiming for a lower point on the neck.

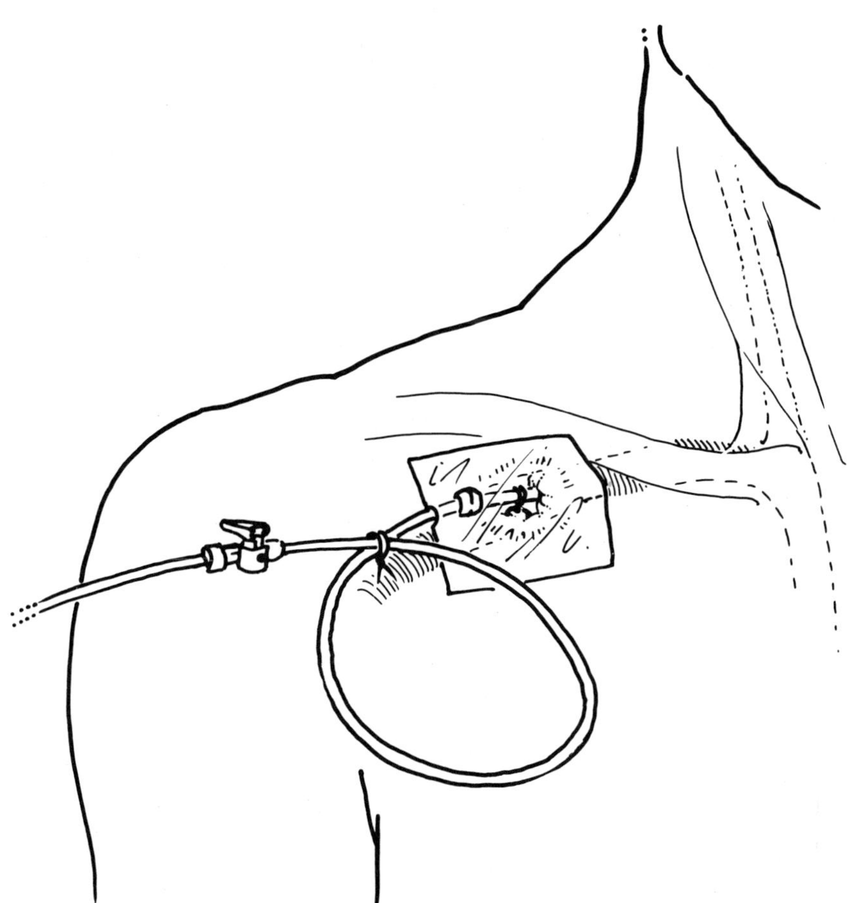

FIGURE 24–28. Securing a subclavian catheter.

5. The 20-gauge, 1½-inch needle used for anesthetic infiltration can be used initially to search for and locate the subclavian vein and thus precisely gauge the angle and depth of insertion of the larger 18-gauge needle. This makes it less likely that you will puncture an undesirable structure such as the lung or subclavian artery with the larger needle.

References

Extensive experience.

Herbst CA: Indications, management, and complications of percutaneous subclavian catheters. Arch Surg 113:1421, 1978.

Sznajder JI, Zvebil FR, Bitterman H, et al: Central vein catheterization failure and complication rate by three percutaneous approaches. Arch Intern Med 146:259, 1986.

Venous Cutdowns

THOMAS TERNDRUP, MD

Indications

Insertion of large-bore catheters or when no other venous access can be obtained and it is urgently needed

Peripheral vein cutdowns can be rapidly performed by inexperienced personnel. The sites for peripheral vein cutdown include the saphenous vein at the ankle, the greater saphenous vein at the groin, and the cephalic vein at the radial side of the wrist.

Contraindications

None

Equipment

Surgical gloves, mask, cap, eye shield
Drapes
Adequate lighting
Betadine solution
Local (infiltration) anesthesia*
Gauze pads (4 × 4-inch)
Scalpel handle and blades (No. 20 for skin and No. 11 for venotomy)
Small curved hemostats
Suture scissors
3-0 silk ties (for vein)
4-0 nylon suture (for skin closure)
Selection of appropriate-size angiocatheters or intravenous extension tubing
Vein lifter*
25-gauge needle*
3-ml syringe*
Intravenous tubing and solution

Universal Precautions

1. Wear mask and gloves.
2. Use an eye shield.

*Nonessential equipment in most circumstances.

Technique

1. If patient status and circumstances allow, explain the procedure to the patient and obtain informed consent.
2. Position patient depending on site.
3. Put on cap, mask, eye shield, and gloves.
4. Prep site with Betadine.
5. Infiltrate incision site with local anesthesia using a 25-gauge needle on 3-ml syringe.
6. Perform the cutdown. The general technique for performance of a peripheral vein cutdown involves the following sequence: Identification of the anatomic landmarks, surgical preparation of the skin (± local anesthesia), skin incision, dissection of the vein (from other subcutaneous structures), introduction of the catheter into the lumen of the vessel, and stabilization of the catheter. The specific steps are as follows:
   a. For peripheral *saphenous vein cutdown at the ankle,* a generous incision with a No. 20 blade can be made from the anterior to the posterior border of the tibia, about 2 fingerbreadths above the medial malleolus (Figure 24–29). Use the curved hemostats to sweep all subcutaneous structures in this incision off the periosteum. Quickly dissect (with the points of the hemostats) the vein from other subcutaneous fat (Figure 24–30*A*). For a formal cutdown the distal vein is ligated with a 3-0 silk tie and the proximal tie is inserted under the vessel (Figure 24–30*B*). A venotomy of about 40% of the diameter of the vein is performed with the No. 11 blade. A vein dilator or lifter may be used to facilitate insertion of the catheter or intravenous extension tubing (Figure 24–31). Following confirmation of venous placement, the proximal tie is set down and the skin is closed.
   b. The *saphenous vein at the groin* can be localized by making an incision starting at the juncture of the labia or the scrotum with the thigh and extending laterally to the vertical line dropped from the midpoint

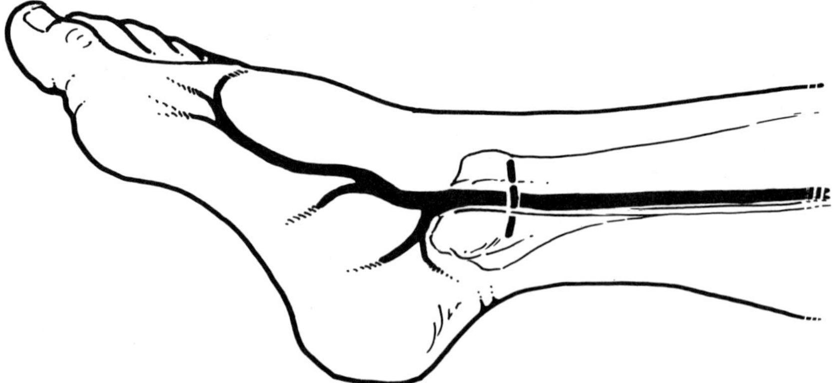

FIGURE 24–29. Site for ankle cutdown.

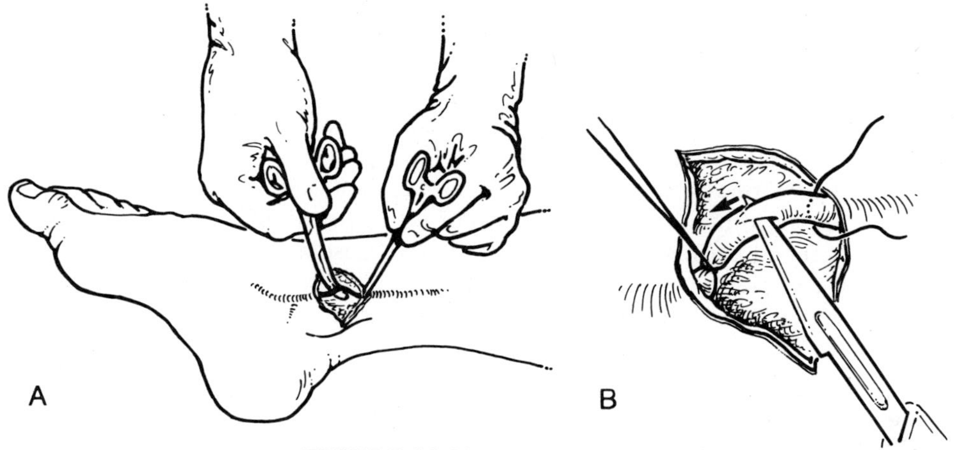

FIGURE 24–30. Ankle cutdown.

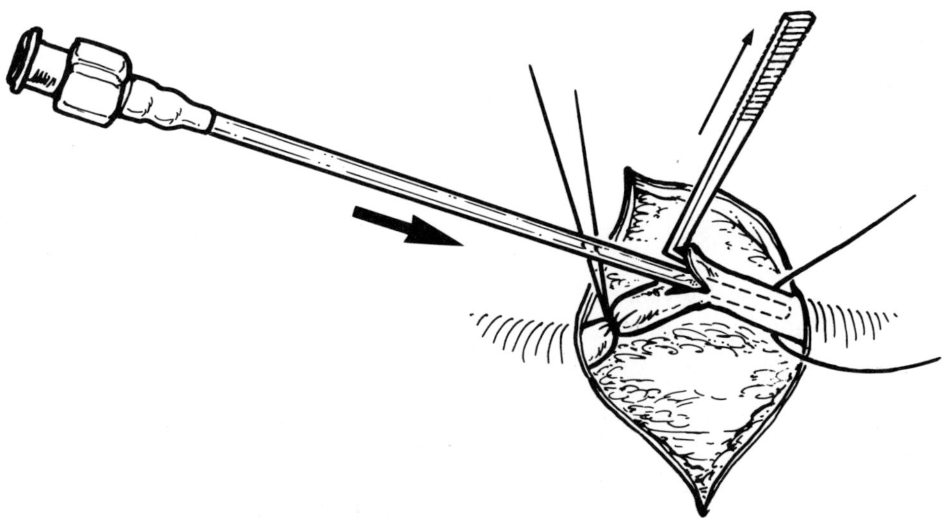

FIGURE 24–31. Ankle cutdown.

between the anterior-superior iliac spine and the pubic tubercle. Blunt dissection is carried out (with gloved fingers), and the vein is located at the midportion of the incision in the superficial subcutaneous fat (Figure 24–32). The introduction and stabilization of the catheter (or intravenous extension tubing) is done in the fashion described for the saphenous vein at the ankle.

c. For the *cephalic vein at the wrist,* the incision is made transversely about 2 fingerbreadths proximal to the radial styloid, on the radial aspect of the wrist (Figure 24–33). The incision should be 1½ to 2 inches in length, just through the dermis. Then hemostats are used to dissect and isolate the cephalic vein. Introduction of the catheter and closure of the skin should be done in the standard fashion.

d. A modified cutdown allows venous cannulation under direct vision, with preservation of peripheral veins for future use. Follow the standard steps outlined earlier for skin incision and vein isolation. At this point, insert a catheter-over-needle unit through the skin into the vein, and then advance the catheter into the lumen of the vessel in the usual fashion. No vein ties are required.

7. Attach intravenous tubing to catheter and begin infusion.
8. Suture catheter to skin with 4-0 nylon suture.
9. Close skin incision with 4-0 nylon sutures.
10. Apply dressing.

Complications

Injury to associated neurovascular structures

Inability to cannulate the vessel

Bleeding

Sclerosis of peripheral veins

Catheter embolism

Infection

Pearls and Pitfalls

1. Rapid, peripheral vein cutdowns can be performed by inexperienced personnel. Using the anatomic locations presented, the success rate is optimized and complications are minimized.
2. Each skin incision should be quite superficial, cut just through the dermis: by using the points of the curved hemostats as the dissection instrument, one can rapidly scoop up all subcutaneous tissue and then isolate the vein from the other subcutaneous fat.
3. Cannulation is facilitated by a generous incision, an adequate venotomy, an appropriate-sized catheter, a distal vein stabilization tie, and the occasional use of a vein lifter.

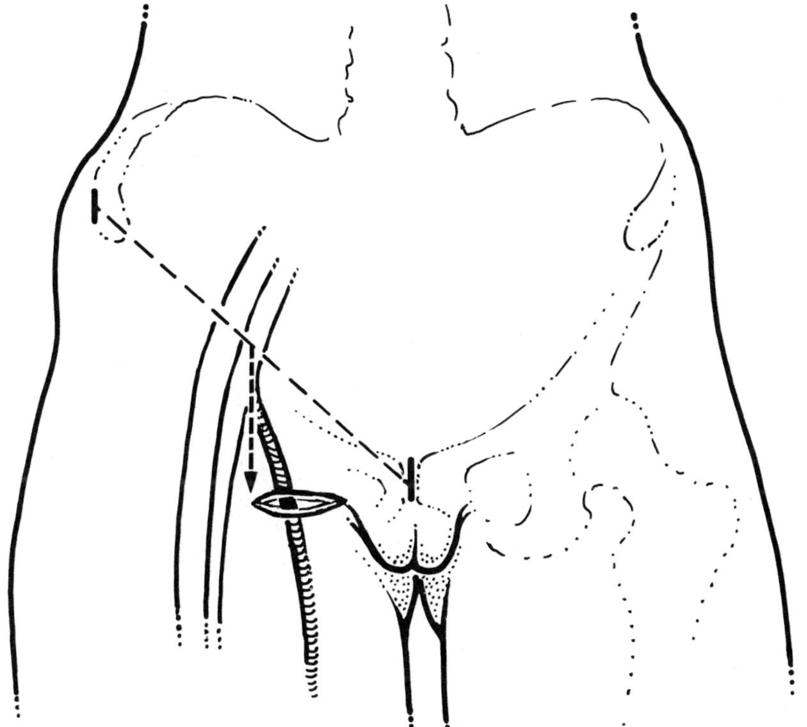

FIGURE 24–32. Femoral vein cutdown.

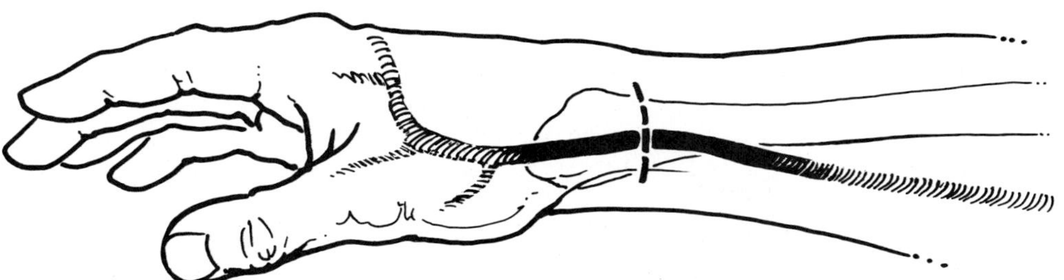

FIGURE 24–33. Wrist cutdown.

References

Simon RR, Hoffman JR, Smith M: Modified new approaches for rapid intravenous access. Ann Emerg Med 16:44–49, 1987.

Talan DA, Simon RR, Hoffman JR: Cephalic vein cutdown at the wrist: Comparison to the standard saphenous vein ankle cutdown. Ann Emerg Med 17:38–42, 1988.

25

Writing Prescriptions

MARCY LAYTON, MD

Indication

To order medications or medical supplies/equipment for your patient

Contraindications

None

Universal Precautions

None

Technique

1. Determine need for medication, supplies, or equipment.
2. Make sure the patient is not allergic to the medication you are considering nor taking any other medication that could result in a serious drug interaction. Consider pregnancy and the safety of the drug you plan to prescribe in women of child-bearing age. Also consider the need for dosage adjustment in major organ system dysfunction (especially renal).
3. Obtain the appropriate prescription form:
   a. Standard—for most drugs and supplies
   b. Triplicate—for controlled substances (list of controlled substances may vary depending on which state you practice in)
   c. Specialized forms for durable medical equipment

4. Legibly complete the form making sure to include the following (Figure 25–1):
   a. Patient's name
   b. Patient's address
   c. Patient's age
   d. Date
   e. Name of medication
   f. Size of pill or concentration of liquid (e.g., mg or mg/ml)
   g. Instructions for use (sig:)
      1) Amount per dose (number of pills or volume of liquid)
      2) Route of administration (e.g., oral, rectal, topical, inhalation)
      3) Frequency of use
      4) Add p.r.n. if medication is to be used only when symptoms occur (e.g., sig: ii puffs p.r.n. wheezing).
   h. Amount to be dispensed (total number of pills or volume of liquid)
   i. Refills (if yes, specify how many)
   j. Specification that brand name must be dispensed if you do not wish the patient to receive generic drug (this may also vary from state to state)
   k. Your signature
   l. Your name printed
   m. If a controlled substance:
      1) Your DEA number
      2) Maximum daily dose
5. Give the prescription to the patient and carefully and clearly explain:
   a. Why the medication or device is being prescribed
   b. Instructions for use
   c. Side effects to watch for and what to do if one occurs

Complications

Drug or dosing error due to illegible writing

Use of a wrong form

Prescribing a medication or device that is not covered by the patient's insurance (a particular problem with Medicaid)

CLINIC ID

PAT # X-REF. # DEPT.# 44 RX-

DISTRIBUTION REFERENCE NO.

PAT. NAME RAISTLIN MAJERE AGE 25

ADDRESS 121 VALLENWOOD SEX

CITY SOLACE STATE ANSALON ZIP m DATE 6/30/90

PHARMACY	AREA C	89842
MED. NUMBER	QUANTITY	CHARGE

INSURANCE #

℞ ONE PRESCRIPTION PER BLANK

TERPIN HYDRATE c̄ CODEINE ELIXIR

SIG: 10cc P.O. q 4H REFILL NO. T

#8oz MAXIMUM DAILY DOSAGE 60cc

Michael S. Jastremski, M.D.

SIGNATURE HERE M.D. ➡ and ➡ PRINT NAME HERE M.D.

THIS PRESCRIPTION WILL BE FILLED GENERICALLY UNLESS PRESCRIBER WRITES "d a w" IN THE BOX BELOW.

DEA REG. NO. AJ7664413 PROVIDER NO.

ALL ℞ FILLED AT UNIVERSITY HOSPITAL WILL BE FILLED GENERICALLY.

Dispense As Written

Mfg.	Type	
Date	Quantity	Signature R PH
2. Date	Quan	R PH
3. Date	Quan	R PH
4. Date	Quan	R PH
5. Date	Quan	R PH
6. Date	Quan	R PH

UNIVERSITY HOSPITAL
SUNY HEALTH SCIENCE CENTER
AT SYRACUSE
750 EAST ADAMS STREET
SYRACUSE, NEW YORK 13210

PHARMACY REGISTRATION NO. 10411
DEA NUMBER AS0552489
MMIS PROVIDER NUMBER 00354590
PHARM. PHONE (315) 473-4210
HOSP. PHONE (315) 473-5540

FIGURE 25–1. Sample prescription.

Pearls and Pitfalls

Prescription Alphabet Soup

Here are some traditional abbreviations that are understood if they can be read:

d—day	b—twice	sig.—label (*signa*)
w—week	t—thrice	p.r.n.—as necessary (*pro re nata*)
q—each	q—four	m.d.d.—maximum daily dose
h—hours	i—times	
	o—every other	
caps—capsules	a—before (*ante*)	po—oral
tabs—tablets	p—after (*post*)	pr—rectal
oz—ounces	c—meals (*cibos*)	sq—subcutaneous
tsp—teaspoon (5 ml)	disp.—dispense	apply—topical
tbsp—tablespoon (15 ml)	M—mix	puff—by inhalation

Prescription Checklist

The Right Drug

1. Have you considered the indications carefully?
2. Have you reviewed the possible side effects?
3. Is there a potential for drug interaction in the patient?
4. Are the benefit/risk and benefit/cost ratios favorable for this particular patient?

The Right Information

5. Does the patient understand why the drug is being given?
6. Does the patient understand the potential side effects and know which of these, if any, might require expeditious action?
7. Does the patient understand how, when, and for how long to take the drug? Are you sure?
8. Are there any specific "dos and don'ts" (e.g., use of alcohol) the patient should be aware of while taking the medication?

The Right Script

9. Is the prescription accurate?
10. Does it conform to what you told the patient?
11. Is it legible?
12. Have you provided for enough of the drug to complete the contemplated therapy? Have you limited the quantity dispensed if you are employing the drug in a therapeutic trial?
13. Did you sign your prescription?
14. Is your BNDD number necessary?
15. Did you use the right form (e.g., triplicate narcotic form, Medicaid)?
16. Can the patient get the medication?
17. Can the patient afford the medication?
18. Have you told the patient whether to refrigerate the medication?

You can save a lot of time if you write a large number of prescriptions by obtaining a hand stamp with your printed name and using this to stamp this portion of the prescription in advance. I do a whole pad at a time while I'm talking on the phone. You can save even more time if you can get someone else to do this for you (e.g., secretary or significant other).

References

Extensive experience.

Gottlieb AJ, Zamkoff K, Jastremski MS, Scalzo A, Imboden K: The Whole Internist Catalog. Philadelphia, WB Saunders, 1980. Prescription Alphabet Soup and Prescription Checklist reproduced with permission.

Index

Note: Page numbers in *italics* indicate figures; those followed by t indicate tables.